CASE REVIEW

Breast Imaging

SECOND EDITION

Series Editor
David M. Yousem, MD, MBA
Professor of Radiology
Director of Neuroradiology
Russell H. Morgan Department of Radiology and Radiological Science
The Johns Hopkins Medical Institutions
Baltimore, Maryland

Other Volumes in the CASE REVIEW Series
Brain Imaging, Second Edition
Cardiac Imaging
Duke Review of MRI Principles
Emergency Radiology
General and Vascular Ultrasound, Second Edition
Gastrointestinal Imaging, Third Edition
Genitourinary Imaging, Second Edition
Musculoskeletal Imaging, Second Edition
Nuclear Medicine, Second Edition
Obstetric and Gynecologic Ultrasound, Second Edition
Pediatric Imaging, Second Edition
Spine Imaging, Second Edition
Thoracic Imaging, Second Edition
Vascular and Interventional Imaging

ELSEVIER
SAUNDERS

Cecilia M. Brennecke, MD
Medical Director
Johns Hopkins at Green Spring
Baltimore, Maryland

CASE REVIEW

Breast Imaging

SECOND EDITION

CASE REVIEW SERIES

ELSEVIER
SAUNDERS

1600 John F. Kennedy Blvd.
Ste 1800
Philadelphia, PA 19103-2899

BREAST IMAGING: CASE REVIEW, SECOND EDITION   ISBN: 978-0-323-08722-3

Notices

Knowledge and best practice in this field are constantly changing. As new research and experience broaden our understanding, changes in research methods, professional practices, or medical treatment may become necessary.

Practitioners and researchers must always rely on their own experience and knowledge in evaluating and using any information, methods, compounds, or experiments described herein. In using such information or methods they should be mindful of their own safety and the safety of others, including parties for whom they have a professional responsibility.

With respect to any drug or pharmaceutical products identified, readers are advised to check the most current information provided (i) on procedures featured or (ii) by the manufacturer of each product to be administered, to verify the recommended dose or formula, the method and duration of administration, and contraindications. It is the responsibility of practitioners, relying on their own experience and knowledge of their patients, to make diagnoses, to determine dosages and the best treatment for each individual patient, and to take all appropriate safety precautions.

To the fullest extent of the law, neither the Publisher nor the authors, contributors, or editors, assume any liability for any injury and/or damage to persons or property as a matter of products liability, negligence or otherwise, or from any use or operation of any methods, products, instructions, or ideas contained in the material herein.

International Standard Book Number
978-0-323-08722-3

Content Strategist: Don Scholz
Content Development Specialist: Gina Donato
Publishing Services Manager: Patricia Tannian
Design Direction: Steven Stave

Printed in the United States of America

Last digit is the print number: 9 8 7 6 5 4

To my mother, Patti R. Brennecke, and
in memory of my father,
Charles N. Brennecke

I have been very gratified by the popularity and positive feedback that the authors of the Case Review series have received on the publication of the first and second editions of their volumes. Reviews in journals and word-of-mouth comments have been uniformly favorable. The authors have done an outstanding job in filling the niche of an affordable, easy-to-read, case-based learning tool that supplements the material in The Requisites series. I have been told by residents, fellows, and practicing radiologists that the Case Review series books are the ideal means for studying for oral board examinations and subspecialty certification tests.

Although some students learn best in a noninteractive study book mode, others need the anxiety or excitement of being quizzed. The selected format for the Case Review series (which consists of showing a few images needed to construct a differential diagnosis and then asking a few clinical and imaging questions) was designed to simulate the board examination experience. The only difference is that the Case Review books provide the correct answer and immediate feedback. The limit and range of the reader's knowledge are tested through scaled cases ranging from relatively easy to very hard. The Case Review series also offers a brief discussion of each case, a link back to the pertinent The Requisites volume, and up-to-date references from the literature.

Because of the popularity of the series, we have been rolling out the second and third editions of the Case Review series volumes. The expectation is that these editions will bring the content up to the current knowledge limits of the field, introduce new modalities and new techniques, and provide new and even more graphic examples of pathology. Personally, I am very excited about the future. Join us.

David M. Yousem, MD, MBA

This second edition of *Case Reviews: Breast Imaging* is an exciting new volume. In the first edition, cases were illustrated with film-screen mammography. In this edition, nearly all cases are digital. This reflects the evolution in mammography to the digital examination. The digital format makes subtle changes of breast disease easier to find on the images compared with film. I hope that you agree and that you enjoy your travels and discovery through the exciting world of breast imaging.

Acknowledgments: I thank the series editor and my Johns Hopkins colleague, Dr. David M. Yousem, and my Elsevier editor, Gina Donato. You always inspire me to do a little better.

I also thank my colleagues at Johns Hopkins Imaging at Green Spring Station: Drs. Susan Harvey, Lisa Mullen, and Bruce Copeland, all superb breast radiologists, and Dr. Fouad Gellad, who is not a breast radiologist but is forgiven for that lapse in judgment. The cases in this book reflect our work at the breast center at Johns Hopkins at Green Spring. Dr. Evelyn May is my colleague at our sister institution, The Johns Hopkins Hospital. She provided images and wrote several of the cases in this book. I thank Evelyn for her expertise.

Cecilia M. Brennecke, MD

Peggy Brennecke was a resident with me in the class of 1984–1988 at Johns Hopkins under the tutelage of Stan Siegelman. Peggy developed an outstanding reputation in breast imaging in the Baltimore-Washington area during the 1990s and was recruited back into the Hopkins fold to lead our outpatient breast imaging center. Knowing what a great job she has done and knowing her interest in teaching, I asked Peggy to work with Emily Conant on the *Breast Imaging Case Review Series*.

I thank Peggy for her hard work and perseverance. I am sure the radiology residents of 2012 and beyond will also appreciate her efforts.

David M. Yousem, MD, MBA

Opening Round

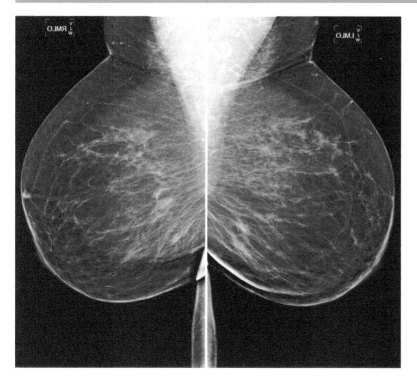

History: A 40-year-old woman presents for a baseline screening mammogram.

1. What is a screening population? (Choose all that apply.)
   A. Asymptomatic women
   B. Patients with a lump that has been assessed as benign by the primary care provider
   C. Patients with a nipple discharge on only one side
   D. Women older than 40 years

2. What is a diagnostic population?
   A. Patients with a strong family history of breast cancer
   B. Patients with a lump or nipple discharge
   C. Patients with chronic cyclic breast pain
   D. Patients who are extremely anxious about breast cancer

3. What is prevalence screening, and what is the approximate cancer detection rate in this population?
   A. Patients who have ovarian cancer; 15/1000
   B. Patients with a family history of breast cancer; 12/1000
   C. First round of screening, no prior mammogram; 6-10/1000
   D. Patients who have had many years of screening

4. What is incidence screening, and what is the approximate cancer detection rate in this population?
   A. Screening in women who have had no prior mammogram; 10/1000
   B. Screening in women undergoing annual mammography; 2-4/1000
   C. Screening in men; 50/1000
   D. Screening in high-risk women

C A S E 1

Incidence and Prevalence

1. A and D
2. B
3. C
4. B

References

Bassett LW, Jackson VP, Jahan R, et al: *Diagnosis of Diseases of the Breast.* Philadelphia: Saunders, 1997.

Smith RA, Duffy SW, Gabe R, et al: The randomized trials of breast cancer screening: what have we learned? *Radiol Clin North Am* 2004;42(5):793-806.

Cross-Reference

Ikeda D: *Breast Imaging: THE REQUISITES*, 2nd ed, Philadelphia: Saunders, 2010, p 39.

Comment

The incidence of breast cancer is an estimate of the number of new cases of breast cancer over a specific period. It can also be stated as the incidence rate, which is the number of people with a diagnosis of breast cancer per 100,000 people. In the United States in 2008, the incidence rate of breast cancer in all women undergoing screening was 3/1000 women. This number reflects new cancers not previously detected.

The prevalence of breast cancer refers to the number of women living with breast cancer at any given time. Prevalence screening is the first mammogram performed in previously unscreened women, and the rate of cancer detected in average-risk women in this first screening event is higher than the incidence rate, at approximately 6 to 10 women with cancer detected per 1000 screens.

Mammography exams are divided into two broad types: screening and diagnostic exams. The screening exam consists of four standard imaging views (mediolateral oblique [MLO] (see the figure) and craniocaudal [CC] view of each breast), and the population is women who have no signs or symptoms of breast cancer. This group includes women who might have an increased risk of breast cancer because of family history. It also includes women with breast pain, which is not considered to be a symptom of breast cancer, particularly if the pain waxes and wanes. Exams of asymptomatic women with implants are also typically considered to be screening. Women with implants have an additional four views performed, with a special maneuver to displace the implants. This is to better visualize the breast tissue anterior to the implant.

Screening mammograms are often read in batches after the patient has left the department. If the exam is considered incomplete, she needs to be recalled for additional evaluation at a later time.

The diagnostic exam is tailored to an abnormality. If a patient presents with a clinical sign or symptom of breast cancer, such as a lump, nipple discharge, or red, swollen breast, the technologist typically marks the area of concern with a radiopaque marker and then performs the standard imaging mammographic views, as well as additional views to better image the area of concern. These views may include spot compression, magnification, tangential, 90-degree lateral, or rolled craniocaudal views. Ultrasound may also be performed for more complete evaluation. The diagnostic exam is directed by the radiologist, and results are given to the patient before she leaves.

Notes

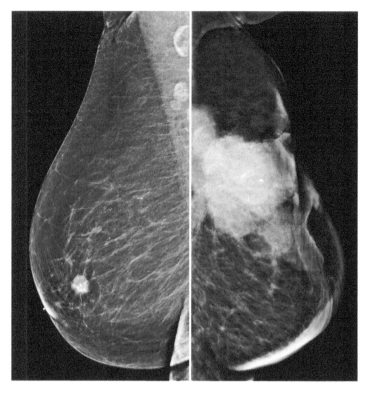

History: A 72-year-old woman presents for her first mammogram because of reduced mobility in her left arm and a draining wound in her left breast.

1. What should be included in the differential diagnosis? (Choose all that apply.)
   A. Bilateral breast cancer
   B. Left breast infection, right breast cancer
   C. Bilateral fibroadenomas
   D. Bilateral metastatic disease

2. What are the American Cancer Society and American College of Radiology guidelines for screening mammography in normal-risk women age 40 and older?
   A. Baseline mammogram at age 35, then annual mammograms thereafter
   B. Begin at age 40, then every other year until age 50, then annual
   C. Begin at age 40, then every year until age 75
   D. Begin annual screening at age 40

3. What is the reported reduction of breast cancer mortality associated with routine screening?
   A. 75%
   B. 50%
   C. 10% to 20%
   D. 20% to 40%

4. What is the incidence of breast cancer for women in the United States?
   A. 1 in 15 women over a woman's lifetime
   B. 1 in 5 women over a woman's lifetime
   C. 1 in 8 women over a woman's lifetime
   D. 1 in 10 women over a woman's lifetime

Screening Guidelines

1. A and B
2. D
3. D
4. C

References

American Cancer Society.

Hendrick RE, Helvie MA: United States Preventive Services Task Force screening mammography recommendations: science ignored. *AJR Am J Roentgenol* 2011;196(2):W112-W116.

Cross-Reference

Ikeda D: *Breast Imaging: THE REQUISITES*, 2nd ed, Philadelphia: Saunders, 2010, p 1.

Comment

The goal of screening mammography is to detect breast cancer as occult disease—before the patient and clinician know it is there. In this patient, her baseline mammogram, performed at age 72, was prompted by the presence of a large, ulcerating mass in her left breast, with bulky left axillary adenopathy. A small cancer is incidentally noted in the contralateral breast. This case illustrates the benefit of screening: The small right breast mass is detected on mammography before it is detected clinically; the locally advanced left breast cancer was detected late (see the figure). Had this patient started routine annual screening mammograms at an earlier age, it is likely that the left mass would have been seen earlier before it was found clinically. This patient had local spread of cancer to the skin and axillary nodes and widespread distant metastases at diagnosis.

Early detection is the attempt to find breast cancer before it has spread beyond the breast, improving morbidity and mortality from breast cancer. Mammography has been shown to decrease mortality from breast cancer by 30%, based on more recent data from the Swedish Two-County trial, including 130,000 women followed for 25 years.

Women in the United States have a slightly less than 1 in 8 lifetime risk for developing invasive breast cancer. The chance of dying from breast cancer is decreasing and is now approximately 1 in 35. The American Cancer Society estimated that there were 230,480 new cases of invasive breast cancer in 2011. This number is increasing and does not include carcinoma in situ. The American Cancer Society estimated that 57,650 new cases of in situ carcinoma were found in 2011. In 2011, 39,520 deaths from breast cancer were estimated to occur. This number is decreasing, likely owing to earlier detection and more effective treatments.

The American Cancer Society more recently updated their recommendations for screening for breast cancer: annual mammograms beginning at age 40 and continuing as long as the woman is in good health. They recommend clinical breast examination about every 3 years for women in their twenties and thirties and annually for women 40 and older. The American Cancer Society added that women should know how their breasts normally look and feel and that they should report any change to their health care provider; this might be termed *breast awareness* rather than *breast self-examination*. Guidelines have been also established for the screening of high-risk women.

Notes

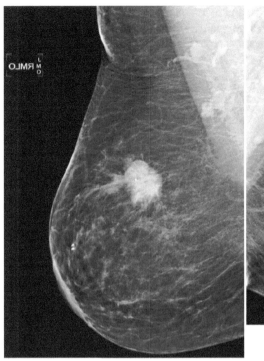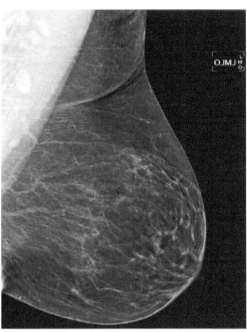

History: A 66-year-old asymptomatic woman presents for routine screening.

1. What are the three most important risk factors for developing breast cancer?
   A. Female gender
   B. Increasing age
   C. Family and personal history of breast cancer
   D. Obesity
   E. Known inherited gene mutation

2. How does estrogen play a role in breast cancer risk?
   A. Estrogen stimulates the development of breast ducts and affects cell division.
   B. Women who have late menarche and early menopause are at greater risk.
   C. There is no role in breast cancer risk. All women have exposure to estrogen, and breast cancer is diagnosed in only a minority.
   D. Taking exogenous estrogen does not increase the risk of breast cancer.

3. What percentage of breast cancers is due to known genetic mutations?
   A. 50%
   B. 1%
   C. 75%
   D. 5% to 10%

4. How do benign breast biopsies affect breast cancer risk?
   A. There is no relation between benign breast biopsy and cancer.
   B. Some lesions that are biopsied contain atypical cells that might be a precursor to cancer.
   C. There is about a 10-fold increase in breast cancer risk with certain benign biopsy results.
   D. Women with a family history of breast cancer and atypical results on biopsy are at no greater risk than women with family history alone.

C A S E 3

Risk Factors

1. A, B, and C
2. A
3. D
4. B

References

Bassett LW, Jackson VP, Jahan R, et al: *Diagnosis of Diseases of the Breast*, Philadelphia: Saunders, 1997, p 308.
Evans DG, Howell A: Breast cancer risk-assessment models. *Breast Cancer Res* 2007;9(5):213.

Cross-Reference

Ikeda D: *Breast Imaging: THE REQUISITES*, 2nd ed, Philadelphia: Saunders, 2010, p 24.

Comment

The most important risk factor for developing breast cancer is being female. Males have a low incidence and have approximately 1% of the total of breast cancers diagnosed. The second most important risk factor is increasing age. Risk steadily increases as the woman ages. Exposure to estrogen is an important risk factor, because estrogen influences cell division and breast duct development. The figure shows a suspicious mass in the right breast seen on a routine screening mammogram.

The longer the exposure to estrogen, the greater the chance of breast cancer, so women who begin menses early and who have a late menopause have higher risk. Women who have no pregnancies are at higher risk. The late timing of the first pregnancy also is thought to increase risk, because the developing breast of the adolescent and young adult has a longer exposure to estrogen. Estrogen supports the growth of estrogen-sensitive tumors.

Family history of breast cancer is an important risk factor, although the majority of women with breast cancer have no family members affected. Family history is present in approximately 25% of cancers diagnosed. The more important family members to assess in risk determination are the first-degree relatives: mother, sister, daughter, father, brother, and son. Second-degree relatives—grandmother, grandfather, aunt, and uncle—also play a role in risk, but to a lesser degree. The age of the relative is also important: The younger the age of the relative at diagnosis, the more significant the risk. Multiple premenopausal women with breast cancer in the family raises the concern for a possible gene mutation. Other factors include the presence of male breast cancer in the family and Ashkenazi Jewish heritage.

The two most common known genetic mutations are *BRCA1* and *BRCA2*. Having one of these two mutations significantly increases the likelihood of developing breast cancer; breast cancer is 50% to 85% more likely to be diagnosed in a woman with either mutation in her lifetime. Recent data suggest that women who have a 20% or greater lifetime risk of breast cancer by a risk-assessment model should be screened with MRI as well as mammography annually. Risk-assessment models are available to practitioners and patients. The Gail, Claus, and Cuzick-Tyrer models are commonly used.

Breast cancer is thought to develop stepwise, through abnormalities in cell proliferation, so that normal cells develop into atypical hyperplasia, then into in situ cancer, then into infiltrative cancer. An abnormality that is detected in screening or by palpation and that is shown to be proliferative on histology confers an increased risk of developing cancer in that patient of 1.5 to 2 times, even though the lesion itself is benign. These lesions include sclerosing adenosis, papillomatosis, complex fibroadenoma, and hyperplasia without atypia. If the lesion is atypical hyperplasia, either lobular or ductal type, the risk increases to 4 to 5 times her normal risk.

Notes

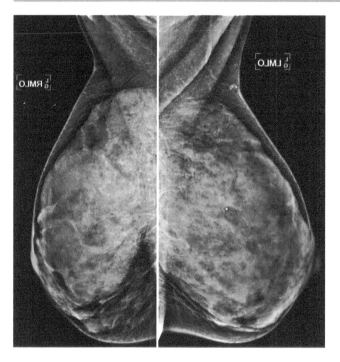

History: An asymptomatic 42-year-old woman presents for a routine screening mammogram.

1. What is in the differential for diagnosis, tissue density, and Breast Imaging Reporting and Data System (BI-RADS) code of the mammogram views presented? (Choose all that apply.)
   A. Normal fatty breast, BI-RADS 1
   B. Indeterminate calcification in left breast, dense, BI-RADS 0
   C. Dense breasts with punctate calcification in both breasts, BI-RADS 2
   D. Normal dense breasts, BI-RADS 1

2. The descriptor of tissue density "scattered fibroglandular densities" corresponds to what percentage of gland tissue on the mammogram?
   A. 10%
   B. 60%
   C. 25% to 50%
   D. There is no percentage of gland tissue in the descriptors; they are meant as subjective assessment only.

3. What is the MQSA?
   A. Mammography Quality Standards Act
   B. A state-by-state law, not federally mandated
   C. A voluntary system for accreditation of mammography centers.
   D. A federal act requiring only free-standing mammography facilities to be accredited. The act does not apply to hospital-based practices.

4. Why is the BI-RADS code important?
   A. It helps patients and referring physicians understand the mammography report, and it is mandated by the MQSA.
   B. Although it is not mandated by law, it is good medical practice.
   C. It helps speed the interpretation of the mammogram.
   D. Although it is good medical practice, it is cumbersome to use, and it makes result tracking more difficult.

CASE 4

The Mammogram Report

1. C and D
2. C
3. A
4. A

References

American College of Radiology: *Breast Imaging Reporting and Data System.* Reston, VA, American College of Radiology, 2003.

Eberl MM, Fox CH, Edge SB, et al: BI-RADS classification for management of abnormal mammograms. *J Am Board Fam Med* 2006;19 (2):161-164.

Liberman L, Abramson AF, Squires FB, et al: The breast imaging reporting and data system: positive predictive value of mammographic features and final assessment categories. *AJR Am J Roentgenol* 1998;171:35-40.

Cross-Reference

Ikeda D: *Breast Imaging: THE REQUISITES,* 2nd ed, Philadelphia: Saunders, 2010, p 39.

Comment

The mammogram report should follow a standard format, which includes the following elements:

1. Reason for exam—screening (routine) versus diagnostic (problem solving)
2. Tissue density (breast composition)
   A. Almost entirely fat (< 25% glandular)
   B. Scattered fibroglandular densities (25% to 50% glandular)
   C. Heterogeneous dense, which could obscure detection of small masses (50% to 75% glandular)
   D. Extremely dense, which might lower the sensitivity of mammography (> 75% glandular) (as in the patient depicted in the figure)

3. Description of any significant findings
   A. Mass
   B. Calcifications (which may be scattered and punctate, as in the figure)
   C. Architectural distortion
4. Comparison to previous exam, if available
5. Impression; include BI-RADS categories
   A. BI-RADS 1—negative
   B. BI-RADS 2—benign finding(s) (as in the mammogram in the figure)
   C. BI-RADS 3—probably benign (< 2% chance of malignancy)
   D. BI-RADS 4—suspicious abnormality, biopsy should be considered
   E. BI-RADS 5—highly suspicious, appropriate action should be taken (> 95% chance of malignancy)
   F. BI-RADS 6—biopsy-proven cancer
   G. BI-RADS 0—incomplete, needs additional evaluation

The inclusion of a recommendation at the end of the report is good medical practice. This should state if the patient is to have her next mammogram at the standard interval, needs a follow-up at a short interval, needs additional views, or needs a biopsy.

Screening mammography results should be limited to normal (BI-RADS 1 or 2) or incomplete (BI-RADS 0), needs more evaluation. BI-RADS 4 or 5 is not given at screening. Suspicious findings should be further evaluated with additional views before rendering a final impression. BI-RADS 3 is used after the full evaluation has been performed and the finding is a small chance of malignancy (< 2%), and a short-interval follow-up is recommended.

Notes

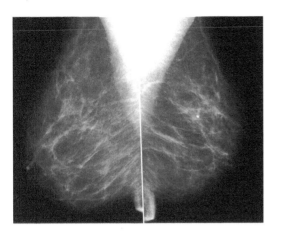
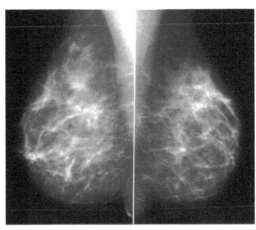
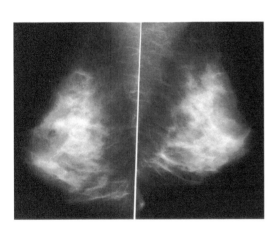
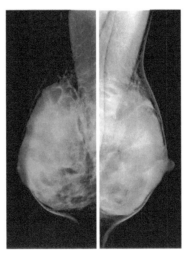

History: Screening mammograms.

1. What is your differential diagnosis for the four different patients? (Choose all that apply.)
   A. No abnormality seen
   B. Normal mammograms with four different tissue densities
   C. Four patients demonstrating different stages of menstrual life (puberty, menstrual, perimenopausal, postmenopausal)
   D. Four normal patients; the differences among the four reflect the timing of the mammogram with the menstrual cycle

2. Why is it important to report the tissue density in the mammogram report?
   A. The breast density reflects your confidence in excluding cancer.
   B. The mammogram is not very sensitive in detecting cancer in the fatty-replaced breast.
   C. It is required by the Mammography Quality Standards Act (MQSA).
   D. It is a very precise way of describing the character of the breast tissue.

3. How does the breast density affect the sensitivity for detecting breast cancer on the mammogram?
   A. Breast cancer sensitivity is highest in the fatty breast.
   B. Sensitivity is highest in the dense breast.
   C. Sensitivity is lower when the density is lower.
   D. Breast density is not related to mammographic sensitivity.

4. Does breast density change over the woman's life?
   A. No, breast tissue density is inherent, and it is stable over time.
   B. Yes, the breast becomes denser as the woman ages.
   C. Yes, there are many changing factors that affect density, such as age, hormonal status, exogenous hormones, and weight.
   D. Yes, density changes only related to the woman's weight. Thinner women have less fat in their breasts.

CASE 5

Breast Tissue Density Examples

1. A and B
2. A
3. A
4. C

References

American College of Radiology : *Breast Imaging Reporting and Data System (BI-RADS)*. Reston, VA: American College of Radiology, 2003.

Kerlikowske K, Carney PA, Geller B, et al: Performance of screening mammography among women with and without a first-degree relative with breast cancer. *Ann Intern Med* 2000;133:855-863.

Lautin EM, Berlin L: Writing, signing, and reading the radiology report: who is responsible and when? *Am J Roentgenol* 2001;177:246-248.

Cross-Reference

Ikeda D: *Breast Imaging: THE REQUISITES*, 2nd ed, Philadelphia: Saunders, 2010, p 29.

Comment

Mammographic density is reported because it tells the referring physician the sensitivity of the mammogram in detecting breast cancer. In the fatty breast, the contrast between the background dark fat and the white tumor is the greatest; therefore, sensitivity for detecting cancer is the highest in this type of breast. In the dense breast, the background density is white, similar to the density of tumor, so a tumor can be missed.

The four-category system of breast density is as follows:

1. Almost entirely fat, $<25\%$ glandular
2. Scattered fibroglandular densities, 25% to 50% glandular
3. Heterogeneously dense, 50% to 75% glandular
4. Extremely dense, $>75\%$ glandular

Dense breasts are seen commonly in young women, and the density can decrease with age. However, many young women do not have dense breasts, and postmenopausal women with no exogenous hormone use can have dense breasts. The density is also affected by lactation. During lactation the breast is commonly very dense. The patient's weight can affect breast density. Typically, thin women have dense breasts, and obese women have fatty-replaced breasts. The sensitivity of the mammogram varies with the patient's age and with breast density.

Notes

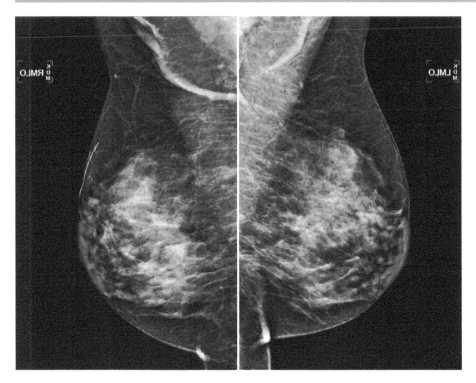

History: Routine mammogram in an 82-year-old asymptomatic woman with no history of breast surgery. She is not taking hormones.

1. What is your differential diagnosis for this patient, including BI-RADS diagnostic code? (Choose all that apply.)
   A. Benign mammogram, BI-RADS 2
   B. Focal asymmetric density in right upper posterior breast, BI-RADS 0
   C. Heterogeneously dense breasts, BI-RADS 2
   D. Dense breasts, advise screening MRI, BI-RADS 0
   E. Suspicious calcifications in left breast, BI-RADS 0

2. Does this breast density confer a higher risk of malignancy?
   A. No, risk is not related to breast density.
   B. No, her only risk factor is her age.
   C. Yes, there is an increased risk of malignancy in women with dense breasts.
   D. No, fatty breasts have the highest risk of malignancy.

3. Is this tissue density seen more often in premenopausal or postmenopausal women?
   A. Dense breasts are more common in postmenopausal women.
   B. There is no relation of breast density to menopausal status.
   C. Breast density is related only to the degree of fat in the breast, not to menopausal status.
   D. Dense breasts are more common in premenopausal women.

4. In the postmenopausal woman, is this density related to hormone therapy?
   A. No, it is not related.
   B. Yes, hormones can increase breast density.
   C. Yes, but hormones cause increased density only in the upper outer quadrant of the breasts.
   D. Yes, but it also always causes pain.

Dense Breast in an 82-Year-Old Woman

1. A and C
2. C
3. D
4. B

References
Harvey JA, Bovbjerg VE: Quantitative assessment of mammographic breast density: relationship with breast cancer risk. *Radiology* 2004;230:29-41.

Stomper PC, D'Souza DJ, DiNitto PA, Arredondo MA: Analysis of parenchymal density on mammograms in 1353 women 25–79 years old. *Am J Roentgenol* 1996;167:1261.

Cross-Reference
Ikeda D: *Breast Imaging: THE REQUISITES*, 2nd ed, Philadelphia: Saunders, 2010, p 29.

Comment
Denser breasts are commonly seen in mammography. This type of mammogram is more difficult to interpret because the radiographic density of the glandular tissue and a mass or cyst is similar, meaning that masses may be obscured in a dense breast. The dense tissue on the mammogram represents the ducts and lobules and also fibrous connective tissue. In a dense breast, there is relatively little fat interspersed between the glandular elements.

Increased density imparted an increased risk of breast cancer in several studies using a quantitative measurement of breast density, with an odds ratio of 4.0 or greater, meaning that women with dense breasts had a fourfold increase in risk of breast cancer compared to those with the least dense breasts. Due to the breast density and advanced age, older women with dense breasts have an even higher risk.

Breast tissue is responsive to hormone changes. Estrogen levels are higher in younger women, and after menopause, estrogen levels diminish and cause the breast lobules to regress. The mammogram then becomes less dense. About 65% of women in their twenties have at least 50% breast density. This decreases to 50% of women in their forties and to 30% of women in their seventies. Therefore, this relatively dense breast is uncommon in older women.

Hormone replacement therapy increases the glandular density of the breast in up to 73% of women, and the greatest increase in density occurs in the first year of use. This increase in density is due to stimulation of the cells of the ducts, lobules, and stroma to proliferate and increase mitotic activity.

The 82-year-old patient reported here is not on hormone replacement therapy, and the mammogram is unchanged compared to previous exams.

Notes

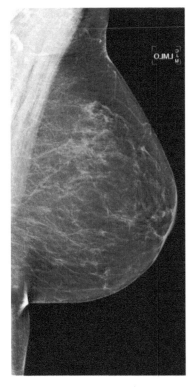 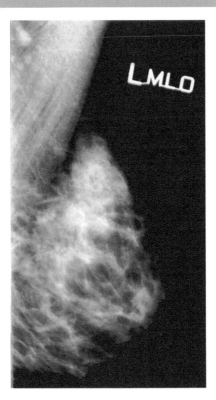

History: Left mediolateral oblique (MLO) mammograms of a 55-year-old woman taken 1 year apart. On the day of the later exam, she complains of bilateral breast tenderness and swelling.

1. What is your differential diagnosis for the change in the mammogram of this patient? (Choose all that apply.)
   A. Weight loss
   B. Edema
   C. Hormone replacement therapy
   D. Typical changes of menopause
   E. Inflammatory breast cancer

2. What personal history question is typically asked of the patient who comes in for a mammogram?
   A. History of hormone use
   B. History of clotting function
   C. Family history of renal and liver disease
   D. History of arthritis

3. What would you do next to work up the patient's symptoms and the change in the mammogram?
   A. MRI is needed for more complete evaluation.
   B. Take a clinical history regarding exogenous hormone use and any focal findings.
   C. Nothing; this is normal for this age.
   D. Ultrasound should be used in both breasts to further evaluate the bilateral breast tenderness and swelling.

4. What is your recommendation for management of this patient?
   A. Exogenous hormone therapy should be stopped because of the change on the mammogram.
   B. The patient should have more frequent mammography, every 6 months for 3 years, to monitor the changes.
   C. Recommend routine mammography.
   D. The patient should have needle biopsy of random sites in both breasts.

CASE 7

Hormones

1. A, B, C, and E
2. A
3. B
4. C

References

Berkowitz JE, Gatewood OM, Goldblum LE, Gayler BW: Hormonal replacement therapy: mammographic manifestations. *Radiology* 1990;174:199-201.

National Cancer Institute: Menopausal hormone replacement therapy use and cancer (factsheet).

Rutter CM, Mandelson MT, Laya MB, Taplin S: Changes in breast density associated with initiation, discontinuation, and continuing use of hormone replacement therapy. *JAMA* 2001;285(2):171-176.

Stomper PC, Van Voorhis BJ, Ravnikar VA, Meyer JE: Mammographic changes associated with postmenopausal hormone replacement therapy: a longitudinal study. *Radiology* 1990;174:487-490.

Cross-Reference

Ikeda D: *Breast Imaging: THE REQUISITES*, 2nd ed, Philadelphia: Saunders, 2010, p 392.

Comment

The breasts bilaterally show an increase in density, although only one view is shown here (see the figures). The density is now "heterogeneously dense," whereas before the density was "scattered fibroglandular densities." The most common cause of bilaterally symmetric increasing density that involves the glandular tissue and not the skin (no edema or skin thickening) is exogenous hormone therapy (HRT), as in this case. The patient had begun taking a combined estrogen and progesterone supplement.

Normally, as a woman enters menopause, involutional changes occur in the breast parenchyma (see the figures). The volume of the mammographically dense areas tends to decrease as the glandular elements involute and are replaced by fat. HRT reverses the normal involution, and histologically the breast epithelium and stromal elements proliferate. This is due to the effects of the estrogen component of the HRT. The progesterone effects include an increase in epithelial mytotic activity and lobular hyperplasia.

These effects have been shown to increase the incidence of breast cancer in the postmenopausal population taking exogenous hormones, particularly combined therapy. In 2002, the Women's Health Initiative (WHI), a study of exogenous hormone use, found an additional eight cases of breast cancer per 10,000 women in women on combined hormonal therapy for 1 year, compared to the placebo group. The choice to remain on hormone therapy is up to the patient and her clinician, and mammography is not typically performed at any different schedule because of this increased risk.

The imaging evaluation is based on the clinical findings. Ultrasound is not indicated when there is a diffuse bilateral increase in density when it can be explained by exogenous hormonal therapy. In our practice, we do not generally perform ultrasound on women who have bilateral diffuse breast pain. If there is a focal area of tenderness or an area of palpable concern, a directed ultrasound is performed. Occasionally, the mammographic and clinical findings are more unilateral and focal, in which case physical exam, directed ultrasound, and possibly MRI may be needed to exclude a developing malignancy.

Notes

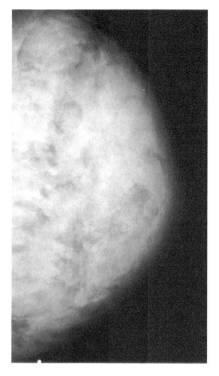
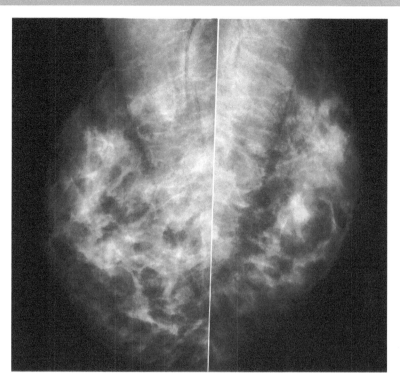

History: A 40-year-old woman presents for routine screening mammogram. The first figure is the right mediolateral oblique (MLO) view 4 years earlier, when she had presented with a palpable lump. The second figure is the current exam.

1. What is your differential diagnosis for the difference in the appearance of the mammogram between the two exams? (Choose all that apply.)
   A. The patient gained weight, causing more fat to develop in the breast.
   B. The patient began taking birth control pills.
   C. The patient was lactating on the earlier exam.
   D. The patient had inflammatory breast cancer on the initial image, which was successfully treated.

2. Can you be sure this is the same patient? What can you do to try to verify the patient's identity when reading mammograms?
   A. Check the patient's name on the image because this will always be correct.
   B. Check for unique patterns of blood vessels and lymph nodes on the image.
   C. Ask the patient if this is her previous mammogram.
   D. When the appearance of the glandular tissue is very different, assume it is not the same patient.

3. Why was only one view performed when the patient presented with a palpable lump?
   A. Mammography is limited during lactation, owing to breast density.
   B. Mammography is dangerous to the infant being nursed, owing to radiation exposure.
   C. Ultrasound alone can be used to evaluate the finding in all cases of palpable masses.
   D. A bilateral four-view mammogram should always be performed in the case of a palpable mass, no matter the circumstances.

4. Why is mammography used at all for a lactating patient?
   A. It should not be used in this situation.
   B. Even though a woman is lactating, she should still have routine screening mammograms.
   C. Mammography is used to evaluate the palpable finding, especially if the ultrasound exam shows a suspicious finding or is negative.
   D. If the ultrasound exam demonstrates a simple cyst, mammography must also be used.

C A S E 8

Lactational Change

1. A, B, and C
2. B
3. A
4. C

Reference

Ahn BY, Kim HH, Moon WK, et al: Pregnancy- and lactation-associated breast cancer: mammographic and sonographic findings. *J Ultrasound Med* 2003;22:491-497.

Cross-Reference

Ikeda D: *Breast Imaging: THE REQUISITES*, 2nd ed, Philadelphia: Saunders, 2010, p 378.

Comment

This 40-year-old woman presented for a routine mammogram. Her prior exam was made available for comparison, yet it is not at all similar to the current exam. It is important to verify the identity of the patient when interpreting studies, because human error can result in the wrong patient's name on the exam. In this case, this *is* her prior exam, and the breast appearance is different because of lactation. This case illustrates the difficulty that can occur in interpreting the mammogram during lactation. During lactation, milk is produced by the lobules and carried in the ducts, which can increase the size and density of the breast, as in this case (see the figures). There is no danger to the nursing infant in performing mammography during lactation.

Ultrasound is often used as the initial exam for evaluating a palpable mass during lactation. If ultrasound demonstrates a simple cyst or a benign-appearing lactating adenoma or other benign mass that corresponds to the palpable finding, no mammogram is indicated. However, if the ultrasound is negative, mammography should be performed for more complete evaluation, essentially to check for a suspicious mass or microcalcifications (which are not present in this patient). If ultrasound demonstrates a suspicious mass, then mammography should be performed to check for extent of disease, such as microcalcifications or additional masses.

Notes

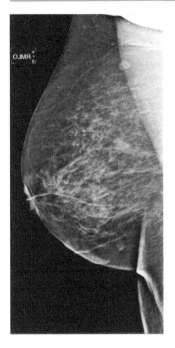 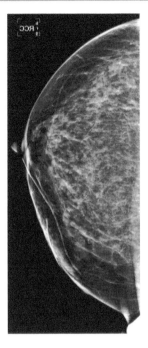 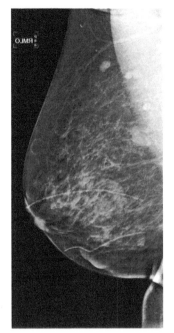 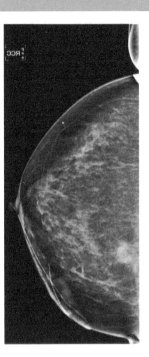

History: A 64-year-old woman with keloids from prior benign surgery presents for a routine screening mammogram. Right mediolateral oblique (MLO) and craniocaudal (CC) views are shown (see the first two figures). The patient returns for a right mammogram when she palpates a lump. Right MLO and CC views are shown from the second mammogram (see the second two figures).

1. What should be included in the differential diagnosis of the two sets of mammograms of the right breast? (Choose all that apply.)
   A. Suspicious mass at 9 o'clock position, not present on first mammogram
   B. Benign-appearing mass in the 4'clock position, new since previous mammogram
   C. Suspicious mass at 1 o'clock position
   D. Benign mass at 1 o'clock position

2. What is the posterior nipple line?
   A. A line connecting the nipples on three views of the same breast
   B. An imaginary line connecting the nipple to the posterior chest wall
   C. A line drawn parallel to the chest wall, at the level of the nipple
   D. A line drawn to measure the distance from the nipple to a lesion

3. If you think that screening mammographic views are not correctly positioned, what is the next step?
   A. The patient should be recalled for proper positioning.
   B. The mammogram should be read, and the radiologist should tell the technologist to do better next time.
   C. The radiologist should make a note in the report that positioning is suboptimal.
   D. Because perfectly positioned films are unreasonable to expect, the radiologist should interpret the images as usual.

4. What is the next step in management of this patient?
   A. MRI
   B. Short-interval follow-up
   C. Ultrasound
   D. Stereotactic biopsy

CASE 9

Poor Positioning, Missed Cancer

1. C and D
2. B
3. A
4. C

References

Eklund GW, Cardenosa G: The art of mammographic positioning. *Radiol Clin North Am* 1992;30(1):21-53.

Majid AS, de Paredes ES, Doherty RD, et al: Missed breast carcinoma: pitfalls and pearls. *Radiographics* 2003;23(4):881-895.

Cross-Reference

Ikeda D: *Breast Imaging: THE REQUISITES*, 2nd ed, Philadelphia: Saunders, 2010, p 6.

Comment

In this patient, a mass was seen only after she presented with a palpable lump. It was not recognized on the routine mammogram performed earlier because of inadequate positioning.

Proper positioning is an important part of breast imaging. It requires constant diligence on the part of the radiologic technologist and cooperation by the patient. Positioning must be evaluated by the radiologist on every examination. If positioning is inadequate, the patient needs to be recalled to have a well-performed mammogram, and the technologist needs to be informed that the positioning was not done to satisfaction.

The posterior nipple line is a way to assess the proper positioning of the mammogram. An imaginary line is drawn from the nipple to the chest wall or edge of the MLO image, perpendicular to the pectoral muscle (see the figures). This line is then drawn on the CC view, from the nipple to the edge of the then image. The length of the line on the CC view should be within 1 cm of the length of the line on the MLO view. In this case, it is not; the CC view is short. The mass present in the medial aspect of the breast was not included on the examination.

Notes

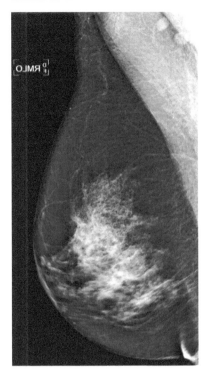 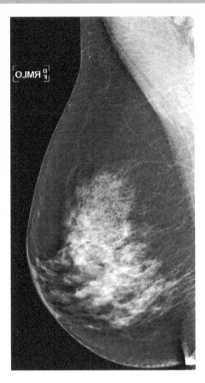

History: An asymptomatic woman presents for a routine screening mammogram.

1. A single right mediolateral oblique (MLO) view is shown in the first figure; repeat right MLO view is shown in the second figure. What is your one best reason for recalling this patient for an additional right MLO view?
   A. The right breast MLO view is poorly positioned.
   B. Microcalcifications in the breast need to be evaluated.
   C. The first view has motion blur.
   D. A possible mass in the central right breast needs to be evaluated.

2. Where is motion blur most likely to occur?
   A. On the craniocaudal (CC) view
   B. In the upper aspect of the breast
   C. On a spot compression view
   D. In the MLO or ML view

3. How can motion blur best be avoided?
   A. Minimize the length of exposure.
   B. Lower the kVp.
   C. Decrease compression.
   D. Perform a "true lateral" view instead of an MLO view.

4. What is a technical recall?
   A. A patient is recalled because the mammogram is not adequate for interpretation, owing to technical reasons.
   B. A patient is recalled for magnifications or spot compression views.
   C. The patient cannot tolerate compression.
   D. The patient has never had a mammogram before.

CASE 10

Motion Unsharpness

1. C
2. D
3. A
4. A

References
Bassett LW: Clinical image evaluation. *Radiol Clin North Am* 1995;33 (6):1027-1039.

Eklund GW, Cardenosa G: The art of mammographic positioning. *Radiol Clin North Am* 1992;30(1):21-53.

Helvie MA, Chan HP, Adler DD, Boyd PG: Breast thickness in routine mammogram: effect on image quality and radiation dose. *AJR Am J Roentgenol* 1994;163:1371-1374.

Majid AS, de Paredes ES, Doherty RD, et al: Missed breast carcinoma: pitfalls and pearls. *Radiographics* 2003;23:881-895.

Taplin SH, Rutter CM, Finder C, et al: Screening mammography: clinical image quality and the risk of interval breast cancer. *AJR Am J Roentgenol* 2002;178(4):797-803.

Cross-Reference
Ikeda D: *Breast Imaging: THE REQUISITES*, 2nd ed, Philadelphia: Saunders, 2010, p 6.

Comment

Technical aspects of a good-quality image of the breast include positioning, compression, exposure, sharpness, noise, artifacts, and contrast. This case demonstrates motion unsharpness in the right MLO view (see the figures). The repeat image (see the figures) reveals sharper detail. Motion unsharpness can result when the patient moves during the exposure, and inadequate compression can contribute to it. This type of motion unsharpness often occurs in the inferior aspect of the breast on the MLO view, and it can be recognized by poor separation and blurriness of the edges of linear structures and tissue borders. This can be difficult to recognize, but it is important, because malignancy can be missed owing to unsharpness of the image. This is particularly true for microcalcifications and small masses. Compression thickness is greater on the MLO view than on the craniocaudal (CC) view, and it is more common to see motion unsharpness on the MLO view. Adequate compression immobilizes the breast and decreases the likelihood of motion unsharpness, reduces breast thickness, and reduces the dose needed for a proper exposure. If blur is seen, mammographic detail is compromised, and the image is not adequate for interpretation. The patient should be recalled for a repeat image ("technical recall").

Notes

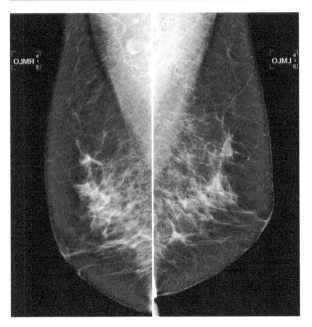
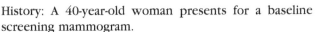
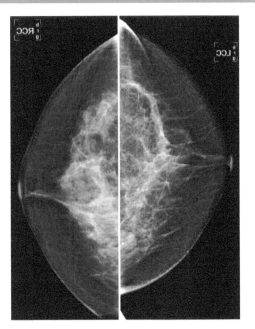

History: A 40-year-old woman presents for a baseline screening mammogram.

1. What should be included in the differential diagnosis, based on the four-view screening mammogram? (Choose all that apply.)
   A. Normal mammogram
   B. Malignant mass in the left medial breast
   C. Benign mass in the left medial breast
   D. Cyst in the left medial breast

2. What is the next step in the evaluation?
   A. Recommend routine screening mammogram in 1 year.
   B. Recall for additional spot compression views and ultrasound.
   C. Perform MRI of the left breast.
   D. Refer patient to a surgeon.

3. Why is the mass seen better on the craniocaudal (CC) view?
   A. The finding is a superimposition of densities, not a true mass.
   B. A mass is typically better seen on the CC view because of better compression of this view compared with the mediolateral oblique (MLO) view.
   C. Typically, the medial breast is not included well on the MLO view.
   D. The CC view is better positioned.

4. What are Tabar's "danger zones"?
   A. Areas of the world in which it is dangerous to practice breast imaging
   B. Areas of the mammogram that are most likely to contain malignancy
   C. Areas of the breast that are more likely to have malignant spread to the lymph nodes
   D. Areas of the breast that are usually normal fat and to which special attention should be paid

Medial Mass

1. B, C, and D
2. B
3. C
4. D

References

Eklund GW, Cardenosa G: The art of mammographic positioning. *Radiol Clin North Am* 1992;30(1):21-53.

Ikeda DM, Birdwell RL, O'Shaughnessy KF, et al: Analysis of 172 subtle findings on prior normal mammograms in women with breast cancer detected at follow up screening. *Radiology* 2003;226(2):494-503.

Cross-Reference

Ikeda D: *Breast Imaging: THE REQUISITES*, 2nd ed, Philadelphia: Saunders, 2010, p 38.

Comment

Masses or densities in the medial breast are in what is termed a "danger zone." Typically, only fat and minimal gland tissue is seen in this area. The other "danger zones" include the retroglandular fat and the edge of the image. This case illustrates two of these "danger zone" findings: a mass in the medial breast (see the figures) and a mass that is just barely seen at the edge of the image on the MLO view (see the figures).

Most of the gland tissue of the breast is in the upper outer quadrant. For this reason, the MLO view was designated a standard view, rather than the orthogonal mediolateral view. The MLO view includes the upper outer quadrant more completely. However, the medial breast is not as well seen on the MLO view. For this reason, the medial breast must be included on the CC view as completely as possible. Medial masses seen on the CC view may not be seen on the MLO view because of the relative limitation of the MLO view in the medial breast. Focal densities seen only on one view, in the medial breast on the CC view, should be viewed with suspicion. Additional imaging should be performed.

This patient was recalled for spot compression views and ultrasound. The mass was seen on both spot compression views, and ultrasound showed a 17-mm solid mass in the 8 o'clock position of the lower inner left breast. The patient underwent a core needle biopsy, and histology showed a fibroadenoma.

Notes

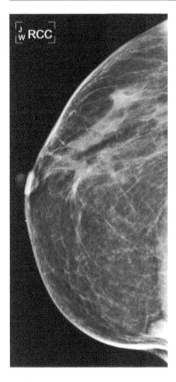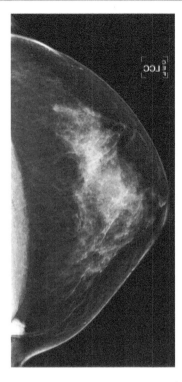

History: Craniocaudal (CC) view from routine mammogram in two different women.

1. What is your differential diagnosis for the finding in the medial aspect of the CC view in these two different patients? (Choose all that apply.)
   A. Abnormality in the pectoralis muscle
   B. Sternalis muscle, a normal variant in some patients
   C. Artifact on the patient
   D. Mass in the medial breast

2. What further work-up is performed next?
   A. Spot compression views
   B. MRI
   C. CT

3. If there is a 5-cm mass in the medial breast on the CC view, does the differential diagnosis still include a sternalis muscle?
   A. No, the sternalis muscle is typically less than 2 cm in cross section.
   B. No, because the sternalis muscle is not located medially.
   C. Yes, the finding could still represent the sternalis muscle.
   D. Yes, whenever a mass is seen only on the CC view, the sternalis muscle should be first in the differential diagnosis.

4. Where is the sternalis muscle?
   A. It is posterior to the pectoralis muscle and runs parallel to the pectoralis.
   B. It is lateral to the sternum, running vertically, perpendicular to the pectoralis.
   C. It is lateral to the pectoralis, running vertically in the mid-axillary line.
   D. It runs parallel to the clavicle, adjacent to the sternum.

CASE 12

Sternalis Muscle

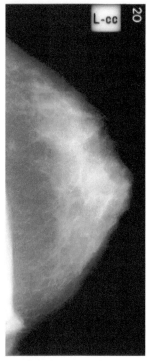

Prior left CC view from patient 2.

1. B and D
2. A
3. A
4. B

References

Bradley FM, Hoover HC Jr, Hulka CA, et al: The sternalis muscle: an unusual normal finding seen on mammography. *AJR Am J Roentgenol* 1996;166(1):33-36.

Zaher WA, Darwish HH, Abdalla AME, et al: Sternalis: a clinically important variation. *Pak J Med Sci* 2009;25(2):325-328.

Cross-Reference

Ikeda D: *Breast Imaging: THE REQUISITES*, 2nd ed, Philadelphia: Saunders, 2010, p 28.

Comment

The sternalis muscle is a variation of the chest wall musculature that is seen in approximately 8% of the population according to cadaveric studies. This muscle is long and narrow and runs vertically along the sternum at 90 degrees to the pectoralis muscle. It may be unilateral or bilateral; more often it is unilateral. It is seen in the far medial aspect of the breast on the CC view only, and it can be mistaken for a medial breast mass. It can have a rounded, triangular, or flame-shaped configuration, and it is usually surrounded by fat. It is typically less than 2 cm in diameter.

It is important to recognize this normal variant muscle (see the figures) and to avoid any additional work-up. Spot compression views and ultrasound are unrevealing, as is the physical exam. If the additional work-up is done and no mass is seen on ultrasound or felt on physical exam, and there is still diagnostic concern, cross-sectional imaging with CT or MR will demonstrate the sternalis muscle running perpendicular to the pectoralis, along the sternum. If prior mammograms are available, comparison can be helpful to observe the stability of the finding (see the figures).

The sternalis should be differentiated from the pectoralis muscle, which is present in nearly all patients, and the technologist should attempt to include the pectoralis on the CC as well as the mediolateral oblique (MLO) views, to demonstrate that the entire breast has been included in the image.

Notes

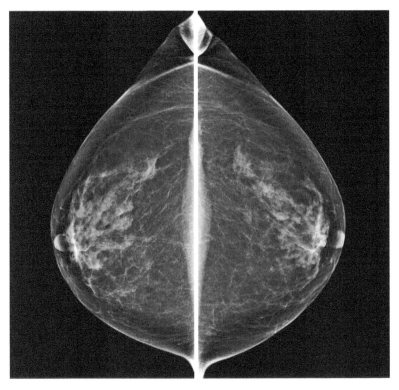

History: Craniocaudal (CC) views from screening mammograms in the same patient are presented.

1. What should be included in the differential diagnosis? (Choose all that apply.)
   A. Normal pectoralis muscle
   B. Mass in the chest wall
   C. Sternalis muscle
   D. Adenopathy

2. What is the next step in the work-up?
   A. MRI to evaluate the chest wall
   B. Breast-specific gamma imaging (BSGI) to evaluate for enhancing lesions
   C. Spot compression views of the denser areas at the chest wall
   D. Referring the patient to a surgeon for a physical examination

3. Is it desirable to position the breast so that the pectoralis muscle is included on the CC view?
   A. No, there is no need to see the pectoralis muscle.
   B. No, it is important only to see the glandular tissue and retroglandular fat.
   C. No, the pectoralis muscle is seen only on the mediolateral oblique (MLO) view.
   D. Yes, it is ideal to see the pectoralis muscle on the CC view.

4. How is the sternalis muscle different from the pectoralis muscle on the CC view?
   A. It is ideal to include the sternalis muscle on every patient.
   B. The sternalis and pectoralis muscles overlap and can be difficult to differentiate.
   C. The sternalis muscle is seen in less than 10% of patients on a mammogram.
   D. The pectoralis muscle is not used to gauge adequate positioning, but including the sternalis muscle indicates a properly positioned image.

Pectoralis Muscle on Craniocaudal View

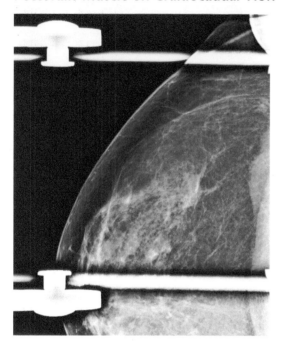

1. A, B, and D
2. C
3. D
4. C

Reference
Eklund GW, Cardenosa G: The art of mammographic positioning. *Radiol Clin North Am* 1992;30(1):21-53.

Cross-Reference
Ikeda D: *Breast Imaging: THE REQUISITES*, 2nd ed, Philadelphia: Saunders, 2010, p 28.

Comment
The pectoralis muscle lies posterior to the breast, the only part of the chest wall that is seen on the mammogram. Positioning the breast to include as much of the breast tissue as possible on the image is one of the most important roles of the mammography technologist. Recognizing that the breast is completely or incompletely imaged is an important responsibility of the radiologist interpreting the mammogram.

The pectoralis muscle is valuable in recognizing the adequacy of breast positioning. It should be seen on the MLO view, extending to the nipple and having a convex anterior margin. On the CC view, it is seen as a convex density at the posterior edge of the image in approximately 25% of patients (see the figures). When the pectoralis muscle is seen, the radiologist can be confident that posterior breast tissue has been adequately included on the image.

The pectoralis muscle may have an undulating contour (see the figures), and this may be confused as a mass. Spot compression views and ultrasound can be used as needed (see the figures) to help evaluate a lumpy contour, but this appearance of the pectoralis muscle is not unusual on the CC view.

Notes

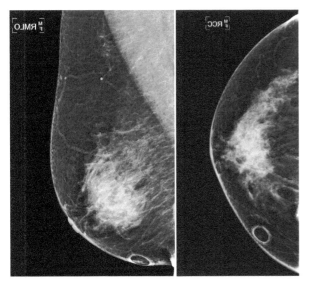
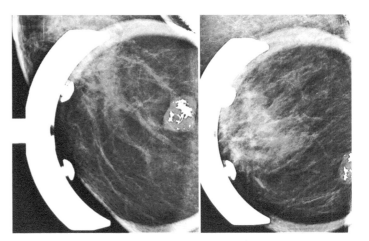
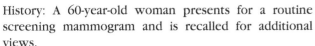

History: A 60-year-old woman presents for a routine screening mammogram and is recalled for additional views.

1. What should be included in the differential diagnosis for the images shown? (Choose all that apply.)
   A. Ductal carcinoma in situ
   B. Calcified fibroadenoma
   C. Fat necrosis
   D. Infiltrating ductal carcinoma

2. Why is the mass not fully seen on the routine views?
   A. It is obscured by surrounding tissue.
   B. It is in the posterior breast.
   C. It is inferior to the central cone of the breast.
   D. It is too far lateral to be included.

3. Which portion of the breast is *not* well seen on the mediolateral oblique (MLO) view?
   A. Lateral aspect
   B. Upper aspect
   C. Medial aspect
   D. Subareolar aspect

4. Where in the right breast is this mass located?
   A. 1 o'clock position
   B. 8 o'clock position
   C. 10 o'clock position
   D. 4 o'clock position

C A S E 1 4

Hidden Mass

1. B, C, and D
2. B
3. C
4. D

References

Harvey JA, Nicholson BT, Cohen MA: Finding early invasive breast cancers: a practical approach. *Radiology* 2008;248(1):61-76.

Majid AS, de Paredes ES, Doherty RD, et al: Missed breast carcinoma: pitfalls and pearls. Radiographics 2003;23(4):881-895.

Singh H: Errors in cancer diagnosis: current understanding and future directions. *J Clin Oncol* 2007;25(31):5009-5018.

Cross-Reference

Ikeda D: *Breast Imaging: THE REQUISITES*, 2nd ed, Philadelphia: Saunders, 2010, pp 29, 408.

Comment

Breast lesions may be missed on mammography for various reasons. This case illustrates a mass that is in the posterior breast, adjacent to the chest wall (see the figures). The posterior breast may be difficult to include on the mammogram. The medial aspect of the breast is another area that may not be well included on both the MLO and craniocaudal (CC) views, so medial lesions can also be missed.

In positioning the breast for the mammogram, the technologist should use the natural features of breast mobility to help include as much breast tissue as possible into the image. The lower portion of the breast is mobile, and the lateral aspect of the breast is mobile. The technologist can mobilize the lateral aspect of the breast medially in positioning the patient for the MLO view. The technologist can mobilize the inferior breast upward for the CC view. In both views, the breast must be pulled gently but firmly away from the chest wall to include as much posterior tissue as possible. Despite these maneuvers, lesions present in the breast may not be included in standard views (see the figures).

The radiologist must pay special attention to the posterior edge of the image to check for the anterior margin of a posterior mass (see the figures). Additional views are needed to try to include this area on the image, such as spot compression (see the figures). If the anterior margin is still not well seen, ultrasound is a useful imaging tool because it is not hampered by the same limitations as mammography.

This patient in this case was aware of the mass in her right breast and knew it was stable by palpation. She reported that a biopsy was performed more than 10 years previously at another institution, and the biopsy finding was a fibroadenoma.

Notes

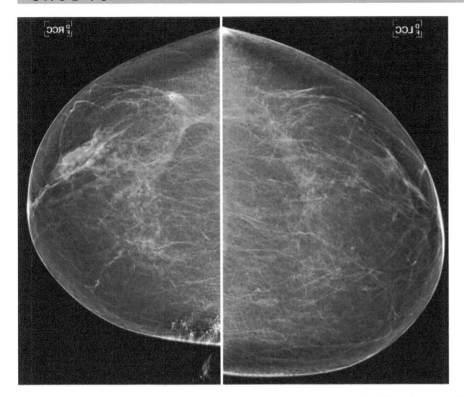

History: A 72-year-old woman presents for a routine screening mammogram. The craniocaudal (CC) views are shown.

1. What should be included in the differential diagnosis of the minus-density finding in the medial right breast? (Choose all that apply.)
   A. Artifact from scratches on the film
   B. Artifact from patient's hair on the image
   C. Linear branching calcifications in the medial right breast
   D. Artifact stuck to the medial aspect of the patient's breast

2. What is the next step in the work-up?
   A. The patient should be recalled for a repeat right CC view.
   B. The patient should be contacted and informed that she should tie back her hair.
   C. Nothing should be done because this is an obvious artifact; there is no breast abnormality.
   D. Spot magnification views of the medial right breast should be obtained.

3. Why is it important to be aware of artifacts?
   A. They are not important because they are obvious when seen.
   B. They can interfere with image interpretation.
   C. They improve image quality.
   D. They can be easily controlled, and there is no excuse for having artifacts.

4. What is an artifact?
   A. An object that is always outside the patient
   B. An object that interferes with interpretation of the image
   C. An object that may mimic a true finding
   D. An object that can be found anywhere along the route of the x-ray beam from source to image receptor
   E. B, C, and D
   F. All of the above

CASE 15

Artifact: Hair

1. B and D
2. A
3. B
4. E

Reference

Hogge JP, Palmer CH, Muller CC, et al: Quality assurance in mammography: artifact analysis. *Radiographics* 1999;19(2):503-522.

Cross-Reference

Ikeda D: *Breast Imaging: THE REQUISITES*, 2nd ed, Philadelphia: Saunders, 2010, p 74.

Comment

Artifacts must be recognized when they are present on an image. There are certain pathognomonic appearances. Once these artifacts are seen, they should be easily recognized when they reappear. Hair artifact is one such finding. The long white curvilinear markings seen at the chest wall aspect of the image should not be confused with breast pathology (see the figures). A hair artifact is typically present on the CC view, as the patient leans in over the image receptor as the exposure is being made. Hair overlying the breast can obscure detail of the tissue underneath, so the image must be repeated.

The radiologist needs to be aware of artifact appearance because the technologist may not recognize the artifact at the time of the examination. If the image is not repeated at the time of the visit, the patient must be recalled for a repeat view that is technically adequate for interpretation.

Notes

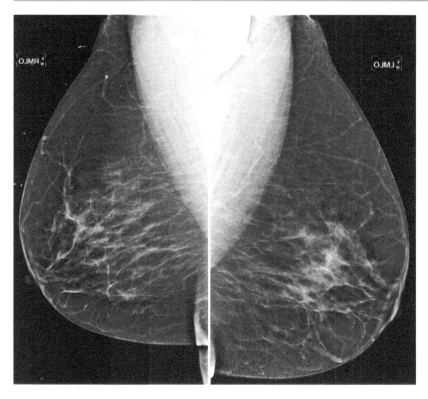

History: Bilateral mediolateral oblique (MLO) views of asymptomatic 85-year-old woman.

1. What is the differential diagnosis for the dense object in the left axilla? (Choose all that apply.)
   A. Large dense lymph node
   B. Pacemaker battery overlying the left upper chest
   C. Patient's chin
   D. Breast mass

2. What Breast Imaging Reporting and Data System (BI-RADS) code should be given to this exam?
   A. BI-RADS 1—normal
   B. BI-RADS 2—benign
   C. BI-RADS 3—probably benign
   D. BI-RADS 0—incomplete

3. What should be done next?
   A. The patient should be recalled for a repeat left view.
   B. The patient should be recalled for an ultrasound of the left axilla.
   C. The patient should be scheduled for an MRI.
   D. A 90-degree lateral view should be performed of the left breast.

4. Why does this common artifact occur?
   A. The patient's head is not held erect during the exposure, so the chin sags down and is superimposed between the x-ray source and the image receptor.
   B. The patient's breast is not positioned deeply enough.
   C. The patient moved during the exposure.
   D. The image receptor was positioned too high into the patient's axilla.

CASE 16

Artifact: Chin

1. B and C
2. D
3. A
4. A

References

Bassett LW, Hirbawi IA, DeBruhl N, Hayes MK: Mammographic positioning: evaluation from the view box. *Radiology* 1993;188:803-806.

Eklund GW, Cardenosa G: The art of mammographic positioning. *Radiol Clin North Am* 1992;30(1):21-53.

Cross-Reference

Ikeda D: *Breast Imaging: THE REQUISITES*, 2nd ed, Philadelphia: Saunders, 2010, p 6.

Comment

This artifact of the chin obscuring the upper portion of the axilla is commonly seen in daily practice, and it is more often seen in elderly patients, like this one. Ideally, this case should not be presented to the radiologist, because the technologist performing the exam should recognize the artifact at the time of the exam and repeat the image. This is particularly true in digital mammography, because the technologist previews the image before accepting it, as she is performing the mammogram at the acquisition work station.

Although the area obscured by the patient's overlying body part is relatively small (see the figures), this film should not be accepted. It should be given a Breast Imaging Reporting and Data System (BI-RADS) 0, and the patient recalled for a repeat left view. It is possible that the chin is obscuring important pathology that could be present in the axilla, and the radiologist is responsible for that area of the anatomy on the mammogram. This additional imaging is a "technical callback" and is performed free of charge.

If the technologist feels that the patient cannot cooperate for improved positioning, as is sometimes the case in extreme kyphosis or in wheelchair-bound patients, for example, then the technologist needs to make that situation clear to the radiologist, and it should be mentioned in the radiology report. If the patient is quite limited, you may instruct your technologists to show the images to the radiologist before the patient leaves, and the radiologist may meet the patient and observe attempts at positioning, to see if improvements can be made.

In this case, the view was repeated, and no abnormality was observed in the axilla.

Notes

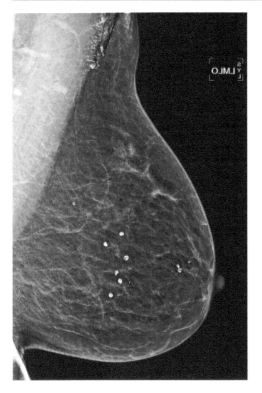 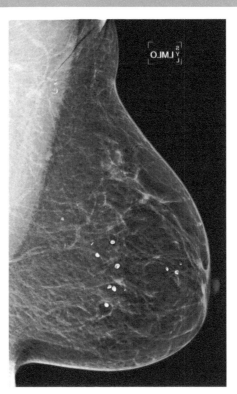

History: A 52-year-old woman presents for routine screening.

1. What is the differential diagnosis for the density in the left axilla in the first figure? (Choose all that apply.)
   A. Artifact from deodorant
   B. Artifact from lotion containing zinc oxide
   C. Artifact from gunshot wound
   D. Calcifications in the breast

2. What is your recommendation and Breast Imaging Reporting and Data System (BI-RADS) based on these images?
   A. Because the density is definitely on the skin, it can be reported as such, BI-RADS 2.
   B. The patient should be recalled for repeat views, and she should be instructed not to apply deodorant or lotion to the skin of the breast or underarm: BI-RADS 0, technical recall.
   C. The patient should return for magnification views of the left axilla, BI-RADS 0.
   D. The patient should return for an ultrasound of the left axilla, BI-RADS 0.

3. What radiographic density is this?
   A. This is metal density.
   B. This is calcium density.
   C. This is fat density.
   D. This is water density.

4. What is the one most important reason for recognizing this artifact?
   A. Patients should always follow instructions not to use deodorant.
   B. Technologists should always see this artifact when performing mammography.
   C. It is necessary to differentiate this from microcalcifications in axillary breast tissue.
   D. A and B are both correct.

CASE 17

Artifact: Deodorant

1. A and B
2. B
3. A
4. C

References

Bassett LW, Jackson VP, Jahan R, et al: *Diagnosis of Diseases of the Breast*. Philadelphia: Saunders, 1997, pp 363-364.

Hogge JP, Palmer CH, Muller CC, et al: Quality assurance in mammography: artifact analysis. *Radiographics* 1999;19:503-522.

Cross-Reference

Ikeda D: *Breast Imaging: THE REQUISITES*, 2nd ed, Philadelphia: Saunders, 2010, p 74.

Comment

Most patients use deodorant, and most facilities instruct their patients not to use deodorant, lotions, powders, and talc on their breasts or underarms on the day of the exam. However, many patients forget this instruction, or they expect to clean the skin before the mammogram and then neglect to do so or do not do so thoroughly enough. Technologists should ask each patient if she has applied any skin product, and if so, should arrange for the patient to remove the product completely.

There may still be residue of the product clinging to skin pores (see the figures) or trapped in the irregular surface of moles or skin keratoses even after cleaning. In that case, the patient needs to return for additional views or to repeat the view after the skin is recleaned (see the figures). If there is a mole or keratosis, this should be marked to help recognize skin product trapped on the lesion's surface. Deodorant or antiperspirant can contain aluminum, and this metal, trapped in skin pores, gives the characteristic appearance seen in the second figure.

The important aspect of this artifact is that such tiny metallic densities can mimic microcalcifications, which need to be evaluated for the possible presence of malignancy.

If the artifact is clearly on the skin, seen tangentially or along skin folds in the axilla, or in a marked mole, the patient might not need to return for technical callback views.

Notes

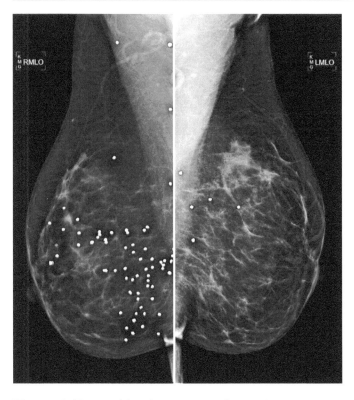

History: A 42-year-old patient presents for routine screening mammogram.

1. What is the differential diagnosis for this mammogram? (Choose all that apply.)
   A. Scattered punctate calcifications
   B. Multiple calcified fibroadenomas
   C. Multiple round metal pellets in the breast, consistent with shotgun injury
   D. Artifact on the patient

2. What is the Breast Imaging Reporting and Data System (BI-RADS) diagnostic code for this mammogram?
   A. BI-RADS 5—highly suspicious
   B. BI-RADS 0—incomplete
   C. BI-RADS 3—probably benign
   D. BI-RADS 2—benign

3. Is there a reason this patient should not have an MRI?
   A. No, the metal in shotgun pellets is nonferromagnetic and does not pose a problem.
   B. No, the motion of the metal pellets within the breast during the scan would not pose a problem.
   C. The material in the pellets would make the MRI scan difficult to interpret, owing to artifact, and may be ferromagnetic.
   D. The patient may choose to have an MRI once she understands the potential problems.

4. Should the metal pellets be removed or biopsied?
   A. No, the metal pellets typically do not cause a health risk.
   B. Yes, as much of the metal should be removed as possible.
   C. If any of the pellets are palpable, they must be removed.
   D. Needle biopsy would be difficult, so excision is recommended.

CASE 18

Artifact: Shotgun Pellets in Breast

1. C and D
2. D
3. C
4. A

References

Frenna TH, Meyer JE, DiPiro PJ, Denison CM: Gunshot residua simulating microcalcifications on mammography. *Breast Dis* 1994; 7:175-178.

Genson CC, Blane CE, Helvie MA, et al: Effects on breast MRI of artifacts caused by metallic tissue marker clips. *AJR Am J Roentgenol* 2007; 188(2):372-376.

Jones RW, Witta RJ: Signal intensity artifacts in clinical MR imaging. *Radiographics* 2000;20:893-901.

Shellock FG: Metallic marking clips used after stereotactic breast biopsy: ex vivo testing of ferromagnetism. *AJR Am J Roentgenol* 1999;172:1417-1419.

Cross-Reference

Ikeda D: *Breast Imaging: THE REQUISITES*, 2nd ed. Philadelphia: Saunders, 2010, pp 403-407.

Comment

Metal artifacts in the breast are relatively common. Needle core biopsies of benign lesions are often performed, and the physician may leave behind a localizing metal clip. Other iatrogenic metal material, including portions of catheters or needle localization devices, can be seen. Surgical clips are common after excision biopsy. Sewing needles and pencil lead fragments can be seen. Shotgun pellets or bullets may be seen.

The important factor in interpreting mammograms with artifacts is to realize that the finding is metal density, not calcification, and thus not native to the breast. Metal artifacts in the breasts are generally well tolerated and do not need to be removed. They do not typically cause symptoms, although superficially located pellets or other artifacts may be palpable.

MR imaging of the breast is best avoided in this patient, because the material in the pellets is unlikely to be known and might contain ferromagnetic material. This material causes two concerns: The pellets could move during the scan and could heat up, and there is an artifact from the metal that would lead to multiple signal-void artifacts on the image in this patient. The signal voids are usually larger than the size of the pellet, and no diagnostic information can be gained in these areas.

Notes

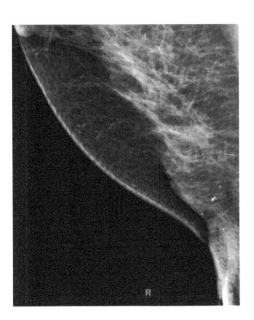
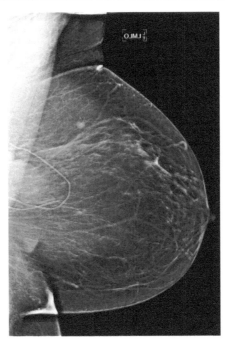
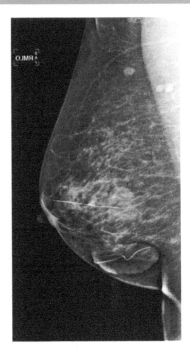

History: Three different women, of different ages, all with history of previous benign breast surgery, present for routine mammograms.

1. What is the differential diagnosis for the three different patients presented here? (Choose all that apply.)
   A. Breast malignancy
   B. Keloids
   C. Neurofibromatosis
   D. Epidermal inclusion cysts

2. Are the calcifications seen in the first image suspicious?
   A. No, calcifications are often seen in keloids.
   B. Yes, they are pleomorphic and should be biopsied.
   C. Yes, magnification views should be performed.
   D. Keloids are scar tissue and should not calcify.

3. Is it important to mark the skin in this condition?
   A. Yes, keloids can mimic a breast mass.
   B. No, it is not important; this condition is obvious on the mammogram.
   C. Yes, as the skin thickening of keloids is indistinguishable from malignant skin thickening.
   D. Yes, keloids are premalignant and must be followed closely.

4. What is the etiology of keloids?
   A. They are always the result of surgical incision.
   B. They are overexuberant scar tissue.
   C. They are more common after burns than after surgical incision.
   D. They are caused by scar tissue that has stretched and thinned.

C A S E 1 9

Keloid

1. B, C, and D
2. A
3. A
4. B

References

Kilkenny TE, Swenson GW: Keloids of the breast: mammographic findings. *AJR Am J Roentgenol* 1995;164(4):1022.

Stigers KB, King JG, Davey DD, Stelling CB: Abnormalities of the breast
caused by biopsy: spectrum of mammographic findings. *AJR Am
J Roentgenol* 1991;156(2):287-291.

Cross-Reference

Ikeda D: *Breast Imaging: THE REQUISITES*, 2nd ed, Philadelphia:
Saunders, 2010, p 407.

Comment

These three women all have the same condition: keloids
formed on the skin after benign breast surgery. Keloids
are composed of overexuberant collagenous scar tissue
that forms in the skin in some patients after trauma from
surgery, needle biopsy, insect bite, infection, or burn.
The new tissue is elevated, rounded, and firm. Young
women and African-Americans are particularly suscepti-
ble to keloid formation. On the mammogram, keloids
are recognized by a smooth area of increased density in
the skin, which typically follows the contour of the scar
on the skin and so is usually tubular. The portion of the
keloid outlined by air has a sharp contour (see the figures). Calcifications can develop within the keloid and
should be superimposed over the area of skin thickening
on both views. If in doubt, the technologist can obtain a
tangential view to show that the calcifications are in the
dermis. The air outline helps in the differentiation of a
skin lesion versus a lesion inside the breast, such as a cyst
or fibroadenoma. Ultrasound is usually not needed for
evaluation, because the keloid should be obvious on
clinical evaluation of the skin. The technologist may mark
the location of the keloid on the skin so that this dermal
lesion is not confused with breast pathology.

Notes

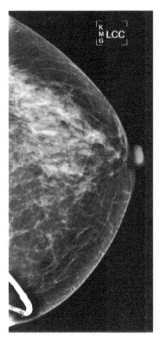

History: A 78-year-old woman presents for routine screening mammogram.

1. What is the differential diagnosis for this left CC mammographic view? (Choose all that apply.)
   A. Normal mammogram view with a catheter superimposed
   B. Tubing on the patient
   C. Normal mammogram view with an artifact from film handling
   D. Vascular calcifications in the breast

2. Nothing is seen on the patient's skin, and the gown is not in the path of the beam. What is the next step?
   A. Ask the patient if there is an indwelling catheter.
   B. Compare prior films.
   C. Call the referring doctor's office for information, if the patient is unaware.
   D. Take an additional view, with spot compression of the area of concern.
   E. All are correct.
   F. A, B, and C are correct.

3. What is the significance of this finding to the mammogram? What is the Breast Imaging Reporting and Data System (BI-RADS) code?
   A. No significance, BI-RADS 2.
   B. The finding obscures breast tissue, and the patient should be recalled, BI-RADS 0.
   C. The finding is of uncertain significance, and the patient should have short-interval follow-up, BI-RADS 3.
   D. The finding is suspicious for malignant calcifications, BI-RADS 4.

4. Is any additional work-up needed?
   A. Yes, spot magnification views of the calcified finding
   B. Yes, ultrasound of the medial right breast
   C. No, no additional work-up needed
   D. Yes, clinical exam to try to palpate the tubular structure

CASE 20

Artifact: Ventriculoperitoneal Shunt

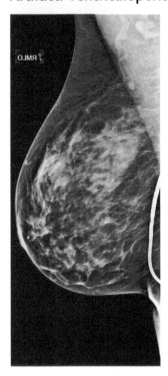

1. A and B
2. F
3. A
4. C

Reference

Hogge JP, Palmer CH, Muller CC, et al: Quality assurance in mammography: artifact analysis. *Radiographics* 1999;19:503-522.

Cross-Reference

Ikeda D: *Breast Imaging: THE REQUISITES*, 2nd ed, Philadelphia: Saunders, 2010, p 74.

Comment

Artifacts are abnormalities in mammographic density that are not native to the breast. Artifacts can occur in any component of the imaging process. Artifacts related to the patient can be due to motion or to superimposed objects, such as deodorant, lotion, hair, jewelry, and implanted medical devices. In this case, the patient has a ventriculoperitoneal shunt for hydrocephalus, and the tubing is seen on the mammogram.

In this patient, the shunt tubing is calcified, but this shunt may be seen without calcification. The figure above shows a different patient with the same history.

Notes

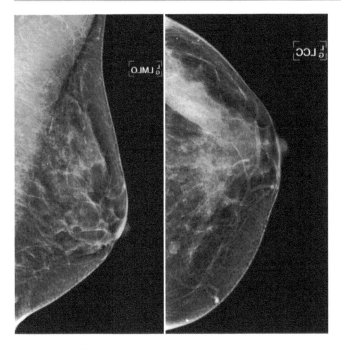

History: A 43-year-old asymptomatic patient has a mass seen in the left breast during routine screening.

1. What should be included in the differential diagnosis? (Choose all that apply.)
   A. Ductal carcinoma in situ
   B. Breast cyst
   C. Mole
   D. Accessory nipple

2. What is the next diagnostic step to differentiate these possibilities?
   A. Examination of the patient's skin
   B. Ultrasound
   C. MRI
   D. Additional mammographic views

3. What is an accessory nipple?
   A. A molelike raised skin lesion that looks like a nipple but is dermatologic, not breast related
   B. An additional nipple that develops only after pregnancy and lactation
   C. A rudimentary, additional nipple along the primitive milk line
   D. A mass of concern for malignancy, owing to abnormal duct formation

4. How common is this entity?
   A. It is very common, seen in at least 50% of women, although it may be tiny.
   B. It is extremely common; nearly all women have one.
   C. It is rare, seen in 2% to 6% of women.
   D. It is common, seen in approximately 20% of women.

CASE 21

Accessory Nipple

1. B, C, and D
2. A
3. C
4. C

References

Bassett LW, Jackson VP, Jahan R, et al (eds): *Diagnosis of Diseases of the Breast*, 6th ed, Philadelphia: Saunders, 1997, p 399.

Grossl NA: Supernumerary breast tissue: historical perspectives and clinical features. *South Med J* 2000;93(1):29-32.

Samardar P, de Paredes ES, Grimes MM, et al: Focal asymmetric densities seen at mammography: US and pathologic correlation. *Radiographics* 2002;22(1):19-33.

Cross-Reference

Ikeda D: *Breast Imaging: THE REQUISITES*, 2nd ed, Philadelphia: Saunders, 2010, p 38.

Comment

Supernumerary nipples (accessory nipples) are located on the embryonic milk line, which extends bilaterally from the upper axilla into the inner thigh. The accessory nipple represents the failure of complete regression of embryonal tissue and is more common in men than in women (about 1.7:1).

More than 75% of accessory nipples are smaller than one-third the size of the normal nipple. Most are below the breast (see the figure), and most are single. Most are found to be unrelated to other disease syndromes and have no clinical significance. The finding may include the nipple alone or be associated with an areola or underlying subareolar gland tissue or both. This gland tissue may produce milk in a lactating woman. The incidence of accessory nipples is estimated to be 2% to 6% of women, but this figure may be low because small accessory nipples may be mistaken for moles.

Notes

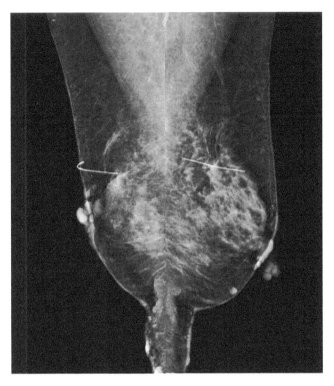

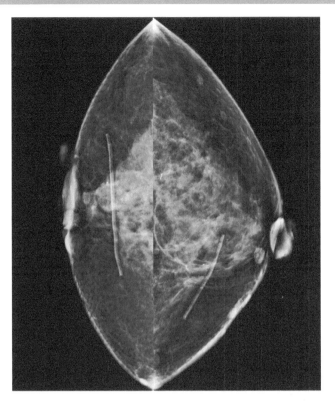

History: A 60-year-old woman presents for a routine mammogram. She has a history of bilateral surgical biopsies.

1. What should be included in the differential diagnosis for this mammogram? (Choose all that apply.)
   A. Multiple breast cysts
   B. Multiple benign solid masses, such as fibroadenomas
   C. Neurofibromatosis (NF)
   D. Bilateral multifocal cancer

2. How can you differentiate if the lesions are on the skin, rather than in the breast?
   A. There is no way to differentiate on the mammogram.
   B. You must be told by the technologist if there are skin lesions.
   C. Ultrasound must be used to determine whether these are cystic versus solid.
   D. Look for air surrounding the lesions on the mammogram, indicating that the masses project out from the skin.

3. Can neurofibromas be found in the breast as well as on the skin?
   A. No, they are only in the cutaneous layer of the breast.
   B. Yes, they are more often found in the breast as well as on the skin.
   C. Yes, but they are very rarely found in the breast compared with skin manifestations.

4. Is there an increased risk of breast cancer in patients with NF?
   A. No, NF is not related to malignancy.
   B. No, the neurofibromas in the breast are never malignant.
   C. No, but there is an increased risk of benign tumors.
   D. Yes, there is an increased risk of breast cancer in these patients.

Neurofibromatosis

1. A, B, and C
2. D
3. C
4. D

References

el-Zawahry MD, Farid M, Abd el-Latif A, et al: Breast lesions in generalized neurofibromatosis: breast cancer and cystosarcoma phylloides. *Neurofibromatosis* 1989;2(2):121-124.

Gokalp G, Hakyemez B, Kizilkaya E, et al: Myxoid neurofibromas of the breast: mammographical, sonographical and MRI appearances. *Br J Radiol* 2007;80(958):e234-e237.

Millman SL, Mercado CL: An unusual presentation of neurofibromatosis of the breast. *Breast J* 2004;10(1):45.

Cross-Reference

Ikeda D: *Breast Imaging: THE REQUISITES*, 2nd ed, Philadelphia: Saunders, 2010, p 408.

Comment

Neurofibromatosis (NF), or von Recklinghausen's disease, is a disorder of the neurocutaneous system. It is relatively common, occurring in 1 in 4000 persons. The disease is characterized by neurofibromas in the skin and nervous system, café-au-lait spots, bone defects, and visual disorders. It is inherited in autosomal dominant fashion.

The mammogram shown is from a woman who has multiple skin neurofibromas (see the figures). She has a history of a malignant cystosarcoma phyllodes removed from the right breast and ductal carcinoma in situ removed from the left breast. This case illustrates the increased risk of breast cancer in patients with NF and the difficulty in finding a breast mass with the overlying multiple skin masses superimposed over the breast. Some of the masses have a rim of air around them, showing that they project outward from the skin rather than being inside the breast.

In patients with NF, not only are breast masses harder to find, but also NF is associated with an increased risk of developing benign and malignant tumors, including breast cancer. A five-times elevated risk of breast cancer has been found in neurofibromatosis patients. If a patient has a palpable mass in the breast, evaluation should proceed with additional mammographic views and ultrasound as needed, the same as in patients who do not carry the NF mutation.

Because no suspicious masses were seen in this mammogram, it was read as benign findings, Breast Imaging Reporting and Data System (BI-RADS) category 2. It was recommended that the patient return for bilateral mammography in 1 year.

Notes

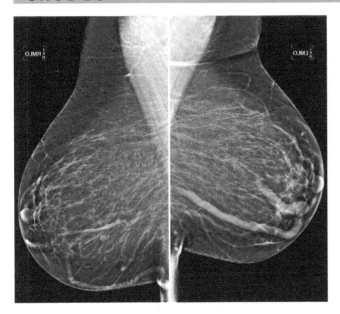 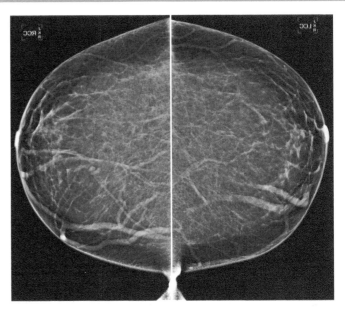

History: A 48-year-old woman with factor V Leiden mutation undergoes routine baseline screening mammogram.

1. What should be included in the differential diagnosis for the images presented? (Choose all that apply.)
   A. Dilated ducts in the left breast
   B. Mondor's disease, left greater than right
   C. Varicose veins secondary to hemodialysis access complication
   D. Chronic superior vena cava obstruction

2. What is the BI-RADS (Breast Imaging Reporting and Data System) code for this mammogram?
   A. BI-RADS 1—normal
   B. BI-RADS 4—suspicious
   C. BI-RADS 2—benign
   D. BI-RADS 3—probably benign

3. What is the next step?
   A. Report the findings to the patient's physician because the venous obstruction may not be known.
   B. The patient should be referred for vascular work-up.
   C. The patient should undergo MRI to evaluate for occult breast malignancy.
   D. Do not include comments about enlarged veins in the mammogram report.

4. What is an etiology of central venous obstruction or stenosis?
   A. Breast malignancy
   B. Mondor's disease
   C. Catheter insertion into a central vein
   D. Phlebitis of a lower extremity superficial vein

Superior Vena Cava Syndrome

1. C and D
2. C
3. A
4. C

References

Krishnan P, Uragoda L, Rao H, et al: Venous dilatation seen on routine mammography: a clue to superior vena cava obstruction. *Chest* 2002;121(4):1361-1363.

Ozdemir A, Ilgit ET, Konuş OL, et al: Breast varices: imaging findings of an unusual presentation of collateral pathways in superior vena caval syndrome. *Eur J Radiol* 2000;36(2):104-107.

Cross-Reference

Ikeda D: *Breast Imaging: THE REQUISITES*, 2nd ed, Philadelphia: Saunders, 2010, p 389.

Comment

Dilated veins may be seen in the breast and are consistent with collaterals that develop to bypass an obstruction or stenosis in a central vein, typically the superior vena cava. This condition may be called *superior vena cava syndrome* or *central venous occlusion*. In patients with chronic central vein obstruction, the presence of collaterals can mean there are no other symptoms of the obstruction. In the patient in this case, who has a hypercoagulable state, involvement of the superior vena cava was unknown. The patient had no clinical symptoms relative to the upper extremities, chest, or neck. No edema was present in the skin or in the breast. The presence of dilated veins in the breast (see the figures) on her baseline screening mammogram led to the discovery of superior vena cava syndrome. In this patient, the obstruction was not due to external compression by a lung or mediastinum mass or from a catheter but rather thrombosis secondary to factor V deficiency.

The collaterals in the breast are not related to breast pathology but are a sign of a systemic process. If the collaterals had not been present, allowing the venous blood to bypass the obstruction and return to the right atrium, one would expect breast edema to be present on the mammogram. Because the presence of collaterals means that no clinical symptoms may be present, it is important to report this finding to the referring physician.

Notes

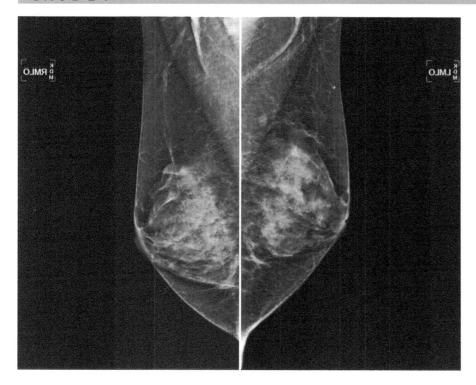

History: A 52-year-old woman, who has a family history of breast cancer in her mother at age 49, presents for routine screening mammogram. The focal density in the upper posterior left breast was not seen on any previous mammogram.

1. What should be included in the differential diagnosis for this mammogram? (Choose all that apply.)
   A. Highly suspicious mass in the left upper breast
   B. Lymph node in the upper left breast
   C. Newly developing fibroadenoma in the left upper breast
   D. Developing cyst in the left upper breast

2. What is the next step in management?
   A. No work-up needed for benign lymph node—recommend annual screening
   B. Scheduling the patient for stereotactic biopsy
   C. MRI of the left breast to check for brisk enhancement
   D. Ultrasound of the left upper breast to evaluate the density further

3. If the ultrasound examination shows a lymph node with thin symmetric cortex, what is the next step?
   A. The patient can return to routine screening.
   B. Short-interval follow-up is needed, to assess for change.
   C. Biopsy is needed, using ultrasound guidance.
   D. Refer the patient for whole-body imaging, preferably with positron emission tomography (PET).

4. What is the anatomic location of this lymph node?
   A. Internal mammary chain
   B. Axilla
   C. Intercostal
   D. Subareolar

CASE 24

Normal Lymph Nodes

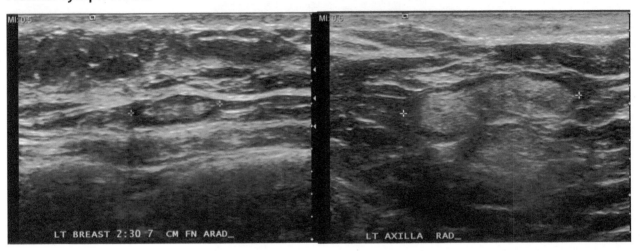

1. B, C, and D
2. D
3. A
4. B

Reference

Leibman AJ, Wong R: Findings on mammography in the axilla. *AJR Am J Roentgenol* 1997;169(5):1385-1390.

Cross-Reference

Ikeda D: *Breast Imaging: THE REQUISITES*, 2nd ed, Philadelphia: Saunders, 2010, pp 135, 152.

Comment

Lymph nodes are commonly seen on mammogram. They are often seen in the axilla and throughout the breast, most often in the upper outer quadrant. Normal nodes have a typical appearance on mammography, and when they are stable and have a characteristic appearance, no further evaluation is necessary. They are characteristically oval with sharp contours and contain a fatty hilum. A notch may be seen where the vessels and lymphatics enter the node. They can be any size, and large nodes with large central fatty hilum are commonly seen, particularly in the axilla. Abnormal nodes may herald otherwise occult breast pathology or systemic illness and require work-up. They become larger and denser and lose the fatty hilum.

If a new finding is seen on a mammogram, a work-up is needed, unless the new finding fits the description of a normal node. Ultrasound is useful in the evaluation of an unknown mass. The ultrasound appearance of the normal node is an oval or reniform mass, parallel to the chest wall, with a thin, concentric cortex and an echogenic central fatty hilum. The abnormal node has an eccentric thickened cortex and loss of the central hilar fat.

In this patient, the oval, circumscribed focal density in the left upper posterior breast had not been previously seen, and she was recalled for additional evaluation. Ultrasound revealed a normal node (see the figures above) with a thin cortex and oval shape, parallel to the chest wall. Also shown is a typical axillary node in the same patient (see the figures), which is larger, owing to an increased size of the fatty hilum. Because of the thin cortex, this node is also classified as benign. Overall size of the nodes in the axilla is irrelevant to the presence of pathology. This patient's mammogram is now BI-RADS (Breast Imaging Reporting and Data System) 1, and she can return to routine screening.

Notes

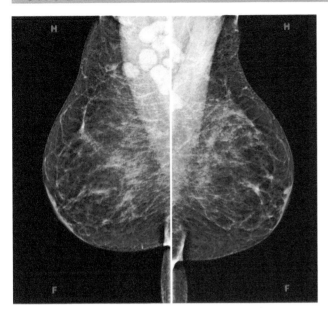
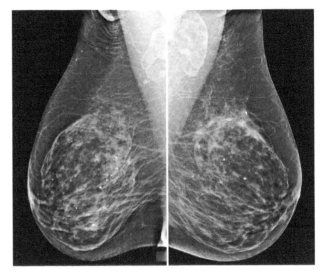

History: An asymptomatic 45-year-old woman presents for baseline screening mammogram; multiple masses are seen in both axillae on the mediolateral oblique (MLO) view. The image at right represents a companion case.

1. What should be included in the differential diagnosis? (Choose all that apply.)
   A. Malignant mass in the lower medial aspect of the right breast
   B. Normal axillary lymph nodes
   C. Enlarged axillary lymph nodes
   D. Lipomas in the axillary tail of Spence

2. Is ultrasound useful in the work-up?
   A. No, because the patient did not note a palpable concern.
   B. No, ultrasound is useful only for distinguishing a cyst from a solid mass.
   C. No, a physical examination can reveal the correct diagnosis.
   D. Yes, ultrasound is useful in the work-up of bilateral axillary adenopathy.

3. What is the next step in management of this patient?
   A. Careful history to elicit evidence of infectious, inflammatory, or lymphoproliferative disorders
   B. Full-body PET scan to check for extent of the disorder
   C. Surgical consultation to excise a node
   D. Image-guided core biopsy of a node

4. What Breast Imaging Reporting and Data System (BI-RADS) category and clinical recommendation should be given for bilateral enlarged axillary nodes seen on a routine baseline screening mammogram?
   A. BI-RADS 4—suspicious, recommend biopsy
   B. BI-RADS 5—highly suspicious for malignancy, biopsy strongly recommended
   C. BI-RADS 1—normal, recommend annual mammography
   D. BI-RADS 0—incomplete, recommend additional evaluation

CASE 25

Enlarged Axillary Lymph Nodes

1. C
2. D
3. A
4. D

References

Alvarez E, Anorbe P, Alcorta F: Role of sonography in the diagnosis of axillary lymph node metastases in breast cancer: a systematic review. *AJR Am J Roentgenol* 2006;186(5):1342-1348.

Orel SG, Weinstein SP, Schnall MD, et al: Breast MR imaging in patients with axillary node metastases and unknown primary malignancy. *Radiology* 1999;212(2):543-549.

Walsh R, Kornguth PJ, Soo MS, et al: Axillary lymph nodes: mammographic, pathologic, and clinical correlation. *AJR Am J Roentgenol* 1997;168(1):33-38.

Cross-Reference

Ikeda D: *Breast Imaging: THE REQUISITES*, 2nd ed, Philadelphia: Saunders, 2010, pp 395-397.

Comment

Bilateral axillary adenopathy is defined as multiple enlarged axillary nodes that do not contain fat (see the figures). The nodes are commonly larger than 2 cm and are typically rounded in contour and denser than normal. The margins may be irregular. Normal axillary nodes can be quite large if they are composed predominantly of fat (see the figures). Abnormal nodes are seen in approximately 0.3% of routine mammograms. The differential diagnosis includes HIV, lymphoma, leukemia, rheumatoid arthitis, scleroderma, lupus, sarcoidosis, and tuberculosis.

In the patient in this case, bilateral axillary adenopathy was due to HIV, and her enlarged nodes are not a new finding. The nodes are symmetric, although more are included in the right mammogram view compared with the left, likely secondary to positioning (see the figures).

Notes

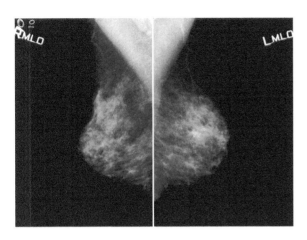

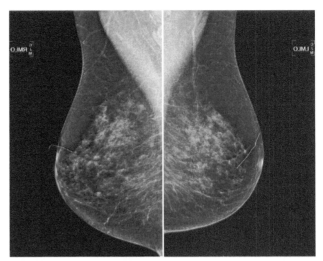

History: A 49-year-old woman presents for routine screening mammogram; two separate screening examinations taken 3 years apart are shown.

1. What advantages does digital mammography have over film-screen mammography? (Choose all that apply.)
   A. Better contrast resolution
   B. Better spatial resolution
   C. Lower noise
   D. Lower dose

2. What did the Digital Mammographic Imaging Screening Trial (DMIST) conclude?
   A. There is no improvement in detection of breast cancer with digital mammography.
   B. There is improvement in detection of breast cancer with digital mammography in all ages of patients.
   C. There is improvement in breast cancer detection with digital mammography in certain groups of patients.
   D. Digital mammography detected more cancers in women with fatty breasts.

3. What is the reason for improvement in sensitivity with digital mammography?
   A. Spatial resolution is improved.
   B. Contrast resolution is improved.
   C. Digital display allows for magnified image.
   D. Soft-copy display is better than hard-copy films.

4. If DMIST showed benefit only in selected groups of women, why are breast centers changing from film-screen to digital mammography?
   A. Equipment is less expensive.
   B. Digital process couples the image acquisition to image display.
   C. Digital acquisition, display, and storage are separated.
   D. Patient satisfaction is much higher.

C A S E 2 6

Digital Mammography

1. A, C, and D
2. C
3. B
4. C

References

Hendrick RE, Pisano ED, Averbukh A, et al: Comparison of acquisition parameters and breast dose in digital mammography and screen-film mammography in the American College of Radiology Imaging Network digital mammographic screening trial. *AJR Am J Roentgenol* 2010;194(2):362-369.

Pisano ED, Gatsonis C, Hendrick E, et al, Digital Mammographic Imaging Screening Trial (DMIST) Investigators Group: Diagnostic performance of digital versus film mammography for breast cancer screening. *N Engl J Med* 2005;353(17):1773-1783.

Pisano ED, Hendrick RE, Yaffe MJ, et al, DMIST Investigators Group: Diagnostic accuracy of digital versus film mammography: exploratory analysis of selected population subgroups in DMIST. *Radiology* 2008;246(2):376-383.

Cross-Reference

Ikeda D: *Breast Imaging: THE REQUISITES*, 2nd ed, Philadelphia: Saunders, 2010, pp 7-15.

Comment

Digital mammography offers advantages over film-screen mammography (see the figures). The elimination of film processing and storage, as was already accomplished with all other radiology applications, is a major advantage. Other advantages include improved contrast resolution and the visualization of the entire dynamic range across the image, out to and including the skin (see the figures). Allowing for the use of computer-aided detection, tomosynthesis, and telemammography is an additional advantage.

Several large studies have been performed, using film-screen mammography as the gold standard, to ensure that digital mammography was at least as good as film in detecting breast cancer. DMIST in the United States, which concluded its recruitment in 2003 and was published in 2005, showed that digital mammography was as sensitive as film across all surveyed groups and had improved sensitivity in the detection of breast cancer in several subgroups, including women younger than 50, premenopausal and perimenopausal women, and women with dense or heterogeneously dense breasts.

In digital mammography, spatial resolution is not as good as in film, but contrast resolution is higher. Spatial resolution is most important in the detection of tiny objects, such as microcalcifications. Studies have shown that digital mammography more accurately characterizes microcalcifications compared with film mammography despite the poorer spatial resolution; this may be due to the higher contrast resolution.

In this patient, the initial mammogram was film-screen (see the figures), and the subsequent mammogram was digital (see the figures). Compare the visualization of the dynamic range of tissue density across the image, which can be attained with digital and not with film technology. This range allows better detection of abnormalities adjacent to the skin compared with film. This case is an example of a woman who was shown in DMIST to benefit from digital mammography because she is younger than 50 with heterogeneously dense breasts.

Notes

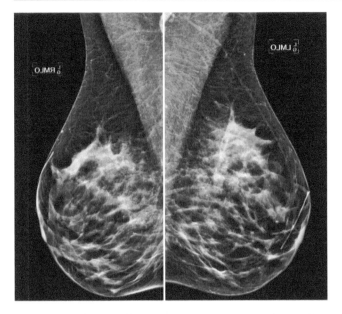
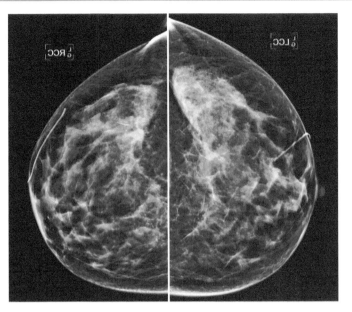

History: A 54-year-old asymptomatic woman who under-went a surgical biopsy previously for papillomas associ-ated with atypical ductal hyperplasia presents for routine screening mammogram.

1. What should be included in the differential diagnosis for the images shown? (Choose all that apply.)
   A. Bilateral suspicious calcifications, possible ductal carcinoma in situ
   B. Bilateral benign fibrocystic calcifications
   C. Bilateral dermal calcifications
   D. Calcifications in multiple tiny bilateral masses such as fibroadenomas or papillomas

2. What is the distribution of these calcifications?
   A. Multiple clusters
   B. Bilateral segmental distribution
   C. Diffuse
   D. Linear

3. What is the risk of malignancy associated with these calcifications?
   A. 0 to 2%
   B. 5% to 10%
   C. 10% to 20%
   D. 25% to 50%

4. What is the Breast Imaging Reporting and Data System (BI-RADS) code for this mammogram?
   A. BI-RADS 2—benign
   B. BI-RADS 3—probably benign
   C. BI-RADS 4—suspicious
   D. BI-RADS 0—incomplete

Punctate Calcifications

1. B, C, and D
2. C
3. A
4. A

References

Burnside ES, Ochsner J, Fowler K, et al: Use of microcalcification descriptors in BI-RADS 4th edition to stratify risk of malignancy. *Radiology* 2007;242(2):388-395.

D'Orsi CJ, Bassett LW, Berg WA, et al: *Breast Imaging Reporting and Data System: ACR BI-RADS—Mammography,* 4th ed, Reston, VA: American College of Radiology, 2003.

Shin HJ, Kim HH, Ko MS, et al: BI-RADS descriptors for mammographically detected microcalcifications verified by histopathology after needle-localized open breast biopsy. *AJR Am J Roentgenol* 2010;195(6):1466-1471.

Cross-Reference

Ikeda D: *Breast Imaging: THE REQUISITES*, 2nd ed, Philadelphia: Saunders, 2010, p 74.

Comment

Many mammograms contain calcifications. It is important to analyze the calcifications to determine if they can be placed into a benign category and dismissed from consideration for possible malignancy. Digital mammography has been shown to identify more calcifications compared with film-screen mammography; in one study, calcifications were seen in 45% of digital mammograms versus 36% of film mammograms.

It is important to determine both the morphology and the distribution of calcifications. The benign morphology category includes round and punctate calcifications. *Round* calcifications differ from *punctate* only by size; round calcifications are larger than 0.5 mm. This morphology is typically benign, but it can be seen in malignant calcifications if they are in a suspicious distribution. Benign calcifications should be in a benign distribution, including stable clusters, regional, multiple clusters, and diffuse distribution (see the figures).

It has been shown in multiple studies that round or punctate calcifications in a benign distribution do not represent malignancy. They are typically due to fibrocystic change or sclerosing adenosis. The calcifications should be noted, and routine follow-up is recommended. If more suspicious calcifications develop in these patients, they should be evaluated further with magnification views.

Notes

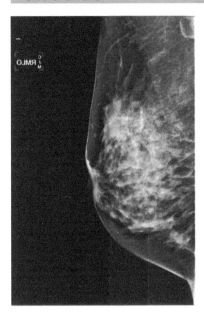
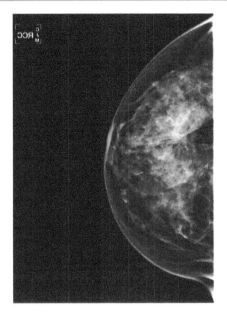

History: A 53-year-old woman who was diagnosed with left breast cancer 13 years ago, in a different state, now presents for routine mammogram after a 3-year delay.

1. What should be included in the differential diagnosis of the right mammogram? (Choose all that apply.)
   A. Distortion in the right breast from prior surgery
   B. Spiculated malignant mass
   C. Radial scar in the right upper breast
   D. Fibroadenoma in the right upper breast

2. Why is it important to know surgical history?
   A. The surgical scar can cause distortion.
   B. The patient's risk of cancer increases markedly if there is a history of previous benign surgery.
   C. Fat necrosis developing at the surgical site increases risk of breast cancer at that site.
   D. Pain at a prior surgery site may affect the decision on imaging needed.

3. What is the best way to work up suspected distortion?
   A. Ultrasound
   B. Spot compression views
   C. MRI
   D. Cleopatra view

4. What is the next best step in management of this finding?
   A. 6-month follow-up
   B. Needle biopsy with imaging guidance
   C. MRI to evaluate for abnormal enhancement
   D. PET/CT to evaluate for distant metastases

CASE 28

Tent Sign

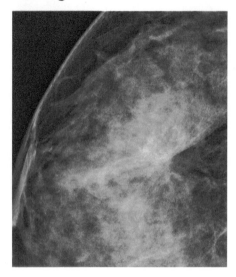 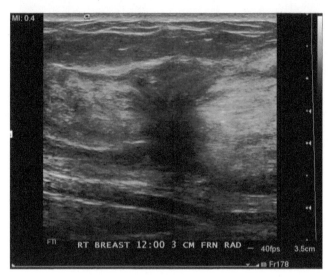

1. A, B, and C
2. A
3. B
4. B

Reference

Bird RE, Wallace TE, Yankaskas BC: Analysis of cancers missed at screening mammography. Radiology 1992;184(3):613-617.

Cross-Reference

Ikeda D: *Breast Imaging: THE REQUISITES*, 2nd ed, Philadelphia: Saunders, 2010, p 34.

Comment

The tent sign is a description of the effect of a spiculated mass on the surrounding tissue. Masses, particularly in the dense breast, can be obscured by surrounding gland tissue. One way to identify a mass is by examining the contour of the glandular tissue. The margins of the anterior and posterior breast should be smooth, scalloped, and adjacent to the subcutaneous and deep posterior fat lobules. Any interruption in this pattern should be examined. The "tenting" of tissue, or the triangular shape of the fat adjacent to the gland tissue, indicates that there is a distortion in the gland tissue. This distortion can be caused by a spiculated mass, scar tissue, radial scar, or fat necrosis. Spot compression or spot magnification views should be obtained to analyze the tenting, when it is seen.

This patient was diagnosed with a mass in the right breast after undergoing a routine mammogram (see the figures on p. 57); the distortion was identified on the craniocaudal (CC) view (see the figures on p. 57). A spot magnification view (see the figure at left above) accentuated the distortion and tenting of the adjacent fat. Ultrasound was performed and showed a spiculated mass (see the figure at right above).

Notes

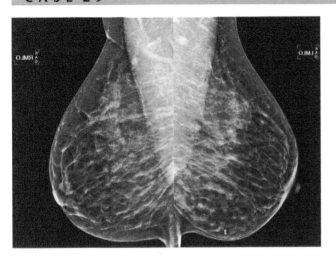

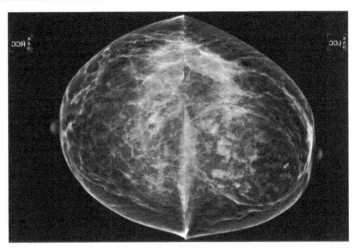

History: A 42-year-old woman undergoes routine baseline mammogram.

1. What should be included in the differential diagnosis of the mammogram shown? (Choose all that apply.)
   A. Fibroadenolipoma
   B. Hamartoma
   C. Steatocystoma multiplex
   D. Lipoma

2. What is the BI-RADS (Breast Imaging Reporting and Data System) code for this mammogram?
   A. BI-RADS 1—normal
   B. BI-RADS 2—benign
   C. BI-RADS 3—probably benign
   D. BI-RADS 4—suspicious

3. This patient was unaware of this mass. How does this finding usually manifest?
   A. A tender mass, fixed to the skin
   B. A firm mass on palpation
   C. A soft mass that is nontender
   D. Skin dimpling and peau d'orange

4. Is biopsy indicated if the mass is palpable?
   A. Yes, biopsy should be performed of any palpable mass.
   B. Yes, the mixed elements in this mass require biopsy to exclude cancer.
   C. No, this mass does not require biopsy, even if palpable.
   D. No, but the mass should be carefully followed because malignant transformation is common.

Hamartoma

1. A and B
2. B
3. C
4. C

References

Georgian-Smith D, Kricun B, McKee G, et al: The mammary hamartoma: appreciation of additional imaging characteristics. *J Ultrasound Med* 2004;23(10):1267-1273.

Helvie MA, Adler DD, Rebner M, et al: Breast hamartoma: variable mammographic appearance. *Radiology* 1989;170(2):417-421.

Cross-Reference

Ikeda D: *Breast Imaging: THE REQUISITES*, 2nd ed, Philadelphia: Saunders, 2010, p 135.

Comment

A hamartoma is a benign overgrowth of fibrous tissue, gland elements, and fat that occurs in women during the reproductive years. A hamartoma can contain different amounts of these three components; fat may predominate, as in this patient (see the figures), or the mass may have relatively little fat and manifest as a dense mass on mammography. The mass is typically well circumscribed and encapsulated. Cancer can arise within a hamartoma but has no special propensity to do so. Hamartoma is coined "breast within a breast" because it contains the histologic elements of normal breast tissue.

If there are no suspicious calcifications within the mass, as in this patient, biopsy may be unnecessary. If biopsy is performed, pathologists may have difficulty distinguishing the mass from normal breast tissue, especially on core biopsy. Ultrasound evaluation is unnecessary in a patient, such as this one, who has a classic presentation. If ultrasound is performed, the mass is oval with heterogeneous internal echoes and circumscribed margins.

Notes

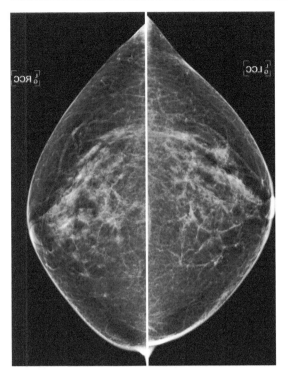

History: A 49-year-old woman underwent a baseline screening mammogram; craniocaudal (CC) views are shown.

1. What should be included in the differential diagnosis for these two views? (Choose all that apply.)
   A. Normal mammogram
   B. Cluster of calcifications in the medial left breast
   C. Dermal calcifications seen on the left CC view
   D. Suspicious mass with associated calcifications in the left breast

2. What is the next step in management?
   A. Recall the patient for magnification views.
   B. Use the digital magnification capability of the workstation to evaluate the calcifications fully.
   C. Recommend routine screening mammogram in 1 year.
   D. Perform ultrasound of the left breast to check for possible mass.

3. Why is it important to know if the calcifications are dermal or in the breast?
   A. Dermal calcifications are suspicious for spread of breast cancer to the skin.
   B. If calcifications can be shown to be within the dermis, they cannot be breast cancer and do not need biopsy.
   C. Dermal calcifications can be related to skin cancer.
   D. Dermal calcifications can be confused with ductal carcinoma in situ because of their lucent centers.

4. How can you show calcifications to be in the skin?
   A. Perform ultrasound of the calcification area and look for calcifications in the skin.
   B. Take repeated images, rotating the breast at 5-degree intervals, until the calcifications are seen in the skin.
   C. Using a fenestrated paddle, compress the area of breast where calcifications are present, then place a BB over the alphanumeric location, retake the image, and perform a tangential view of the BB.
   D. Perform stereotactic biopsy.

Dermal Calcifications Localization

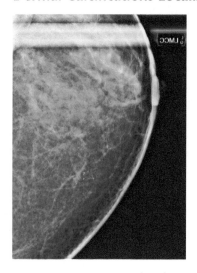 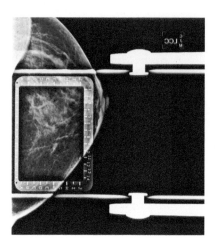 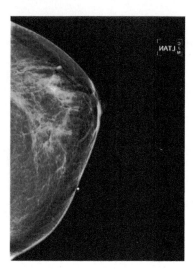

1. B and C
2. A
3. B
4. C

References

Berkowitz JE, Gatewood OM, Donovan GB, et al: Dermal breast calcifications: localization with template-guided placement of skin marker. *Radiology* 1987;163(1):282.

Homer MJ, D'Orsi CJ, Sitzman SB: Dermal calcifications in fixed orientation: the tattoo sign. *Radiology* 1994;192(1):161-163.

Cross-Reference

Ikeda D: *Breast Imaging: THE REQUISITES*, 2nd ed, Philadelphia: Saunders, 2010, p 76.

Comment

Dermal calcification is very common, with individual calcifications typically 1 to 2 mm in size and having a smooth, round contour. Calcifications that are in the skin never represent primary breast malignancy. They are of no clinical significance and do not need follow-up. They arise from sebaceous glands and often have lucent centers. This appearance may be characteristic, and the calcifications may be dismissed easily on screening mammogram, without the need for further characterization. Skin calcifications may be grouped and may have a fixed relationship within the group, a finding termed the *tattoo sign,* which may also help in differentiation from breast calcifications. When calcifications are seen for the first time and are near the skin surface, as in this patient (see the figures), further evaluation can be done to determine if the calcifications are in the skin and can be dismissed, rather than performing a biopsy.

Magnification views are performed first (see the figures). If there is a possibility the calcifications are dermal, skin localization views can be performed. The technologist places the breast in compression using an alphanumeric fenestrated paddle, such as is used for a needle localization procedure (see the figures). The image is viewed, and the location of the calcification within the fenestration is marked on the skin with a BB, and this is confirmed with another image. The breast is removed from that compression paddle, and the BB marker is imaged in tangent (see the figures). If the calcifications are in the skin, this view confirms them in the dermal layer. In this patient, the calcifications are superficial in the breast but are not in the dermis, and biopsy is recommended.

Skin calcifications are seen much more easily with digital mammography than with film-screen mammography because the tissue density is equalized out to the skin.

Notes

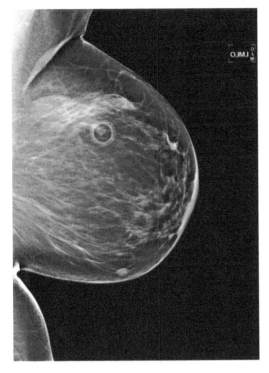 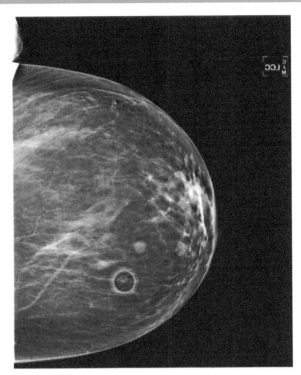

History: A 55-year-old woman undergoes routine screening mammogram. She had a left breast fibroadenoma diagnosed by core needle biopsy 14 years ago.

1. What should be included in the differential diagnosis of the two mammogram views shown? (Choose all that apply.)
   A. Three benign masses in the left breast
   B. A fibroadenoma, an oil cyst, and a mole on the skin
   C. A cyst, an oil cyst, and a mole on the skin
   D. A suspicious solid mass, an oil cyst, and a mole on the skin

2. In what quadrant is the structure marked with a ring marker?
   A. Upper outer quadrant
   B. Lower inner quadrant
   C. Upper inner quadrant
   D. Lower outer quadrant

3. In what quadrant are the two lesions in the left breast?
   A. The oil cyst is in the upper inner quadrant; the fibroadenoma is in the lower inner quadrant.
   B. The oil cyst is in the upper inner quadrant; the fibroadenoma is in the lower outer quadrant.
   C. The oil cyst is in the upper outer quadrant; the fibroadenoma is in the lower outer quadrant.
   D. You cannot tell which quadrant the lesions are in without a true mediolateral view.

4. Why are moles marked before mammogram views are performed?
   A. Moles can become malignant.
   B. Moles can be confused for masses in the breast.
   C. Moles do not have to be marked because they always have air around them and a cobblestone surface.
   D. The patient may palpate the mole as a suspicious breast lump.

Triangulation

1. B and C
2. C
3. A
4. B

References

Park JM, Franken EA Jr: Triangulation of breast lesions: review and clinical applications. *Curr Probl Diagn Radiol* 2008;37(1):1-14.

Sickles EA: Practical solutions to common mammographic problems: tailoring the examination. *AJR Am J Roentgenol* 1988;151(1):31-39.

Cross-reference

Ikeda D: *Breast Imaging: THE REQUISITES*, 2nd ed, Philadelphia: Saunders, 2010, p 49.

Comment

Triangulation is the determination of the location of a mass in the breast by assessing its appearance on the standard views. In this patient, both lesions are seen in both views, but this may not always be the case. Triangulation can also refer to locating a lesion that is seen only on one view.

In this patient, there is a known fibroadenoma in her left breast, a calcified oil cyst in the left breast, and a mole on the skin (see the figures). When a lesion is seen in two projections of the mammogram, the location can be known, even though the mediolateral oblique (MLO) view is not orthogonal to the craniocaudal (CC) view. Not all lesions that project above the nipple on the MLO view are truly above the nipple. A mass in the upper inner breast may project below the nipple, and a mass in the lower outer breast may project above the nipple. It is important to understand triangulation, based on the MLO and CC views, so that you can be certain you are locating the same lesion on ultrasound.

First, assess the location of the lesion on the CC view: medial or lateral to the nipple? How far medial or lateral? Then look at the MLO view, and try to judge where the lesion would be on the mediolateral (ML) view, which is the true location in the breast. If the lesion is lateral on the CC view, it appears higher on the MLO view than it truly is. The further lateral on the CC view, the more discrepant the location on the MLO view. Conversely, if the lesion is in the medial breast, it appears lower on the MLO view than it truly is. If the lesions are close to the nipple on the CC view, as these two lesions are (see the figures), the location in the breast is similar to the location on the MLO view.

The calcified oil cyst is in the upper inner quadrant and about 1 to 2 cm medial to the nipple. This means that the location would not be very different on the ML view compared with the MLO view, and you would expect to find this lesion at the 11 o'clock position. The solid oval mass is also in the medial breast, about 1 to 2 cm from the nipple. However, on the MLO view, it is at the inferior aspect of the breast, so its location is at the 7 o'clock position in the left breast. The mole can be found easily by inspecting the skin, but it can be confused for a mass inside the breast, so it is good practice to mark moles before performing mammography.

Notes

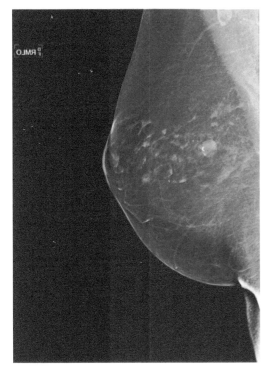 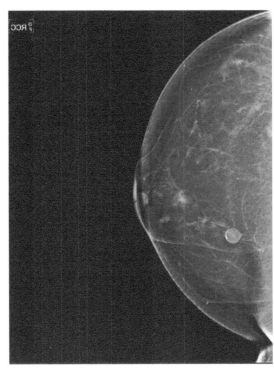

History: A 75-year-old woman presents for routine mammogram.

1. What is the differential diagnosis for the finding in the right breast? (Choose all that apply.)
   A. Mass suspicious for malignancy
   B. Lipoma
   C. Oil cyst
   D. Fibroadenoma

2. What is the likely cause of this finding?
   A. Trauma
   B. Infection
   C. Lactation
   D. Associated malignancy

3. Is any further work-up needed? What Breast Imaging Reporting and Data System (BI-RADS) score would you give?
   A. No additional work up is needed: BI-RADS 2.
   B. Yes, spot magnification views are needed for the calcifications: BI-RADS 0.
   C. Yes, ultrasound is needed to confirm the suspected benign diagnosis: BI-RADS 0.
   D. Yes, ultrasound is needed to guide needle core biopsy: BI-RADS 4.

4. What are the characteristic mammographic findings of this condition?
   A. Round or oval shape
   B. Fat density
   C. Thick, irregular radiodense rim
   D. A and B are correct.
   E. A and C are correct.

C A S E 3 2

Oil Cyst

1. C
2. A
3. A
4. D

References

American College of Radiology : *Illustrated BI-RADS*, 4th ed, Reston, VA: American College of Radiology, 2004, pp 76-81.

Sickles EA: Breast calcifications: mammographic evaluation. *Radiology* 1986;160:289-293.

Cross-Reference

Ikeda D: *Breast Imaging: THE REQUISITES*, 2nd ed, Philadelphia: Saunders, 2010, p 137.

Comment

The calcified oil cyst is one of the common benign calcifications seen on the mammogram. It is caused by trauma, which results in focal tissue death, with necrosis of the fat, which is then surrounded by a thin wall that can calcify.

The oil cyst is recognized by the central fat lucency and the thin, often calcified wall. This thin calcification is referred to as *eggshell calcification* and is diagnostic of an oil cyst. The trauma is typically caused by surgery to the breast, from either excisional biopsy or reduction mammoplasty, and it can occur in a motor vehicle accident. In the case of trauma from surgery, the oil cysts are typically in the area of scar. In a motor vehicle accident, the seat belt tightening against the breast can cause bruising and subsequent fat necrosis. This may be seen in a typical linear pattern across the chest, tracing the path of the shoulder harness of the seat belt. In this patient (see the figures), the oil cyst was likely caused by a benign surgical biopsy many years before. It is not palpable. This was seen on routine screening mammogram, and no further work-up is needed.

Patients may present with a palpable mass that is an oil cyst. You may be able to elicit a history of trauma or surgery. The mass is usually superficial and in the area of the scar or the seat belt. If the typical findings of an oil cyst are seen on mammogram, no further work-up is needed. If ultrasound is performed, the appearance can be variable and can cause some doubt about the diagnosis. The mass will be round on ultrasound, and the central fat portion can have varying degrees of echogenicity. If the rim is calcified, it can shadow on ultrasound, giving it a more ominous appearance. If the typical findings of fat lucency and thin rim are seen on mammography, ultrasound is not needed.

Notes

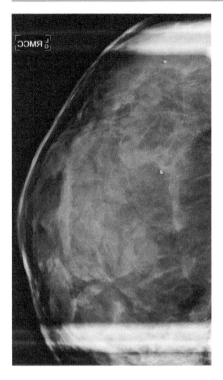
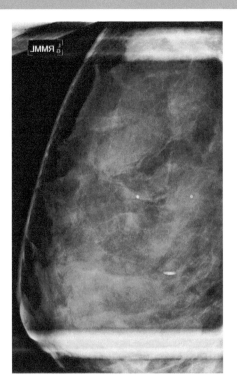

History: An asymptomatic woman having a routine mammogram had calcifications in the lateral right breast on standard images. She was recalled for magnification views, which are shown.

1. What is the differential diagnosis based on the magnification views? (Choose all that apply.)
   A. Ductal carcinoma in situ (DCIS)
   B. Amorphous, indeterminate calcifications
   C. Milk of calcium
   D. Rod-shaped calcifications typical of secretory type

2. How do the magnification views give you the diagnosis?
   A. The calcifications remain linear in two projections.
   B. The calcifications are pleomorphic on the craniocaudal (CC) view.
   C. The calcifications are indistinct on both views.
   D. The calcifications have a different appearance on the CC and mediolateral (ML) magnification views.

3. What is the next step in follow-up?
   A. The calcifications should be biopsied.
   B. The patient should return in 6 months for follow-up magnification views.
   C. Routine annual mammogram should be scheduled.
   D. Diagnostic mammogram should be done in 1 year, with magnification views repeated.

4. What is milk of calcium?
   A. It is calcium in ducts, related to lactation.
   B. It is calcium sediment in a cyst, which layers to the bottom.
   C. It is often seen adjacent to DCIS.
   D. Also called "secretory type," it is calcium in milk ducts.

CASE 33

Milk of Calcium

1. C
2. D
3. C
4. B

Reference

Linden SS, Sickles EA: Sedimented calcium in benign breast cysts: the full spectrum of mammographic presentations. *AJR Am J Roentgenol* 1989;152(5):967-971.

Cross-Reference

Ikeda D: *Breast Imaging: THE REQUISITES*, 2nd ed, Philadelphia: Saunders, 2010.

Comment

This patient demonstrates the common condition of milk of calcium calcifications in the breast. In this case (see the figures) the calcifications are clustered on the CC view and layer in a meniscus shape on the ML view. This is characteristic of sedimented calcifications that are present in a macrocyst. The ML view is of utmost importance, with the x-ray beam perpendicular to the breast cyst, to display the calcifications dependent in the cyst. If this view is not performed, the dependent layering can be missed, and the calcifications are seen only as clustered and may be suspected to be malignant. The calcifications have a very different appearance on the ML magnification view (layering or linear) and the CC magnification view (smudgy or punctate). If the typical appearance is seen on the magnification views, the calcifications can be correctly assigned to Breast Imaging Reporting and Data System (BI-RADS) category 2, benign, and no biopsy or follow-up is needed.

Milk of calcium can also manifest as a single calcification in each of many tiny imperceptible cysts. In such cases, many layering separate calcifications are seen on the ML magnification view.

Notes

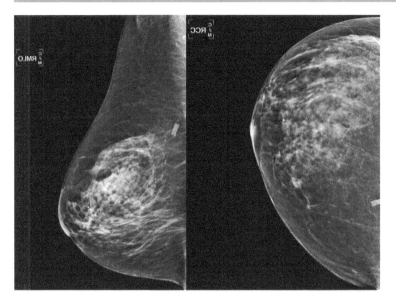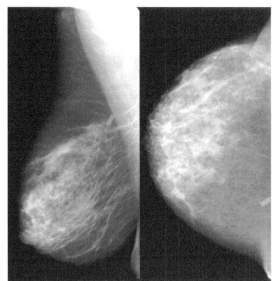

History: A 64-year-old woman undergoes routine screening mammogram.

1. What should be included in the differential diagnosis of the right mammogram shown? (Choose all that apply.)
   A. Normal mammogram with artifact from retained catheter cuff in the right upper inner chest
   B. Suspicious mass in the right upper inner breast
   C. Evidence of infection around a retained sheath from a removed catheter
   D. Evidence of previous placement and removal of central venous catheter with no evidence of other abnormality

2. What BI-RADS (Breast Imaging Reporting and Data System) would you give this mammogram?
   A. BI-RADS 1—normal
   B. BI-RADS 2—benign
   C. BI-RADS 3—probably benign
   D. BI-RADS 4—suspicious

3. Which statement is *not* related to the origin of this artifact?
   A. The patient had a central line placed.
   B. The central line catheter was removed by traction.
   C. The central line was removed by cutting down on the catheter surgically.
   D. The sheath is in a subcutaneous tunnel.

4. What side effect of the retained sheath is most commonly seen on the mammogram?
   A. Breakage of the sheath into smaller pieces
   B. Migration of the sheath
   C. Infection of the sheath
   D. Hematoma formation around the catheter

C A S E 3 4

Retained Catheter Cuff

1. A and D
2. B
3. C
4. C

References

Beyer GA, Thorsen MK, Shaffer KA, et al: Mammographic appearance of the retained Dacron cuff of a Hickman catheter. *AJR Am J Roentgenol* 1990;155(6):1203-1204.

Ellis RL, Dempsey PJ, Rubin E, et al: Mammography of breasts in which catheter cuffs have been retained: normal, infected, and postoperative appearances. *AJR Am J Roentgenol* 1997;169(3):713-715.

Kohli MD, Trerotola SO, Namyslowski J, et al: Outcome of polyester cuff retention following traction removal of tunneled central venous catheters. *Radiology* 2001;219(3):651-654.

Cross-Reference

Ikeda D: *Breast Imaging: THE REQUISITES*, 2nd ed, Philadelphia: Saunders, 2010, p 404.

Comment

Central venous catheters are placed for many reasons—chiefly to supply a patient with long-term delivery of parenteral nutrition, chemotherapy, antibiotic therapy, or hemodialysis. The catheters are tunneled under the skin and have a Dacron cuff. The purpose of the cuff is to help maintain the catheter in position, as fibrous tissue is stimulated to grow around it. The cuff is positioned in the subcutaneous tunnel.

Catheters are removed most commonly by pulling, or "traction." According to one report, in about 10% of cases, the cuff remains inside the subcutaneous tunnel when the catheter is pulled out. This retention does not occur if the catheter is removed by cutting down on the catheter surgically. Most catheters are placed into the central venous system on the right side, so the retained cuffs are most commonly seen in the right upper inner breast on the mammogram, as in our patient (see the figures).

Catheters are removed either because the function is no longer needed or because the catheter becomes infected. If the cuff is retained after the catheter is removed, it does not need to be removed. Infection of the retained cuff is unusual. If this occurs, there is usually a palpable, erythematous mass in the area of the subcutaneous tunnel. The infection may be recognized on the mammogram with an area of increased density and spiculation around the cuff. However, these findings are not exclusive to infection; many noninfected cuffs have an area of increased density around them owing to fibrosis from scarring. When density is seen around a retained cuff, correlation with patient symptoms should be made.

Notes

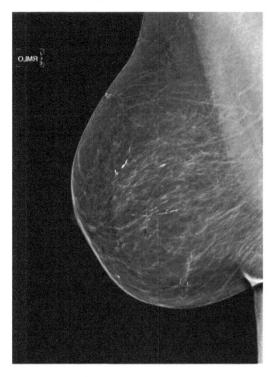

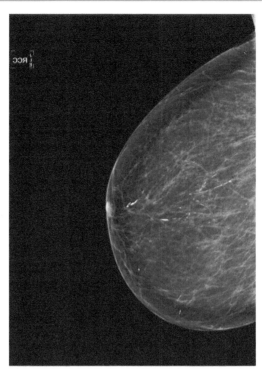

History: A 68-year-old woman presents for routine mammogram.

1. What is the differential diagnosis for the right breast calcifications? (Choose all that apply.)
   A. Ductal carcinoma in situ (DCIS)
   B. Fibrocystic change
   C. Secretory-type calcifications
   D. Fat necrosis

2. Are any additional mammographic images needed?
   A. Yes, magnification views are needed to assess these calcifications.
   B. Yes, spot compression views are needed.
   C. No additional views are needed for this finding.
   D. Yes, the patient should have true lateral (ML) projections to check for layering.

3. What is your recommendation and Breast Imaging Reporting and Data System (BI-RADS) category?
   A. Routine annual mammogram: BI-RADS 2
   B. Recall for additional views: BI-RADS 0
   C. Short-interval follow-up: BI-RADS 3
   D. Recommend biopsy: BI-RADS 4

4. Is this condition in a spectrum of ductal carcinoma or in a spectrum of benign disease?
   A. Because this condition involves the duct, it is related to ductal carcinoma.
   B. Calcifications in a ductal distribution are always of concern for ductal carcinoma.
   C. This is a benign condition of the ducts.
   D. There is overlap between this condition and ductal carcinoma in situ.

CASE 35

Secretory Calcifications

1. C
2. C
3. A
4. C

References

Bassett LW, Jackson VP, Jahan R, et al: *Diagnosis of Diseases of the Breast*, Philadelphia: Saunders, 1997.

Cardenosa G: *The Core Curriculum. Breast Imaging*, Baltimore: Lippincott Williams & Wilkins, 2004.

Cross-Reference

Ikeda D: *Breast Imaging: THE REQUISITES*, 2nd ed, Philadelphia: Saunders, 2010, pp 81–83.

Comment

Secretory-type calcifications are one of the benign types of calcification commonly seen on the mammogram. The calcifications are located histologically in the periductal cells and are associated with chronic inflammation. The ducts are dilated and may be filled with secretions. This process develops over time, and the calcifications are more commonly seen in the older population. A condition termed *plasma cell mastitis,* described in the literature of the early 20th century, described this condition when it manifests as a palpable mass due to the inflammatory response.

If the calcifications have the typical smooth, rodlike forms, usually greater than 1 mm in diameter, such as seen here (see the figures), then no further work-up is needed. These calcifications can have lucent centers, can taper (cigar-shaped), and can branch. This is a benign condition, the condition does not typically produce symptoms, and it is given a BI-RADS score of 2, with routine annual mammography recommended.

Occasionally, there can be some doubt about the etiology of linear calcifications, with concern for possible DCIS. The calcifications of DCIS are typically thinner and more irregular, with a crushed-stone or snakeskin appearance. The calcifications of DCIS can also follow a ductal or segmental distribution. If the etiology is in doubt, magnification views can be performed.

Notes

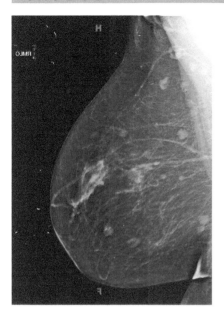
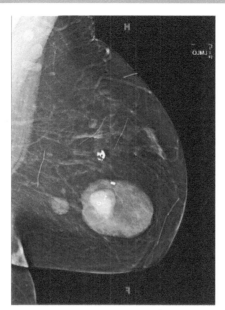
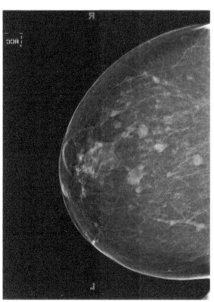
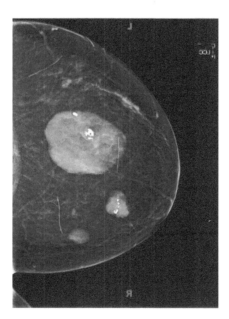

History: A 56-year-old asymptomatic patient presents for a routine baseline screening mammogram.

1. What is the differential diagnosis in this patient? (Choose all that apply.)
   A. Multiple bilateral fibroadenomas
   B. Multiple bilateral cysts
   C. Multiple suspicious masses
   D. Multiple lipomas

2. What work-up is indicated?
   A. Bilateral ultrasound must be performed to confirm whether the bilateral masses are cystic or solid.
   B. MRI is needed to evaluate for the typical enhancement pattern of fibroadenomas.
   C. Biopsy of the largest mass should be performed.
   D. No work-up is needed.

3. What type of calcifications is seen on this mammogram?
   A. Suspicious pleomorphic calcifications
   B. Indeterminate, coarse heterogeneous calcifications
   C. Benign popcorn-type calcifications
   D. Clustered calcifications typical of fat necrosis

4. How often is this finding multiple or bilateral?
   A. Nearly always, about 90%
   B. Rarely, approximately 2%
   C. Approximately 10% to 20%
   D. About 50%

Multiple Fibroadenomas

1. A and B
2. D
3. C
4. C

References

Campbell RE: Image interpretation session: 1993. Fibroadenoma of the breast. *Radiographics* 1994;14(1):209-210.

Feig SA: Breast masses: mammographic and sonographic evaluation. *Radiol Clin North Am* 1992;30(1):67-92.

Cross-Reference

Ikeda D: *Breast Imaging: THE REQUISITES*, 2nd ed, Philadelphia: Saunders, 2010, pp 117-120.

Comment

This asymptomatic patient has multiple bilateral benign masses (see the figures). The fibroadenoma is the most common solid mass of the breast and is benign. Characteristically, fibroadenomas are round or oval, with sharply circumscribed, smooth borders. The contour can be macrolobulated. The density is equal to that of breast tissue on the mammogram. They are composed of stromal (fibrous) and epithelial (adenoma) elements. Some of the masses contain the classic calcifications seen in fibroadenomas, termed *popcorn* calcifications. The calcifications are thought to look like popped kernels of corn. The calcifications can reflect sclerosis and hyalinization of the mass.

Calcifications commonly form in fibroadenomas and help in characterizing the mass as benign, Breast Imaging Reporting and Data System (BI-RADS) 2. They can form initially in the periphery of the mass, and then become large and dense. In the early stage of the calcifications' development, they may be faint and irregular and difficult to differentiate from malignant calcifications. In that case, they should be biopsied. Malignancy in a fibroadenoma is rare, occurring in about 1 in 1000 cases.

Fibroadenomas can be multiple and bilateral. In the dense breast, they may be difficult to distinguish from the background fibroglandular tissue, because the density is the same. Ultrasound can be used for further evaluation. On ultrasound, the mass is typically hypoechoic or isoechoic to the surrounding fat and is oval, with the long axis of the mass parallel to the skin (wider than tall) and a thin capsule.

Notes

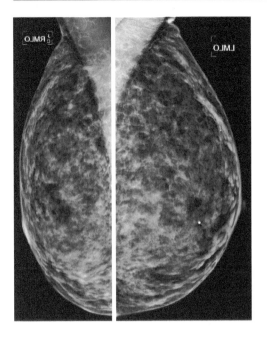
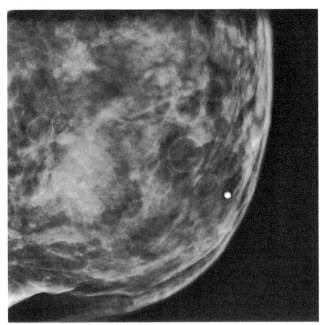
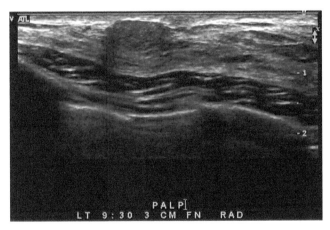

History: A 41-year-old woman presents for a routine screening mammogram.

1. What should be included in the differential diagnosis of the mammogram and ultrasound images shown? (Choose all that apply.)
   A. Normal mammogram with multiple lipomas
   B. Normal mammogram with multiple oil cysts
   C. Normal mammogram in a woman with steatocystoma multiplex
   D. Benign mammogram with multiple simple breast cysts

2. Where are the lesions of steatocystoma multiplex located?
   A. In the subcutaneous fat
   B. In the mid to deep dermis
   C. In the epidermis
   D. In the breast stroma

3. How does a patient acquire steatocystoma multiplex?
   A. It is the sequela of a skin infection.
   B. It is the result of trauma, such as a burn.
   C. It either arises spontaneously or is an inherited skin condition.
   D. It is a reaction to one of many allergens.

4. What is the BI-RADS (Breast Imaging Reporting and Data System) code and recommendation for this mammogram?
   A. BI-RADs 1—normal, routine screening recommended
   B. BI-RADS 2—benign, routine screening recommended
   C. BI-RADS 3—probably benign, short-interval follow-up recommended
   D. BI-RADS 4—suspicious, biopsy of one of the lesions recommended

Steatocystoma Multiplex

1. A, B, and C
2. B
3. C
4. B

References

Cao MM, Hoyt AC, Bassett LW: Mammographic signs of systemic disease. *Radiographics* 2011;31(4):1085-1100.

Kim HS, Cha ES, Kim HH, et al: Spectrum of sonographic findings in superficial breast masses. *J Ultrasound Med* 2005;24(5):663-680.

Park KY, Oh KK, Noh TW: Steatocystoma multiplex: mammographic and sonographic manifestations. *AJR Am J Roentgenol* 2003;180(1): 271-274.

Cross-Reference

Ikeda D: *Breast Imaging: THE REQUISITES*, 2nd ed, Philadelphia: Saunders, 2010, p 137.

Comment

Steatocystoma multiplex is a rare skin disorder that is a malformation of the pilosebaceous unit of the mid to deep dermis. The result of this malformation is the development of keratin-filled cysts, which are recognized on a mammogram as oval radiolucent masses with a thin high-density rim. In 40% of cases, the condition is inherited as an autosomal dominant trait. It is seen in men and women. Typically, the cysts involve the upper anterior chest and axilla but can also involve the groin.

The differential diagnosis of a fatty cyst includes lipoma, oil cyst, fat necrosis, and galactocele. The differentiation of this condition from other fatty lesions is not difficult because the others listed do not involve the skin, and they are usually not so numerous. A sebaceous cyst or epidermal inclusion cyst is located in the dermis and can contain fat, but it is unusual to have so many lesions (see the figures).

This condition can lead to palpable findings, and if the patient presents with a palpable finding, ultrasound should be performed. Ultrasound of the lesions of steatocystoma multiplex shows an oval hypoechoic or anechoic mass in the skin, with smooth, sharp margins. Deeper cystic masses may extend into the subcutaneous fat (see the figures).

Patients should be followed routinely because there is no association with breast disease. No work-up is needed.

Notes

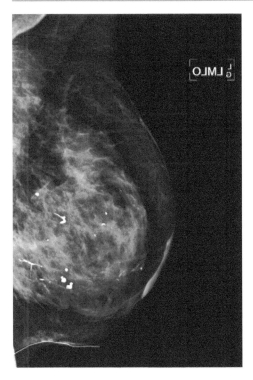
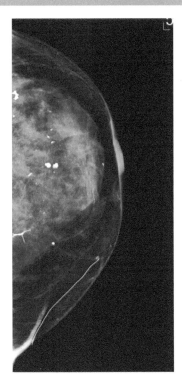

History: A 70-year-old woman with a history of surgery in the left breast.

1. What is the differential diagnosis of the branching calcification in the center of the breast?
(Choose all that apply.)
   A. Vascular calcifications
   B. Recurrent malignancy, ductal carcinoma in situ (DCIS)
   C. Secretory-type calcifications
   D. Suture calcifications

2. Why is it important to recognize suture calcification?
   A. The calcification can mimic recurrence at a lumpectomy site.
   B. The surgeon should be alerted to remove this calcification.
   C. Calcified suture often explains the clinical finding of palpable mass at the surgical site.
   D. It must be differentiated from secretory-type calcifications, which are suspicious.

3. What other types of calcifications are seen on this patient's mammogram?
   A. There are suspicious calcifications near the lumpectomy site.
   B. There are coarse, benign calcifications scattered in the breast.
   C. There are extensive vascular calcifications in the breast.
   D. There are calcifications diagnostic of fat necrosis in this breast.

4. What is the most important consideration in evaluating the mammogram of a patient who has had breast conservation therapy for cancer?
   A. To assess for the presence of benign findings and report them
   B. To recognize signs of recurrent or residual disease in the breast
   C. To report any evidence of fat necrosis.
   D. To recommend adjunct ultrasound and MRI for these high-risk patients

C A S E 3 8

Suture Calcifications

1. B, C, and D
2. A
3. B
4. B

Reference

Davis SP, Stomper PC, Weidner N, Meyer JE: Suture calcification mimicking recurrence in the irradiated breast: a potential pitfall in mammographic evaluation. *Radiology* 1989;172:247-248.

Dershaw DD: Mammography in patients with breast cancer treated by breast conservation (lumpectomy with or without radiation). *AJR Am J Roentgenol* 1995;164:309-316.

Cross-Reference

Ikeda D: *Breast Imaging: THE REQUISITES*, 2nd ed, Philadelphia: Saunders, 2010, pp 404-407.

Comment

The importance of suture calcification lies in the need to differentiate it from recurrent disease at the lumpectomy site. Recurrence often takes the form of calcifications, which should be recognized as linear, branching, or clustered, as DCIS is recognized anywhere in the breast. It is common for developing calcifications to be seen at the lumpectomy site, especially punctate calcifications or calcifications typical of fat necrosis (rim calcifications and coarse irregular forms). Suture calcification is relatively rare. Benign calcifications at the lumpectomy site can develop early or can take years to develop, and they most often result from fat necrosis due to microvascular damage caused by surgery and radiation.

Suture material is an artifact and causes an abnormal density in the breast. It does not usually calcify, but the shape of the calcification should suggest the diagnosis, especially when a knot is seen (see the figures). In the early stage of development of calcifications, there can be doubt about the etiology, and magnification views should be performed if there is any question about the calcifications, to exclude DCIS from the differential diagnosis. If the calcifications are considered indeterminate after magnification views, a decision needs to be made if they are low suspicion (Breast Imaging Reporting and Data System [BI-RADS] category 3, 6-month follow-up recommended) or higher suspicion (BI-RADS 4, biopsy should be considered). In these patients stereotactic biopsy should be considered as the first choice for biopsy method, rather than re-excision.

Notes

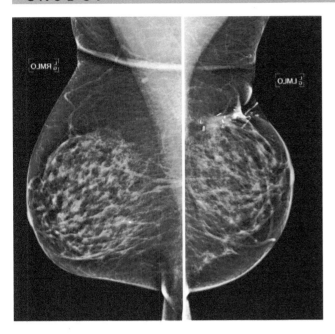

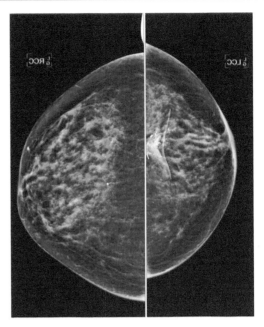

History: A 60-year-old woman who had lumpectomy for breast cancer 4 years ago now presents for routine bilateral mammogram.

1. What should be included in the differential diagnosis for the mammogram? (Choose all that apply.)
   A. Normal postlumpectomy mammogram
   B. Evidence of left lumpectomy, with expected changes after treatment
   C. Evidence of left lumpectomy, with calcifications consistent with fat necrosis
   D. Recurrent malignancy at the lumpectomy site

2. What is the next step in management?
   A. MRI to check for enhancement at the lumpectomy site
   B. Ultrasound to check for evidence of mass at the lumpectomy site
   C. Magnification views of the lumpectomy site
   D. Short-interval follow-up in 6 months

3. If image-guided biopsy is chosen, how is the finding targeted?
   A. Stereotactic biopsy
   B. Ultrasound-guided biopsy
   C. MRI-guided biopsy
   D. Needle localization for surgical excision

4. If the histology of the needle biopsy is fat necrosis, what is the next step?
   A. Routine annual follow-up because the finding is concordant
   B. Referral for surgery because the biopsy histology is nonconcordant
   C. Short-interval follow-up in 6 months for concordant histology
   D. MRI of the breast to check for abnormal enhancement

Postlumpectomy Fat Necrosis

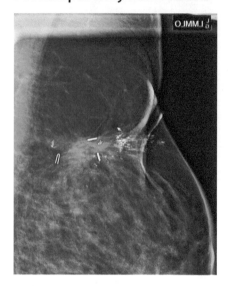 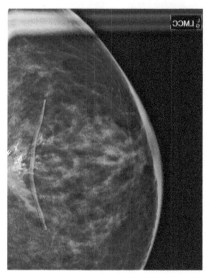

1. C and D
2. C
3. A
4. C

References

Geiss CS, Keating DM, Osborne MP, et al: Comparison of rate of development and rate of change for benign and malignant breast calcifications at the lumpectomy bed. *AJR Am J Roentgenol* 2000;175(3):789-793.

Gunhan-Bilgen A, Oktay A: Management of microcalcifications developing at the lumpectomy bed after conservative surgery and radiation therapy. *AJR Am J Roentgenol* 2007;188(2):393-398.

Cross-Reference

Ikeda D: *Breast Imaging: THE REQUISITES*, 2nd ed, Philadelphia: Saunders, 2010, p 313.

Comment

Breast conservation therapy is a common treatment for breast cancer. Surgery to remove the cancer (lumpectomy) and radiation therapy to the whole breast or as a partial-breast irradiation constitute one local therapy for breast malignancy. This therapy causes changes in the breast—initially a seroma and hematoma, followed by scarring, retraction, and skin thickening and breast edema (see the figures). Calcifications may develop at the lumpectomy site, which may represent recurrence of the malignancy or fat necrosis.

It can be difficult to differentiate fat necrosis from malignancy. The timing of development of the calcifications may suggest an etiology. Studies have shown that benign calcifications typically develop earlier; in one study, the median time was 23 months, and the median time for development of malignant calcifications was 39 months. The morphology is also important: Punctate, or coarse, curvilinear calcifications are typically benign shapes, whether associated with a normal patient or a patient following lumpectomy. Pleomorphic, faint, linear, and branching calcifications are suspicious whether they are seen in a breast that has had surgery or one that has not. If developing calcifications are suspicious or indeterminate, stereotactic biopsy should be performed.

The calcifications developing in this patient 4 years after treatment are pleomorphic and in linear configuration and were thought to be indeterminate (see the figures). Stereotactic biopsy was performed, and the histology was fat necrosis. Two biopsy clips seen on the images were placed at the time of biopsy. The tissue diagnosis was believed to be concordant, and 6-month follow-up magnification views were recommended because there are remaining calcifications that were not sampled.

Notes

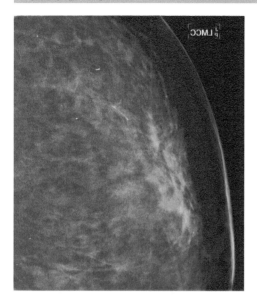
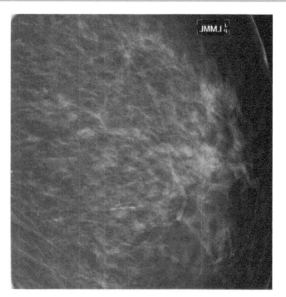
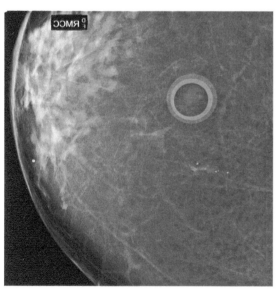
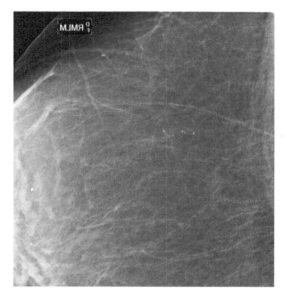

History: Magnification views of microcalcifications in two patients, discovered on screening mammogram, recalled for additional views.

1. What is the differential diagnosis for these calcifications? (Choose all that apply.)
   A. Arterial calcifications
   B. Milk of calcium
   C. Ductal carcinoma in situ (DCIS)
   D. Atypical ductal hyperplasia

2. What is the BI-RADS (Breast Imaging Reporting and Data System) designation for these two cases?
   A. BI-RADS 2—benign
   B. BI-RADS 5—highly suspicious
   C. BI-RADS 3—probably benign
   D. BI-RADS 4—suspicious

3. Is any additional work-up needed prior to biopsy in these two cases?
   A. Yes, ultrasound should be performed.
   B. Yes, MRI should be performed.
   C. Yes, both ultrasound and MRI should be performed.
   D. No, biopsy is the next step.

4. You perform the stereotactic biopsy, and the result is DCIS. What is the next step?
   A. Nothing. Your diagnosis is complete.
   B. You must inform the patient and her referring physician of the diagnosis.
   C. You must inform the patient and direct the definitive management of her cancer.
   D. Nothing. DCIS is not invasive cancer, so it can be managed expectantly with follow-up mammograms.

Suspicious Microcalcifications

1. A, C, and D
2. D
3. D
4. B

References

Berg WA, Arnoldus CL, Teferra E, Bhargavan M: Biopsy of amorphous breast calcifications: pathologic outcome and yield at stereotactic biopsy. *Radiology* 2001;221:495-503.

Dershaw DD, Abramson A, Kinne DW: Ductal carcinoma in situ: mammographic findings and clinical implications. *Radiology* 1989; 170:411-415.

Sickles EA: Breast calcifications: mammographic evaluation. *Radiology* 1986;160:289-293.

Cross-Reference

Ikeda D: *Breast Imaging: THE REQUISITES*, 2nd ed, Philadelphia: Saunders, 2010, p 65.

Comment

In evaluating calcifications, magnification views are essential. When performed with a proper technique, the views provide information to help determine whether the calcifications are more likely to be benign or malignant. If microcalcifications are seen on a conventional screening mammogram, it is important to recall the patient for additional magnification views rather than to try to make a diagnosis on the standard screening images.

Magnification views are often performed in the 90-degree lateral view to check for layering. If the calcifications layer on this view (milk of calcium), they can be reliably characterized as benign, needing no further evaluation.

Differentiating benign from suspicious calcifications is a step-by-step process. The first step is to analyze the magnification views and determine if the calcifications fall into any of the definitely benign categories (round, eggshell, coarse linear, and popcorn). The next step is to decide if the calcifications are suspicious for malignancy. Suspicious calcifications are pleomorphic and can have irregular margins or broken-glass shapes. Calcifications of ductal carcinoma in situ (DCIS) form inside the duct, making casts, and can branch, following the course of the duct (see the figures). In patient one, these cast-type calcifications are seen.

Calcifications that are neither definitely benign nor suspicious may be termed indeterminate for malignancy. In this category are coarse, heterogenous, and amorphous forms, which are faint, small, hazy calcifications. If their distribution is linear or segmental, which are more suggestive of malignancy, biopsy is recommended. In patient two, although the calcifications were not casting, their somewhat linear configuration on both views was considered suggestive for DCIS, and biopsy was performed.

The distribution of the calcifications, as well as the individual morphology, is important. Distribution is categorized as follows (in order of increasing level of suspicion):

1. Diffuse, distributed throughout most of the breast
2. Regional, distributed in an area at least 2 cm of the breast, not in ductal distribution
3. Grouped or clustered (at least five calcifications in less than 1 cm^3 of tissue)
4. Linear, forms suggestive of ducts
5. Segmental, distributed in a lobe or segment of the breast, suspicious for involving a duct and its branches

The casting-type calcifications in the first patient are DCIS (see the first and second figures). She went on to surgical and oncologic management. The calcifications in patient two (see the third and fourth figures) were benign and were not related to the duct. No further treatment was needed.

Notes

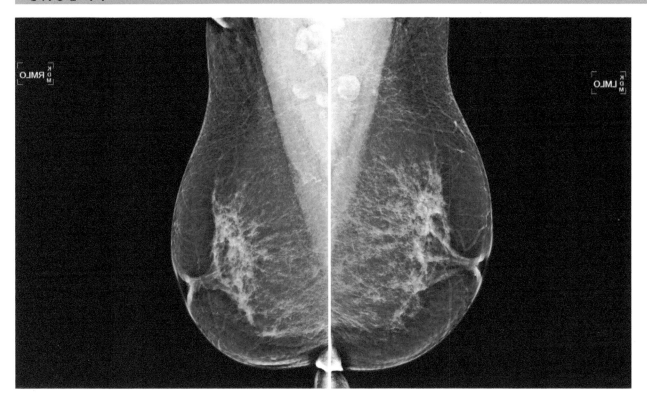

History: A 60-year-old woman presents for routine screening mammography.

1. What should be included in the differential diagnosis based on the images provided? (Choose all that apply.)
   A. Pathologically unilateral retracted nipple
   B. Bilateral benign nipple inversion
   C. Subareolar spiculated masses
   D. Normal mammogram

2. If a patient presents with chronically inverted nipples, what is the next diagnostic step?
   A. Spot compression views of both breasts, subareolar area
   B. Ultrasound of the nipples
   C. No further imaging needed
   D. MRI to exclude a mass

3. If a patient presents with new retraction of one nipple, what is the next diagnostic step?
   A. Spot compression views of the retracted nipple
   B. Ductography of the retracted nipple
   C. MRI should be performed before any additional mammographic views
   D. Surgical consultation for duct excision

4. Why is new nipple retraction a concern?
   A. The retracted nipple can interfere with lactation.
   B. Cancer may be present in the retroareolar breast, tethering the nipple.
   C. A retracted nipple is predominantly a cosmetic concern.
   D. Paget disease of the nipple is the most common reason for retracted nipple.

Nipple Inversion

1. B and D
2. C
3. A
4. B

References

An HY, Kim KS, Yu IK, et al: Image presentation. The nipple-areolar complex: a pictorial review of common and uncommon conditions. *J Ultrasound Med* 2010;29(6):949-962.

Nicholson BT, Harvey JA, Cohen MA: Nipple-areolar complex: normal anatomy and benign and malignant processes. Radiographics 2009;29 (2):509-523.

Cross-Reference

Ikeda D: *Breast Imaging: THE REQUISITES*, 2nd ed, Philadelphia: Saunders, 2010, pp 26 36.

Comment

Bilateral nipple inversion is a benign condition, in which the nipples are completely beneath the level of the skin (see the figures). The nipples may evert on pressure and then resume the inverted position. This condition may interfere with lactation but is not otherwise of clinical concern and is often long standing or congenital. Benign inversion may also manifest as a slitlike area of the nipple pulled in. Nipple inversion is better seen on digital mammography than on film-screen mammography because tissue equalization algorithms allow better visualization of the skin and nipples.

A benign inverted nipple must be differentiated from a pathologically retracted nipple. The terms *retraction* and *inversion* are used interchangeably, which may cause confusion. When nipple retraction is new, it may be caused by duct ectasia, periductal mastitis, or malignancy. Cancer that develops in the retroareolar breast is typically invasive ductal carcinoma or invasive lobular carcinoma and, particularly if it develops close to the nipple, may cause the nipple to pull in, or retract. A pathologically retracted nipple does not evert on clinical examination, as a benign inverted nipple does. Paget disease of the nipple manifests as an erythematous area on the nipple-areolar complex and may cause nipple retraction. It has an association with ductal carcinoma in situ in the subareolar ducts. Inflammatory cancer of the breast can manifest with nipple retraction, but additional findings are present, with larger areas of thick, erythematous skin and peau d'orange.

The patient shown here had long-standing bilateral nipple inversion, and the mammographic appearance was stable. No further work-up is needed.

Notes

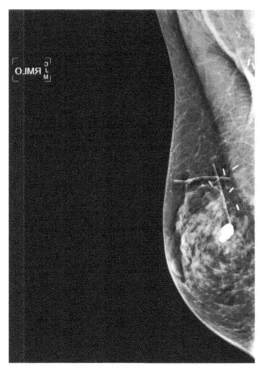

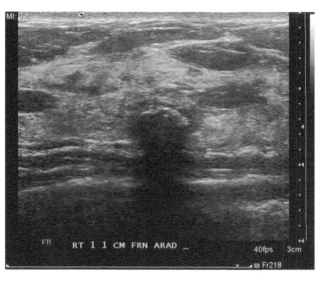

History: A 60-year-old woman presents for routine mammography. She has a personal history of breast cancer, which was occult on mammography and seen only on ultrasound. She was treated with breast conservation therapy. Because of her history, she requests ultrasound of both breasts annually, in addition to mammography.

1. What should be included in the differential diagnosis of the mammogram and ultrasound images shown? (Choose all that apply.)
   A. Calcified fibroadenoma
   B. Breast conservation therapy with calcified fat necrosis
   C. Breast conservation therapy with calcification suspicious for recurrence
   D. Calcification in the right breast related to radiation therapy

2. If you find a dense shadowing mass on ultrasound, how should you proceed?
   A. All dense shadowing masses are suspicious, and biopsy should be performed.
   B. Correlate the ultrasound finding with the mammogram.
   C. Further work-up should be based on clinical examination.
   D. Evaluate further with MRI, looking for abnormal enhancement.

3. What is the BI-RADS (Breast Imaging Reporting and Data System) for this mammogram and ultrasound?
   A. BI-RADS 1—normal
   B. BI-RADS 2—benign
   C. BI-RADS 3—probably benign
   D. BI-RADS 4—suspicious

4. If this mammogram was the patient's first mammogram in your office, which statement regarding prior examinations is *not* correct?
   A. It can be expensive to obtain prior mammograms.
   B. No prior examinations are needed to evaluate the coarse calcification.
   C. A patient who has a history of breast cancer should always have her mammogram compared with prior examinations.
   D. Prior mammograms are not needed for this benign mammogram.

CASE 42

Calcification on Ultrasound

1. A, B, and D
2. B
3. B
4. D

Reference

Stavros AT: *Breast Ultrasound*, Philadelphia: Lippincott Williams & Wilkins, 2004.

Cross-Reference

Ikeda D: *Breast Imaging: THE REQUISITES*, 2nd ed, Philadelphia: Saunders, 2010, p 83.

Comment

Fibroadenoma is a common breast lesion. It is often seen in all types of patients, including patients who develop malignancy. In this patient, the dense, calcified fibroadenoma existed for many years before the malignancy was detected (see the figures). Calcifications in the breast that has undergone lumpectomy need to be evaluated because recurrence may calcify. However, a large, coarse calcification such as this is benign and needs no further evaluation. This case illustrates how such a benign calcification can have a worrisome appearance on ultrasound (see the figures).

To distinguish a shadowing large calcification from a shadowing suspicious mass, look for the curvilinear dense rim along the anterior wall. This rim is the anterior margin of the calcification, which causes acoustic shadowing. The soft tissue mass of the fibroadenoma surrounding the calcification may also be seen on ultrasound. Also look at the mammogram to correlate the location of the shadowing structure with the location of the calcification on the mammogram. If the shadowing mass corresponds to the location of a coarse calcification on the mammogram, no further evaluation is needed for the shadowing mass.

Notes

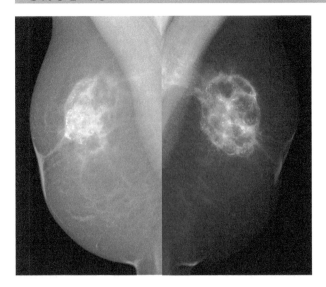

History: A 60-year-old woman had subglandular silicone implants placed 30 years ago. A mammogram obtained 6 years ago showed possible rupture, which was confirmed with MRI. She had the implants surgically removed. The routine screening mammogram following this surgery is shown.

1. What should be included in the differential diagnosis of the mammogram shown? (Choose all that apply.)
   A. Fat necrosis in both breasts
   B. Bilateral, locally advanced breast cancer
   C. Bilateral retained implant capsule
   D. Ductal carcinoma in situ

2. What is the next step in management?
   A. Stereotactic biopsy
   B. Referral to plastic surgeon
   C. MRI
   D. Physical examination

3. What is the "retained capsule"?
   A. Free silicone that has extravasated from the implant
   B. The envelope of the silicone implant that was left behind in the surgical bed
   C. The fibrous capsule, formed by the patient, surrounding the implant was not removed
   D. It is the same as "retained siliconoma"

4. Can saline implants also show calcification on the mammogram?
   A. No, only silicone implants calcify
   B. Yes, because the fibrous capsule calcifies, not the implant
   C. Yes, because saline implants have a silicone envelope
   D. Yes, but only in the subglandular position

Implant Removal with Retained Capsule

1. A and C
2. B
3. C
4. B

References

Caskey CI, Berg WA, Hamper UM, et al: Imaging spectrum of extra-capsular silicone: correlation of US, MR imaging, mammographic, and histopathologic findings. *Radiographics* 1999;19(Spec No): S39-S51.

Frazer CK, Wylie EJ: Mammographic appearances following breast prosthesis removal. *Clin Radiol* 1995;50(5):314-317.

Hardt NS, Yu L, LaTorre G, et al: Complications related to retained breast implant capsules. *Plast Reconstr Surg* 1995;95(2):364-371.

Rockwell WB, Casey HD, Cheng CA: Breast capsule persistence after breast implant removal. *Plast Reconstr Surg* 1998;101(4):1085-1088.

Sinclair DS, Spigos DG, Olsen J: Case 2. Retained silicone and fibrous capsule in the right breast and retained fibrous capsule in the left breast after removal of implants. *AJR Am J Roentgenol* 2000;175 (3):862-864.

Stewart NR, Monsees BS, Destouet JM, et al: Mammographic appearance following implant removal. *Radiology* 1992;185(1):83-85.

Cross-Reference
Ikeda D: *Breast Imaging: THE REQUISITES*, 2nd ed, Philadelphia: Saunders, 2010, p 343.

Comment

Implants are placed in the breast to augment the size of the breast. The implants are composed of a silicone elastomer shell and contain either silicone gel or saline as the filler. They are placed either in front of the pectoral muscle (see the figures), termed *subglandular,* or behind the pectoral muscle, termed *subpectoral.*

A complication of implants is the formation of the fibrous capsule. The fibrous capsule is the body's immune response to the foreign material—an attempt to "wall off" the implant. This fibrous capsule can calcify, which often has a bizarre appearance on mammogram, as it forms plaques over the curved sheet of fibrous tissue surrounding the implant (see the figures).

When silicone implants rupture, the implant may be removed surgically. Removing the fibrous capsule was thought to be unnecessary in the past because this added morbidity and expense to the surgical procedure. There was evidence that because the capsule formed as a response to the implant, it would resorb spontaneously after the implant was removed. More recent evidence showed that spontaneous resorption did not always occur, and potential problems could arise from the retained capsule, including serous effusion, expansile hematoma, and siliconomas.

Mammography of the retained capsule most commonly shows masses at the site where the implant had been present, often with unusual calcifications (see the figures). These calcified forms have been termed "gold leaf" and "tin foil." These calcified masses may be confused with carcinoma, so it is important to obtain the history of explantation from the patient to avoid unnecessary concern and biopsy. Free silicone and silicone granulomas are also commonly seen as well as silicone in the axillary nodes, not present in this patient. The retained capsule was excised as a separate surgical procedure in this patient.

Notes

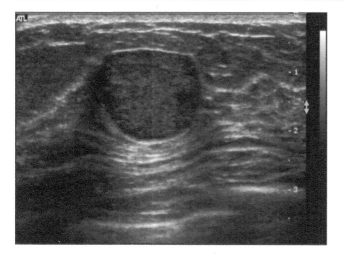

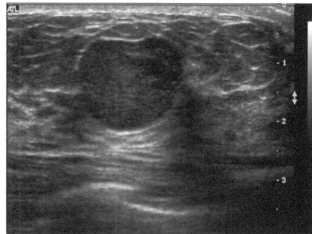

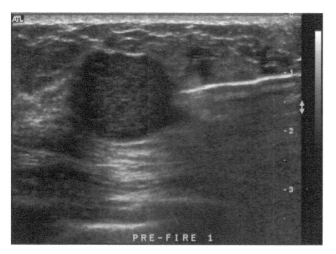

PRE-FIRE 1

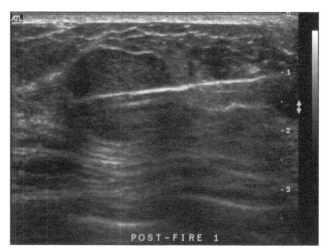

POST-FIRE 1

History: A 23-year-old woman feels a palpable mass in her left breast.

1. What should be included in the differential diagnosis for the images shown? (Choose all that apply.)
   A. Complex cyst
   B. Fibroadenoma
   C. Hamartoma
   D. Mucinous carcinoma

2. What is the BI-RADS (Breast Imaging Reporting and Data System) for this mass?
   A. BI-RADS 2—benign
   B. BI-RADS 3—probably benign
   C. BI-RADS 4—suspicious
   D. BI-RADS 5—highly suspicious

3. What is the next step in management of this palpable mass?
   A. Biopsy must be performed because the mass is palpable.
   B. Biopsy should be performed because the mass is not a BI-RADS 3.

C. The patient should be followed with ultrasound in 6 months.
D. The patient should have clinical follow-up; no further imaging follow-up is needed.

4. What are the features of a solid mass that allow follow-up rather than biopsy?
   A. Elliptical shape, wider than tall, and complete thin capsule
   B. Round shape with microlobulations
   C. Elliptical, taller than wide, thin complete capsule
   D. Elliptical, with thin capsule interrupted by one or two angular margins

CASE 44

Myxoid Fibroadenoma with Biopsy

1. B, C, and D
2. C
3. B
4. A

References

Santamaría G, Velasco M, Bargalló X, et al: Radiologic and pathologic findings in breast tumors with high signal intensity on T2-weighted MR images. *Radiographics* 2010;30(2):533-548.

Stavros AT: *Breast Ultrasound,* Philadelphia: Lippincott Williams & Wilkins, 2004.

Cross-Reference

Ikeda D: *Breast Imaging: THE REQUISITES,* 2nd ed, Philadelphia: Saunders, 2010, pp 163, 212.

Comment

Fibroadenoma is a very common mass in young women. When a patient presents with a palpable mass or a mammographic mass, and the classic features of a fibroadenoma are seen on ultrasound, the mass can be given a BI-RADS 3 designation. The patient has the following options: 6-month follow-up, core needle biopsy, or surgical excision. The BI-RADS 3 designation means that the mass has a less than 2% chance of malignancy. To have this designation, the mass must be elliptical, wider than tall, with a complete thin capsule. Two or three gentle lobulations are allowed.

Because of its round shape (see the figures), this mass is not a classic fibroadenoma and does not meet the strict BI-RADS 3 classification, and biopsy was performed (see the figures). Needle core biopsy was performed with a 14-gauge, spring-activated sampling device and ultrasound guidance. The pathology was "myxoid fibroadenoma."

Fibroadenomas are composed of gland and stromal elements. The stromal elements can undergo myxoid change, sclerosis, hyalinization, and calcification. None of these changes affect the malignant potential; all are benign changes. However, the abundant mucin accumulated in the stroma of this lesion can be confused with a mucinous carcinoma on core needle sampling.

On ultrasound, myxoid fibroadenomas are more likely to be round and compressible. On MRI, they are bright on T2-weighted images.

There is a syndrome of myxoid lesions in the skin and heart, called Carney's syndrome; however, most patients with a myxoid fibroadenoma do not have this syndrome. In the present case, the mass can be followed and does not need to be excised.

Notes

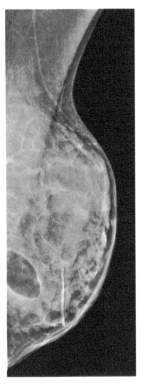 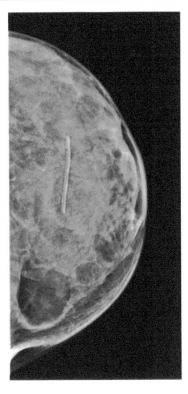

History: A 59-year-old woman presents for routine mammogram.

1. What is the differential diagnosis of the mass in the left breast? (Choose all that apply.)
   A. Air in a cyst after aspiration
   B. Oil cyst
   C. Hamartoma
   D. Lipoma

2. What additional studies are needed to make the diagnosis?
   A. Ultrasound, to evaluate cystic versus solid
   B. MRI, to evaluate for extent of disease
   C. Physical exam, to check if this is palpable
   D. None

3. Why is this lesion so clearly seen on this mammogram?
   A. The fat density of the mass blends in with the subcutaneous fat.
   B. The mass is the same density as the surrounding fatty breast tissue.
   C. The mass is fat, and it contrasts with the surrounding dense breast tissue.
   D. It is palpable.

4. What is the Breast Imaging Reporting and Data System (BI-RADS) code and recommendation for this lesion?
   A. BI-RADS 2—benign, routine follow-up
   B. BI-RADS 3—probably benign, short-interval follow-up
   C. BI-RADS 4—suspicious, recommend biopsy
   D. BI-RADS 0—incomplete, need additional evaluation

Lipoma

1. B, C, and D
2. D
3. C
4. A

References

Lanng C, Eriksen BO, Hoffmann J: Lipoma of the breast: a diagnostic dilemma. *Breast* 2004;13(5):408-411.

Stavros AT: *Breast Ultrasound*, Philadelphia: Lippincott Williams & Wilkins, 2004, p 569.

Cross-Reference

Ikeda D: *Breast Imaging: THE REQUISITES*, 2nd ed, Philadelphia: Saunders, 2010, p 137.

Comment

Lipomas are benign tumors composed of mature fat. They are the most common soft-tissue tumor of the body. They can occur in many areas of the body, including the GI tract and spine, but they are commonly found in the subcutaneous tissues. In the breast, the lipoma is likely a variation of hamartoma, containing mostly fat, with negligible amounts of stroma and gland elements. If the mass contains a more equal distribution of fat and glandular tissue, it is an adenolipoma. The masses are slow growing and soft and have a thin fibrous capsule. The patient can present with a palpable mass, unlike the patient represented here (see the figures), who has dense, lumpy breasts and did not appreciate this mass on clinical exam.

If the mass is palpable, ultrasound can be performed to evaluate the clinical finding. This is helpful if the mass is not apparent on the mammogram, which is commonly the case. Because the lipoma may be surrounded by fat, it is often not recognized on the mammogram. Ultrasound can be done to assess the palpable finding and ensure that no suspicious mass is present. The ultrasound appearance of the lipoma is typically isoechoic with the surrounding fat or slightly hyperechoic. The mass is often in the subcutaneous fat, oval, and wider than tall. The margins can be difficult to appreciate. The mass is soft and easily deformed.

However, if the mass is not palpable and is of fat density easily seen on the mammogram, as in this patient, no further work-up is needed.

Notes

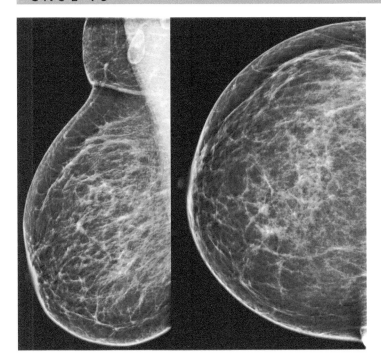

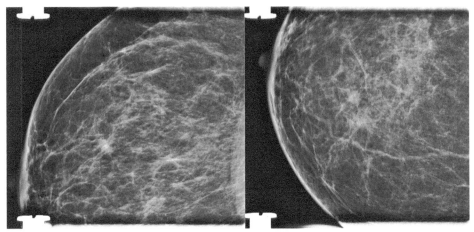

History: A 68-year-old woman undergoes a routine mammogram. She has a family history of breast cancer in a sister at age 40.

1. What should be included in the differential diagnosis of the standard views of the right breast? (Choose all that apply.)
   A. Radial scar in upper inner breast
   B. Normal mammogram
   C. Infiltrating ductal carcinoma
   D. Suspicious calcifications in the posterior right breast

2. What is the next step in management?
   A. Perform routine mammogram in 1 year.
   B. Recall patient for ultrasound.
   C. Recall patient for MRI.
   D. Recall patient for additional views with spot compression.

3. What is the spot compression view?
   A. A view of the entire breast in which more compression is applied to displace tissue better
   B. A view that uses magnification to visualize microcalcifications better
   C. A smaller paddle is used to image a focal area better
   D. A larger paddle is used to image the entire breast better

4. What is the purpose of the spot compression view?
   A. To separate true lesions from superimposition of normal structures
   B. To visualize microcalcifications better
   C. To determine if a mass is cystic or solid
   D. To visualize better the lateral aspect of the breast on the craniocaudal (CC) view

CASE 46

Spot Compression View

1. A and C
2. D
3. C
4. A

References

Ikeda DM, Andersson I, Wattsgard C, et al: Interval carcinomas in the Malmo Mammographic Screening Trial: radiologic appearance and prognostic considerations. *AJR Am J Roentgenol* 1992;159 (2):287-294.

Majid AS, de Paredes ES, Doherty RD, et al: Missed breast carcinoma: pitfalls and pearls. Radiographics 23(4):881–895.

Cross-Reference

Ikeda D: *Breast Imaging: THE REQUISITES*, 2nd ed, Philadelphia: Saunders, 2010, p 42.

Comment

When a lesion is suspected on review of screening mammogram views, the patient is recalled for additional evaluation. The most common reason for missed cancer at screening mammography is the developing density. In a review of interval cancers, 22% were found to have subtle signs of malignancy on the previous mammogram, and most of these were developing densities. Comparison with previous mammograms is important, and if a density is new, particularly in a postmenopausal patient, the mammogram should be given a BI-RADS 0, and the patient should be recalled.

When the patient returns, it is often best to perform spot compression views first when evaluating a possible developing density. The finding is often normal, and the spot compression view can efface the lesion. When the lesion is effaced, no further work-up may be needed.

The spot compression view is performed with a small paddle applied directly over the area of concern. The greater compression applied makes a true lesion stand out from the surrounding normal tissue because the malignancy mass is denser, firmer, and less likely to compress compared with normal gland tissue.

In this patient, there was a subtle neodensity in the upper right breast on the mediolateral oblique (MLO) view (see the figures). She was recalled for additional views, and the spot compression views confirmed a true spiculated mass, seen on both views (see the figures). Ultrasound was performed for ease of biopsy. Biopsy was performed with ultrasound guidance and needle core technique and confirmed an infiltrating ductal carcinoma, grade II, 6 mm in size.

Notes

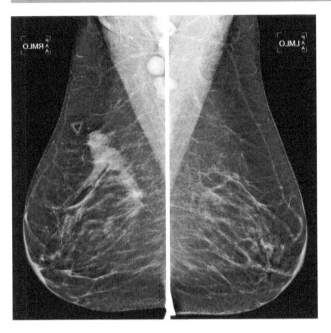

History: A 41-year-old woman presents for evaluation of a palpable mass in the right breast.

1. What should be included in the differential diagnosis? (Choose all that apply.)
   A. Right breast mastitis with enlarged axillary nodes
   B. Lactating adenoma
   C. Invasive ductal carcinoma
   D. Invasive lobular carcinoma

2. What is the next step in management?
   A. MRI to evaluate enhancement
   B. Stereotactic biopsy
   C. Ultrasound of the breast
   D. Surgical referral

3. What are the ultrasound features of suspicious lymph nodes?
   A. Oval shape, with large fatty hilum
   B. Round, anechoic
   C. Round and echogenic
   D. Greater than 2 cm in size

4. Can the axillary node be sampled with imaging guidance?
   A. No, biopsy of the axilla is too difficult with imaging guidance.
   B. No, it is difficult to position the axilla for stereotactic guidance.
   C. No, there is no reason to biopsy the nodes because they will be removed with sentinel node biopsy.
   D. Yes, the axillary nodes should be evaluated with ultrasound and sampled with needle biopsy.

C A S E 4 7

Mass and Axillary Node

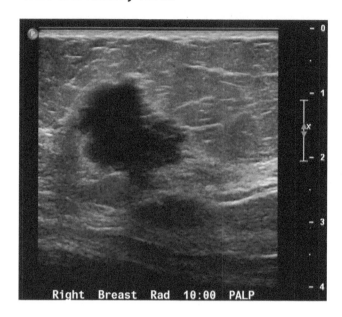

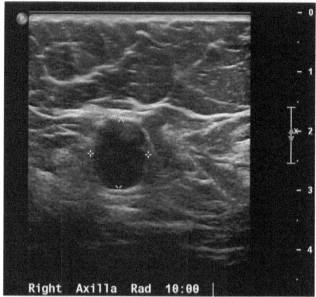

1. C and D
2. C
3. B
4. D

References

Abe H, Schmidt RA, Sennett CA, et al: US-guided core needle biopsy of axillary lymph nodes in patients with breast cancer: why and how to do it. *Radiographics* 2007;27(Suppl 1):S91-S99.

Feu J, Tresserra F, Fabregas R, et al: Metastatic breast carcinoma in axillary lymph nodes: in vitro US detection. *Radiology* 1997;205 (3):831-835.

Yang WT, Chang J, Metreweli C: Patients with breast cancer: differences in color Doppler flow and gray-scale US features of benign and malignant axillary lymph nodes. *Radiology* 2000;215 (2):568-573.

Cross-Reference

Ikeda D: *Breast Imaging: THE REQUISITES*, 2nd ed, Philadelphia: Saunders, 2010, pp 214, 395.

Comment

Breast cancer may manifest as a palpable mass. Most palpable breast masses are benign tumors, such as fibroadenomas or cysts; however, malignancy should always be foremost in the differential diagnosis. The features on mammography of a suspicious mass include irregular shape, microlobulation, indistinct or spiculated margins, and high density (see the figures). Ultrasound features of a suspicious mass are similar, including round or irregular shape, microlobulated or spiculated margins, echogenic halo boundary, and hypoechoic internal echotexture (see the figures).

When a suspicious mass is seen, the surrounding breast tissue should be evaluated for the presence of satellite lesions, and all suspicious findings should be included in the biopsy planning. To evaluate extent of disease further, the axilla should be evaluated with mammography and ultrasound. The axilla should be included on a mediolateral oblique mammographic view, but if it is not well seen, a spot compression view can be obtained.

The axilla is easily evaluated with ultrasound. Malignant nodes have a characteristic appearance on ultrasound. In cases of obvious infiltration, the node is round, and the hilum is absent (see the figures). In earlier stages of infiltration, the hilum is present but may be slit-like. In even earlier infiltration, the hilum may appear normal, but there may be a focal thickening of the node cortex. Size is not an independent factor; normal nodes may be quite large, with a large fatty hilum and thin cortex. Malignant nodes may be small. Color flow Doppler should be performed of axillary nodes; increased blood supply on Doppler verifies the malignant tissue in the node. Doppler can also help map the location of axillary blood vessels before node biopsy.

If a lymph node is suspected to contain metastatic disease, needle biopsy can be performed with ultrasound guidance. Core technique or fine-needle aspiration biopsy is acceptable, although core technique is less operator dependent and has a higher success rate compared with fine-needle aspiration biopsy, and the evaluation of the material obtained does not depend on experienced cytologists. If lymph node metastasis is established before surgery, the patient need not undergo sentinel node biopsy.

Notes

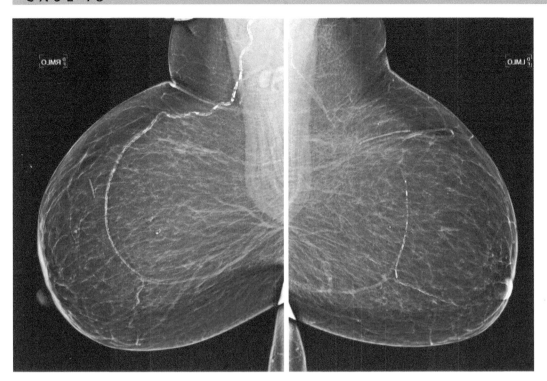

History: A 64-year-old woman presents for a routine screening mammogram. Health history includes a renal transplant 10 years ago.

1. What should be included in the differential diagnosis of the mammogram shown? (Choose all that apply.)
   A. Normal mammogram
   B. Benign mammogram with benign calcifications present
   C. Suspicious linear calcifications in both breasts, possible ductal carcinoma in situ
   D. Vascular calcifications

2. What management is needed for this patient?
   A. Recall for magnification views
   B. Short-interval follow-up
   C. Routine mammogram in 1 year
   D. Doppler ultrasound to check for stenosis in the calcified arteries

3. Which patients are at risk for this condition?
   A. Young and healthy patients
   B. Patients with chronic renal failure
   C. Patients who are on dialysis only
   D. Patients with diabetes if untreated

4. This mammographic finding may be a marker for what condition?
   A. Acute renal failure
   B. Atherosclerotic disease
   C. Ductal carcinoma in situ
   D. Mondor disease

C A S E 4 8

Vascular Calcifications

1. A, B, and D
2. C
3. B
4. B

References

Cao MM, Hoyt AC, Bassett LW: Mammographic signs of systemic disease. *Radiographics* 2011;31(4):1085-1100.

Duhn V, D'Orsi ET, Johnson S, et al: Breast arterial calcification: a marker of medial vascular calcification in chronic kidney disease. *Clin J Am Soc Nephrol* 2011;6(2):377-382.

Kataoka M, Warren R, Luben R, et al: How predictive is breast arterial calcification of cardiovascular disease and risk factors when found at screening mammography? *AJR Am J Roentgenol* 2006;187(1):73-80.

Zgheib MH, Buchbinder SS, Abi Rafeh N, et al: Breast arterial calcifications on mammograms do not predict coronary heart disease at coronary angiography. *Radiology* 2010;254(2):367-373.

Cross-Reference

Ikeda D: *Breast Imaging: THE REQUISITES*, 2nd ed, Philadelphia: Saunders, 2010, p 84.

Comment

Vascular calcifications typically do not cause difficulty in diagnosis. Characteristically, they are seen as parallel lines of calcification, often with amorphous calcification within the parallel lines indicating the vessel wall en face. This condition is much more commonly seen in patients older than 60 years. These typical calcifications need no further work-up. They are found in approximately 7% to 34% of mammograms, increasing with age in one study; the prevalence exceeds 50% in women older than 65.

Vascular calcifications seen on mammography are in the media of the smaller vessel walls and the arterioles and not in the intima of the wall. The risk of the development of this calcification is increased in diabetes and chronic renal failure, and there may be an increased risk factor for coronary artery disease. The calcifications are not related to breast disease. The presence of arterial calcifications (see the figure) may be a useful marker for the presence of medial vascular calcification elsewhere in the body.

Notes

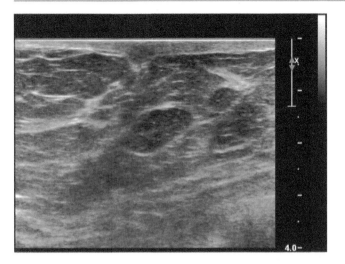

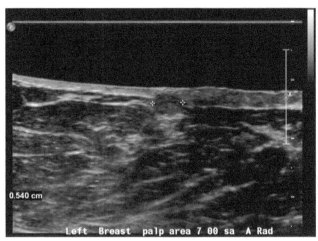

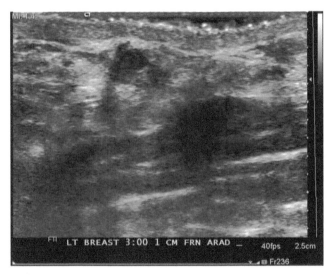

History: A 66-year-old woman presents with a palpable mass near the nipple. Mammography was negative (not shown). The third image represents a companion case.

1. What should be included in the differential diagnosis for the ultrasound images shown? (Choose all that apply.)
   A. Benign papillary lesion
   B. Invasive papillary cancer
   C. Sebaceous cyst
   D. Simple cyst

2. If mammogram and ultrasound are negative, but a superficial mass is clearly palpable, what examination could be performed next?
   A. MRI to check for abnormal enhancement
   B. Surgical consultation
   C. Use of a standoff pad to optimize the ultrasound evaluation
   D. Needle aspiration, guided by palpation

3. What is the next step in management for this lesion?
   A. Surgical excision
   B. Needle core biopsy
   C. Annual mammogram
   D. Short-interval follow-up

4. Why does a standoff pad help in imaging superficial structures on ultrasound?
   A. The standoff pad allows visualization of the outer layer of the dermis.
   B. The standoff pad allows the focal zone and the lesion to be farther away from the transducer face.
   C. The focal point of an ultrasound transducer is too shallow for superficial structures.
   D. The standoff pad increases the volume-averaging artifact.

CASE 49

Standoff Pad

1. A, B, and C
2. C
3. B
4. B

Reference

Stavros AT: *Breast Ultrasound*, Philadelphia: Lippincott Williams & Wilkins, 2004.

Cross-Reference

Ikeda D: *Breast Imaging: THE REQUISITES*, 2nd ed, Philadelphia: Saunders, 2010, p 149.

Comment

Palpable masses are of increased concern for breast cancer. Ultrasound is an important tool in the evaluation of a palpable mass. Ultrasound is typically the tool used to supplement mammography except in patients younger than 30 years and nursing or pregnant patients. In these subgroups, ultrasound is the first imaging tool.

If the mass palpated by the patient is small and superficial, as in this patient (see the figures), ultrasound may not characterize the mass adequately because of constraints in the near field of the transducer. The short-axis resolution, which refers to the resolution in the superficial-to-deep plane, or elevation plane, must be optimized. For lesions in the shallowest 1 cm of the breast, a standoff pad or thicker layer of gel can yield better imaging analysis of the lesion.

The standoff pad improves resolution and decreases volume averaging of superficial structures (see the figures). There is improved margin sharpness and improved contrast resolution of the mass in the second figure compared with the same mass on the same day in the first figure. The focus zones, as adjusted by the sonographer for optimal imaging, are appropriately positioned for both images. The lesion is too small and too superficial to be adequately seen without a standoff pad. However, the standoff pad is useful only in this narrow application. It is not practical to use in evaluating the entire breast because deep lesions would be outside the focal zone and may be missed. It is also awkward to palpate the lesion while scanning with a standoff pad. The third figure demonstrates the application of a thicker layer of gel, in a different patient, to visualize a superficial palpable mass better.

Notes

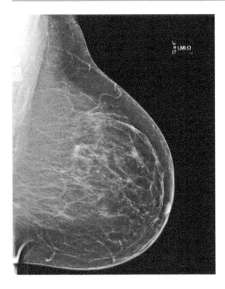

History: A 50-year-old woman presents for her baseline mammogram. A focal density is seen in the posterior left breast, but only on the mediolateral oblique (MLO) view.

1. What is the differential diagnosis for this single view of the routine mammogram? (Choose all that apply.)
   A. Cyst at the edge of the image, posteriorly in the left breast
   B. Highly suspicious mass at the edge of the image
   C. Benign solid mass at the posterior edge of the image
   D. Blood vessel at the edge of the image

2. What is the work-up?
   A. No work-up is needed; the mammogram is normal.
   B. Additional views with spot compression and mediolateral (ML) view are needed to help triangulate.
   C. Initially, perform ultrasound.
   D. Perform MRI.

3. How does the mediolateral (ML) view help triangulate the location of the density?
   A. If the lesion is seen to move superiorly in the breast on the ML view, compared to the MLO view, it is in the lateral breast.
   B. If the lesion is seen to move inferiorly in the breast on the ML view, as compared to the MLO view, it is in the lateral breast.
   C. The ML view does not help if the lesion is seen in the same location on both the ML and MLO views.
   D. The ML view does not help in locating the lesion.

4. Is MRI needed in the evaluation of this patient?
   A. Yes, MRI is important for complete evaluation.
   B. Yes, the MRI is needed to prove that the mass is a looped blood vessel.
   C. No, the MRI is unnecessary.
   D. Yes, MRI should be performed next when a mass that can be seen on the mammogram cannot be seen on ultrasound.

CASE 50

Blood Vessel Presenting as a Mass at the Posterior Edge of an Image

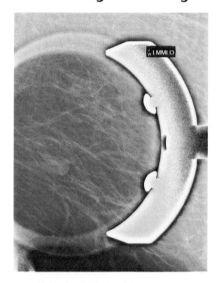
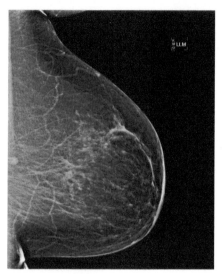

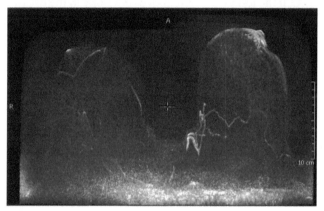

1. A, C, and D
2. B
3. B
4. C

References

Park JM, Franken EA Jr: Triangulation of breast lesions: review and clinical applications. *Curr Probl Diagn Radiol* 2008;37(1):1-14.

Sickles EA: Practical solutions to common mammographic problems, tailoring the examination. *AJR Am J Roentgenol* 1988;51:31-39.

Cross-Reference

Ikeda D: *Breast Imaging: THE REQUISITES*, 2nd ed, Philadelphia: Saunders, 2010, pp 42-51.

Comment

This asymptomatic patient had a routine screening mammogram, her baseline. The masslike structure was seen at the posterior edge of the image, on the left MLO view (see the figures). A spot compression view (see the figures) was performed, and the diagnosis is now apparent: The "mass" is a looped blood vessel. Blood vessels are seen on mammograms; they can loop, and the apex of the loop can be perceived as a mass. The proper diagnosis can usually be made with routine imaging, such as a spot compression view, angled views (for instance, 15 degrees from the view that showed the finding, or step-oblique images), or a rolled view if the mass is seen on the craniocaudal (CC) view.

If the additional views do not help, and the lesion is seen only on the MLO view, as in this case (see the figures), then an ML view can be helpful to locate the lesion in the breast. This is called *triangulation*. By comparison of the MLO view to the ML view, the lesion can be determined to be in the medial or lateral breast on the CC view. Medial lesions, such as this one (see the figures) will be seen to "move up" on the ML view relative to the position on the MLO view.

MRI is not necessary to evaluate this mammographic lesion, because it is seen to be a looped blood vessel on the spot compression view (see the figures). Further work-up with ultrasound is not likely to be helpful, and MRI, although it confirms the diagnosis in this case (see the figures), is an expensive tool for this purpose in this case. If the mass had been suspicious in appearance on mammographic images and not seen on ultrasound or felt on palpation, then stereotactic biopsy should be the next consideration. In this case, the radiologist recommended MRI for this density because stereotactic biopsy was felt to be not possible owing to the far posterior location of the density. It was not recognized as a blood vessel at the time of imaging.

Notes

Fair Game

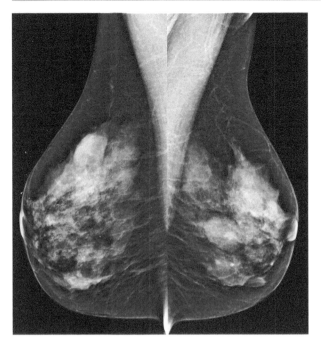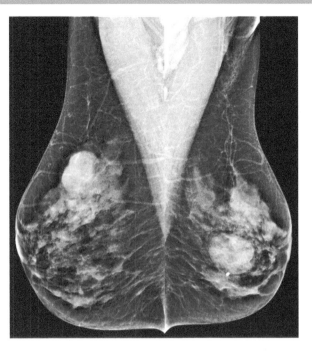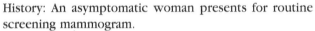

History: An asymptomatic woman presents for routine screening mammogram.

1. What should be included in the differential diagnosis based on the images shown? (Choose all that apply.)
   A. Multiple bilateral fibroadenoma
   B. Multiple bilateral cysts, with a suspicious mass in the upper left breast
   C. Bilateral breast cysts
   D. Multiple bilateral complicated cysts

2. What is the next step in management of this patient?
   A. Recall for bilateral ultrasound
   B. Bilateral breast MRI
   C. Routine screening mammogram in 1 year
   D. Aspiration of largest cyst

3. What is the cancer rate in women with bilateral circumscribed masses?
   A. Slightly higher than the national average because of proliferative change
   B. Approximately double the normal rate
   C. Approximately the same as the normal population
   D. Slightly higher, unless the cysts are palpable

4. What is the BI-RADS (Breast Imaging Reporting and Data System) for this finding on a baseline mammogram?
   A. BI-RADS 2—benign
   B. BI-RADS 3—probably benign
   C. BI-RADS 4—suspicious
   D. BI-RADS 0—incomplete

CASE 51

Changing Pattern of Multiple Bilateral Masses

1. A, C, and D
2. C
3. C
4. A

References

Berg WA, Campassi CI, Ioffe OB: Cystic lesions of the breast: sonographic-pathologic correlation. *Radiology* 2003;227(1):183-191.

Hines N, Slanetz PJ, Eisenberg RL: Cystic masses of the breast. *AJR Am J Roentgenol* 2010;194(2):W122-W133.

Leung JWT, Sickles EA: Multiple bilateral masses detected on screening mammography: assessment of need for recall imaging. *AJR Am J Roentgenol* 2000;175(1):23-29.

Cross-Reference

Ikeda D: *Breast Imaging: THE REQUISITES*, 2nd ed, Philadelphia: Saunders, 2010, pp 137, 381.

Comment

The simple cyst is a round or oval space, filled with fluid and lined by epithelium. It is the most common mass in the female breast and has no malignant potential. It develops and regresses spontaneously, and cysts may increase when estrogens are taken.

On mammography, simple cysts are usually round or oval but may be lobulated and are typically water density, the same as the surrounding parenchyma. They are often multiple and bilateral. Although a cyst cannot be differentiated from a solid mass on mammography, the presence of multiple bilateral circumscribed masses can be considered benign. There should be at least three circumscribed or partially circumscribed masses, with at least one in each breast, to be considered a benign finding. There should be no suspicious findings, such as distortion or suspicious microcalcifications. The masses are most commonly cysts or fibroadenomas. When the masses change in size, location, and number on successive mammograms, they can be considered cysts (see the figures). Ultrasound is not needed if the patient is asymptomatic and all of the above-mentioned conditions are met. The rate of malignancy in a large study of women with bilateral circumscribed masses was approximately 0.1%, lower than the incident rate of breast cancer in the normal age-matched population. If one mass is disproportionately larger or denser or has poorly defined margins, the patient should be recalled.

This patient with bilateral, similar, circumscribed masses is at no increased risk of malignancy, and her mammogram is benign, BI-RADS 2. Assigning the patient to a BI-RADS 3 category, with short-interval follow-up, is unnecessary.

Notes

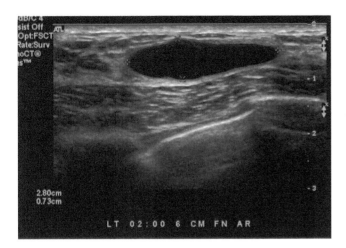

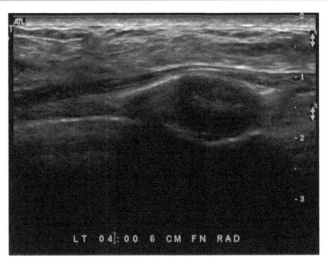

History: A 21-year-old woman presents with two palpable masses in her left breast—one in the upper outer quadrant and one in the lower outer quadrant.

1. What should be included in the differential diagnosis for the two ultrasound images shown? (Choose all that apply.)
   A. Suspicious mass in the lower outer breast
   B. Simple cyst in the upper outer breast
   C. Rib in the lower outer breast
   D. Fibroadenoma in the lower outer breast

2. How is a rib distinguished from a breast mass on ultrasound?
   A. The rib is posterior to the chest muscle.
   B. The breast mass should be posterior to the chest muscle.
   C. The rib never looks oval, and masses are often oval.
   D. Masses are typically more hypoechoic than the rib.

3. What is the BI-RADS (Breast Imaging Reporting and Data System) code for the ultrasound examination of this patient?
   A. BI-RADS 0—incomplete
   B. BI-RADS 1—normal
   C. BI-RADS 2—benign
   D. BI-RADS 3—probably benign

4. How reliable is the negative ultrasound examination when evaluating a palpable mass?
   A. Not reliable—a mammogram must be performed for more complete evaluation.
   B. Not reliable—the patient must be seen by a surgeon for consideration for biopsy.
   C. Relatively reliable—the radiologist may correlate the palpable finding with the ultrasound.
   D. Somewhat reliable—the patient should return for a short-interval follow-up.

CASE 52

Ultrasound of Rib

1. B and C
2. A
3. C
4. C

References

Dennis MA, Parker SH, Klaus AJ, et al: Breast biopsy avoidance: the value of normal mammograms and normal sonograms in the setting of a palpable lump. *Radiology* 2001;219(1):186-191.

Soo MS, Rosen EL, Baker JA, et al: Negative predictive value of sonography with mammography in patients with palpable breast lesions. *AJR Am J Roentgenol* 2001;177(5):1167-1170.

Cross-Reference

Ikeda D: *Breast Imaging: THE REQUISITES*, 2nd ed, Philadelphia: Saunders, 2010, pp 100, 150, 175.

Comment

Patients often present with a palpable finding. They may note cysts (see the figures), solid masses, or normal parenchyma. Patients may confuse normal anatomy with pathology; the normal rib may be perceived as a mass. Ultrasound is an important tool in the evaluation of a breast lump because the area of concern can be addressed in a precise manner. One method of evaluating the lump is to place your finger or a cotton-tipped swab over the lump, as pointed out by the patient. Apply the ultrasound transducer to the finger or swab, then withdraw the finger and scan directly underneath.

The beginner ultrasonographer may confuse the rib in cross section with a breast mass (see the figures). To differentiate the rib from a breast mass, note the position of the finding relative to the pectoralis muscle, note the periodicity of the ribs, and note that turning the transducer 90 degrees elongates the rib.

Notes

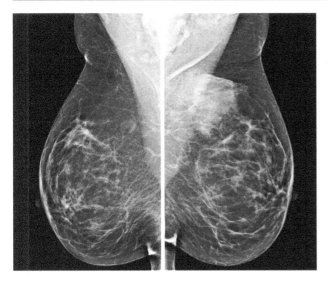

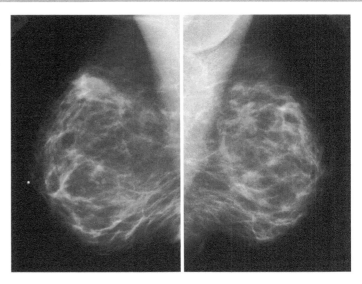

History: A 55-year-old woman presents for a screening mammogram. Her last mammogram was obtained 4 years ago and is available for comparison.

1. What should be included in the differential diagnosis for the finding in the left breast? (Choose all that apply.)
   A. Invasive ductal carcinoma
   B. Pseudoangiomatous stromal hyperplasia
   C. Ductal carcinoma in situ
   D. Asymmetric glandular tissue

2. What is the BI-RADS (Breast Imaging Reporting and Data System) category?
   A. BI-RADS 0—incomplete
   B. BI-RADS 2—benign
   C. BI-RADS 3—probably benign
   D. BI-RADS 4—suspicious

3. Which of the following imaging tools is *inadequate* for further work-up?
   A. Additional mammographic views
   B. Ultrasound
   C. MRI
   D. PET/CT

4. Which of the following statements regarding focal asymmetry is *false*?
   A. According to the BI-RADS lexicon, a focal asymmetry is a space-occupying lesion seen in two different views.
   B. It is not a very rare finding on screening mammogram.
   C. A new focal asymmetry requires further work-up.
   D. Biopsy is useful in differentiating a benign from a malignant process.

Developing Asymmetry

1. A, B, and D
2. A
3. D
4. A

References

Leung JW, Sickles EA: Developing asymmetry identified on mammography: correlation with imaging outcome and pathologic findings. *AJR Am J Roentgenol* 2007;188(3):667-675.

Samardar P, de Paredes ES, Grimes MM, et al: Focal asymmetric densities seen at mammography: US and pathologic correlation. *Radiographics* 2002;22(1):19-33.

Sickles EA: The spectrum of breast asymmetries: imaging features, work-up, management. *Radiol Clin North Am* 2007;45(5):765-771.

Youk JH, Kim EK, Ko KH, et al: Asymmetric mammographic findings based on the fourth edition of BI-RADS: types, evaluation, and management. *Radiographics* 2009;29(1):e33.

Cross-Reference

Ikeda D: *Breast Imaging: THE REQUISITES*, 2nd ed, Philadelphia: Saunders, 2010, p 410.

Comment

The breasts are usually fairly symmetric in density and architecture. Nevertheless, asymmetries are not an unusual finding on routine mammogram (see the figures), reportedly seen in 3% of healthy women. According to the BI-RADS lexicon, *asymmetric findings* constitute an area of tissue with fibroglandular density that is more extensive in one breast compared with the corresponding region of the contralateral breast. Asymmetries are planar, lack convex borders, usually contain interspersed fat, and lack the conspicuity of a three-dimensional mass.

There are three types of asymmetric findings: global asymmetry, focal asymmetry, and developing asymmetry. *Global asymmetry* involves a large portion of the breast (at least a quadrant), *focal asymmetry* corresponds to a density with similar shape in two views but lacking convex outward borders, and *developing asymmetry* is focal asymmetry that is new or increasing. A developing asymmetry may be a normal variant but can also constitute a sign of malignancy and must be viewed with caution and evaluated thoroughly.

It is important to review all previous mammograms, with at least a 2-year interval, because an area of increasing density may not be apparent over a shorter interval (see the figures). If the previous mammograms are at a different site, there is value in obtaining them. If the area is stable compared with prior films, no further work-up is needed. However, a new, larger or denser asymmetry and a palpable abnormality require additional evaluation. Additional mammographic views help to determine if the tissue spreads out or if there is interspersed fat, which is a benign feature. Additional views may include spot compression views, rolled craniocaudal views, and a true lateral view.

Ultrasound is a very good tool for evaluating focal asymmetries. The classic ultrasound appearance of an island of normal breast tissue is that of a hyperechoic area with ducts coursing through. There should be no mass, distortion, or abnormal shadowing.

A core biopsy can be performed if concern is expressed by the patient or if the asymmetry is palpable. The histology is often benign breast tissue, stromal fibrosis, or pseudoangiomatous stromal hyperplasia. MRI can be done instead of needle biopsy, although the role of MRI for assessment of asymmetric breast findings has not yet been established. With administration of contrast material, the enhancement of the asymmetric tissue should be the same as that of the rest of the glandular tissue, with no abnormal enhancement.

Notes

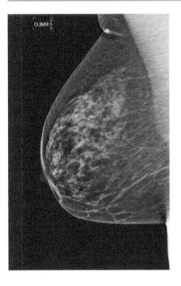
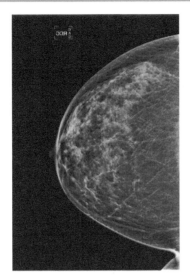

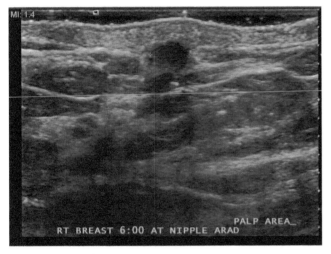

History: A 61-year-old woman of normal risk palpated a tiny mass just below her right nipple. Mammogram views of the right breast are shown.

1. What is the differential diagnosis of the mammogram of the right breast? (Choose all that apply.)
   A. There is a suspicious mass near the nipple at the 6 o'clock position.
   B. There is no suspicious finding.
   C. There is a focal masslike density in the upper outer quadrant, but there is no abnormality in the nipple area.
   D. Suspicious clustered microcalcifications are seen near the nipple.

2. What is the next step in the management of this patient?
   A. The mammogram is normal, so she can return in 1 year.
   B. The patient should seek a surgical consultation, because the mammogram is abnormal.

C. The patient should be evaluated with ultrasound of the palpable mass.
D. The patient should be asked to return in 6 months.

3. How accurate is the normal mammogram in the setting of a palpable mass?
   A. Very accurate: 80% to 100%
   B. Not very accurate: 20% to 40%
   C. The accuracy depends on the glandular density.
   D. The mammogram is nearly 100% accurate in the patient with a dense breast.

4. What should be the next step if ultrasound reveals a simple cyst at the palpable area?
   A. All palpable cysts must be aspirated.
   B. All simple cysts should be referred to a surgeon for excision or aspiration.
   C. All simple cysts should be followed with an ultrasound exam in 6 months.
   D. Simple cysts can be aspirated if the patient desires; otherwise, the patient should receive routine follow-up.

Importance of Ultrasound in a Palpable Mass

1. B
2. C
3. C
4. D

References

Berg WA, Gutierrez L, Ness Aiver MS, et al: Diagnostic accuracy of mammography, clinical examination, US, and MR imaging in preoperative assessment of breast cancer. *Radiology* 2004;233(3):830-849.

Seidman H, Gelb SK, Silverberg E, et al: Survival experience in the Breast Cancer Detection Demonstration Project. *CA Cancer J Clin* 1987;37:258-290.

Stavros AT, Thickman D, Rapp CL, et al: Solid breast nodules: use of sonography to distinguish between benign and malignant lesions. *Radiology* 1995;196:123-134.

Cross-Reference

Ikeda D: *Breast Imaging: THE REQUISITES*, 2nd ed, Philadelphia: Saunders, 2010, pp 100, 137.

Comment

Patients often present with a palpable mass noted either on self-exam or on a clinician's exam. The mammogram is not a perfect study for the detection of cancer. A 10% false-negative rate is published, based on early studies (Seidman et al, 1987). Depending on the density of the breast tissue, the false-negative rate may be higher. Conversely, when the breast is entirely fatty, the mammogram has a very low false-negative rate. If a patient presents with a palpable finding, and the mammogram shows glandular density in the area (see the figures), then a mass may be obscured by the surrounding gland tissue, and ultrasound should be performed. In this case, the patient failed to mention the palpable concern to the technologist before the mammogram views were performed, so no marker was placed to locate the site of concern. The patient decided to mention the concern after the views, and the exam was converted from screening to diagnostic because of the concern.

Ultrasound was performed (see the figures) and demonstrates a tiny mass in the subcutaneous tissues inferior to the nipple. The mass is indeterminate for the presence of malignancy. Although it is roughly oval and wider than tall (both benign features), the borders are microlobulated. This is a suspicious feature, and the presence of one suspicious feature means that biopsy should be performed. Needle core biopsy was performed with ultrasound guidance, and histology was invasive mammary carcinoma with duct and lobular features.

Ultrasound should be performed in the setting of the normal mammogram and a palpable mass. The ultrasound should be correlated with a physical exam, while scanning, to ensure that the palpable concern is evaluated. If ultrasound demonstrates a simple cyst, no further work-up is needed. A simple cyst on ultrasound is anechoic, with imperceptible walls, a sharp back wall, and increased through transmission posteriorly. If a complex cyst is seen (mass within the cyst, or cyst with irregular, thickened wall), then biopsy should be performed. If a solid mass is seen, biopsy is typically performed, particularly if there is a suspicious feature on ultrasound, such as in this patient.

Notes

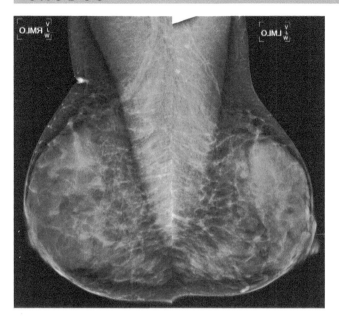

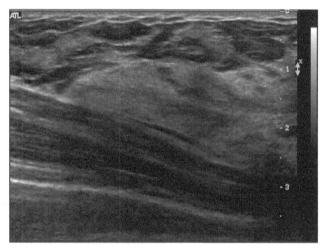

History: A 38-year-old woman who feels a lump in the right upper outer breast undergoes a baseline mammogram.

1. What should be included in the differential diagnosis for the images shown? (Choose all that apply.)
   A. Focal masslike density in the right breast on mammogram and normal ultrasound
   B. Normal mammogram and ultrasound
   C. Normal mammogram and dense, focal fibrosis on ultrasound
   D. Dense glandular tissue on mammogram with fibrous ridge on ultrasound

2. What is the negative predictive value of a normal mammogram and normal ultrasound in the setting of a palpable mass?
   A. The negative predictive value is less than 50%.
   B. This has not been determined; if a patient has a palpable mass and negative imaging, she should see a surgeon for clinical evaluation.
   C. Published studies reveal nearly 100% negative predictive value in a normal mammogram and ultrasound.
   D. The negative predictive value is approximately 75%; needle core biopsy should be performed for all palpable masses.

3. What is the management of this patient after normal standard imaging?
   A. The imaging report should state that a dense area of fibrosis is seen, explaining the palpable finding, and she should be followed clinically.
   B. The patient should be referred for mandatory surgical evaluation.
   C. Needle biopsy of the echogenic tissue seen on ultrasound should be offered.
   D. The patient should be recommended to return in 6 months to follow the palpable area closely with mammogram and ultrasound.

4. What is the BI-RADS (Breast Imaging Reporting and Data System) of this study?
   A. BI-RADS 1—normal
   B. BI-RADS 3—probably benign
   C. BI-RADS 4—suspicious
   D. BI-RADS 5—highly suspicious

CASE 55

Predictive Value of Negative Imaging

1. B, C, and D
2. C
3. A
4. A

References

Dennis MA: Breast biopsy avoidance: the value of normal mammograms and normal sonograms in the setting of a palpable lump. *Radiology* 2001;219(1):186-191.

Moy L, Slanetz PJ, Moore R, et al: Specificity of mammography and US in the evaluation of a palpable abnormality: retrospective review. *Radiology* 2002;225(1):176-181.

Shetty MK, Shah YP, Sharman RS, et al: Prospective evaluation of the value of combined mammographic and sonographic assessment in patients with palpable abnormalities of the breast. *J Ultrasound Med* 2003;22(3):263-268.

Soo MS, Rosen EL, Baker JA, et al: Negative predictive value of sonography with mammography in patients with palpable breast lesions. *AJR Am J Roentgenol* 2001;177(5):1167-1170.

Cross-Reference

Ikeda D: *Breast Imaging: THE REQUISITES*, 2nd ed, Philadelphia: Saunders, 2010, p 174.

Comment

When a patient older than 30 years presents with a palpable finding, a mammogram should be performed as the initial study. Ultrasound is particularly helpful in the setting of a normal dense mammogram, with no evidence of a mass or suspicious microcalcifications (see the figures). Ultrasound may reveal an occult mass or cyst or may be normal. A normal mammogram and normal ultrasound in a patient who feels a lump are quite common. Often the reason for the palpable finding can be seen on ultrasound as an isolated dense, echogenic area surrounded by fat or a dense ridge (see the figures). The dense tissue is adenosis or fibrosis but is a normal variation and should be communicated as such to the patient and the referring physician.

Several studies have shown that the positive predictive value of a negative mammogram and negative ultrasound in the setting of a palpable finding is nearly 100%. The normal findings are reliable, the report is given a BI-RADS 1, and no imaging follow-up is needed. The patient and the physician may choose to follow up with a surgical consultation based on clinical grounds alone.

It is important that the radiologist personally correlate the clinical and imaging findings in this situation. The technologist performing the ultrasound may miss a subtle finding or may believe that the clinically apparent lump is quite suspicious on palpation. If the clinical finding is suspicious, and no abnormality is seen on standard imaging, MRI can be performed to evaluate further.

Notes

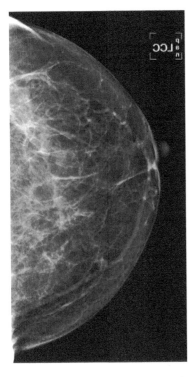
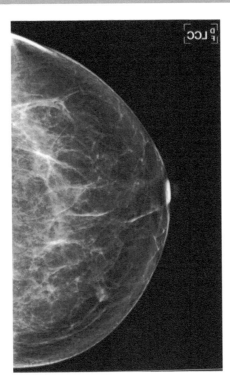
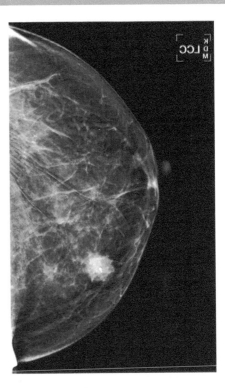

History: A 66-year-old woman presents with a palpable mass in her left breast, 6 weeks after a screening mammogram that was interpreted as normal.

1. What should be included in the differential diagnosis for the three mammogram images shown? (Choose all that apply.)
   A. Rapid growth of a breast malignancy
   B. Abscess developing in left breast
   C. Benign mass was excised; mass represents palpable surgical site
   D. Rapid growth of a benign fibroadenoma

2. Why are cancers missed at screening mammography?
   A. The breast tissue is fatty.
   B. The missed cancer is spiculated and associated with calcifications.
   C. The radiologist incorrectly interpreted the mammogram.
   D. There are prior mammograms for comparison.

3. What is an interval cancer?
   A. A cancer that develops between routine screening examinations
   B. A cancer that is intermediate grade
   C. A cancer that develops in a woman who has a family history of breast cancer in her daughter
   D. A cancer that develops in the same breast as cancer was diagnosed earlier

4. What are "minimal signs" or "nonspecific signs" on mammography?
   A. A visible lesion on mammogram, not worrisome enough to warrant recall
   B. Tissue density that is 25% to 50% dense
   C. Lesions that are suspicious for malignancy
   D. Secondary signs of malignancy, such as skin thickening

C A S E 5 6

Interval Cancer

1. A, B, and C
2. C
3. A
4. A

References

Cho N, Kim SJ, Choi HY, et al: Features of prospectively overlooked computer-aided detection marks on prior screening digital mammograms in women with breast cancer. *AJR Am J Roentgenol* 2010;195(5):1276-1282.

Hofvind S, Skaane P, Vitak B, et al: Influence of review design on percentages of missed interval breast cancers: retrospective study of interval cancers in a population-based screening program. *Radiology* 2005;237(2):437-443.

Ikeda DM, Andersson I, Wattsgard C, et al: Interval carcinomas in the Malmo Mammographic Screening Trial: radiologic appearance and prognostic considerations. *AJR Am J Roentgenol* 1992;159(2):287-294.

Roubidoux MA, Bailey JE, Wray LA, et al: Invasive cancers detected after breast cancer screening yielded a negative result: relationship of mammographic density to tumor prognostic factors. *Radiology* 2004;230(1):42-48.

Cross-Reference

Ikeda D: *Breast Imaging: THE REQUISITES*, 2nd ed, Philadelphia: Saunders, 2010, p 408.

Comment

An interval cancer is one that is detected between routine screening mammograms. It is typically found on clinical examination by the patient's physician at a routine clinical visit or felt by the patient on breast self-examination. The incidence of interval cancer relates to the sensitivity of mammography, which is variably reported as 80% to 90%—that is, some cancers are missed on mammography, no matter how skilled the radiologist.

When the patient presents with a clinical finding, and the previous screening mammogram is reviewed, a suspicious lesion may be seen that was clearly overlooked by the interpreting radiologist. This situation may be due to a perception error or a misinterpretation error. A smaller percentage of findings on the previous screen are termed "minimal" or "nonspecific," meaning that although a lesion is present, it does not meet the threshold for recall. It may be low density, with smooth margins, as in the patient in this case (see the figures). Other cases are truly occult on the previous screening mammogram and are typically aggressive, rapidly growing tumors (see the figures).

Several studies have shown that women with interval cancers have higher stage disease and more often have positive lymph nodes compared with women with cancers detected on screening examination. Interval cancers are more often well-defined masses, which are uncommon and which may have a nonspecific appearance, such as the special types of infiltrating ductal carcinoma, including medullary, mucinous, invasive papillary, and tubular cancers. This patient had the much more common infiltrating ductal carcinoma, not otherwise specified, grade II/III. She had a positive axillary lymph node.

To attempt to reduce the number of overlooked cancers, the radiologist should be alert to subtle changes in lesions, including change in size or density (see the figures), and should judge a lesion by its most suspicious feature.

Notes

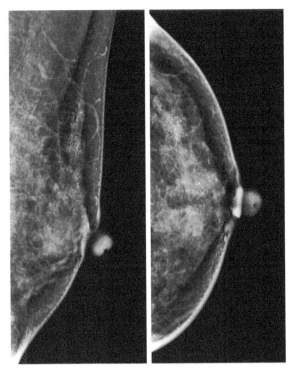

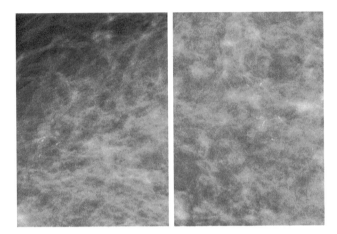

History: Two patients present for routine screening mammography. The first figure shows the left mammogram in a 40-year-old asymptomatic woman. The second figure shows the magnification views performed as additional views after routine mammogram in a 58-year-old asymptomatic woman.

1. What should be included in the differential diagnosis for the two patients shown? (Choose all that apply.)
   A. Lobular carcinoma in situ (LCIS)
   B. Fibrocystic change
   C. Invasive ductal carcinoma
   D. Ductal carcinoma in situ (DCIS)

2. What are the descriptive terms used for the calcifications in patient 1?
   A. Coarse, heterogeneous, and segmental
   B. Amorphous and linear
   C. Coarse, linear, and rodlike
   D. Clusters of punctate calcifications

3. What are the descriptive terms used for the calcifications in patient 2?
   A. Snakeskin, filling the ducts
   B. Coarse and heterogeneous
   C. Fine, linear, and branching
   D. Indistinct and clustered

4. Why is it important to recognize the location of calcifications within the breast?
   A. Calcifications *not* in ducts, lobules, or masses are typically benign.
   B. Calcifications in ducts are almost always malignant.
   C. Calcifications in masses are typical of fibroadenoma.
   D. Calcifications in lobules are typical of LCIS.

Ductal Carcinoma In Situ

1. C and D
2. A
3. C
4. A

References
Evans A: The diagnosis and management of pre-invasive breast disease: radiological diagnosis. *Breast Cancer Res* 2003;5(5):250-253.

Holland R, Hendriks JH: Microcalcifications associated with ductal carcinoma in situ: mammographic-pathologic correlation. *Semin Diagn Pathol* 1994;11(3):181-192.

Holland R, Hendriks JH, Vebeek AL, et al: Extent, distribution, and mammographic/histological correlations of breast ductal carcinoma in situ. *Lancet* 1990;335(8688):519-522.

Cross-Reference
Ikeda D: *Breast Imaging: THE REQUISITES*, 2nd ed, Philadelphia: Saunders, 2010, p 64.

Comment

Mammography is the primary tool for the detection and biopsy of DCIS. Calcifications develop in ducts and have characteristic appearances. Calcifications are present in 80% to 90% of cases of DCIS that have a mammographic abnormality (see the figures). The remaining 10% to 20% of cases manifest as a noncalcified mass or developing asymmetric density.

DCIS is classified as low grade, intermediate grade, and high grade. The histopathologist uses the terms *comedocarcinoma, micropapillary, solid,* and *cribriform* to describe the DCIS architecture on histology. The individual calcifications form in the necrotic portions of the intraductal tumor. The shapes of calcifications are termed *pleomorphic, fine linear,* and *branching* (see the figures); *coarse* and *fine heterogeneous* or *granular* (see the figures); amorphous; and indistinct. The term *pleomorphic* means the calcifications within the group vary in shape, size, and density, which is common in DCIS. The distribution of the calcifications is very important. Terms for DCIS distribution include *clustered, linear,* and *segmental.* The first figure shows segmental distribution, and the second shows clustered distribution.

In the assessment of breast calcifications, it is important to consider the worst-appearing calcifications within the group. In the second figure, there are some punctate forms, which are typical of benign fibrocystic change. This patient's histology report described cancerization of the lobules. In cancerization, tumor spreads from the duct into the adjacent lobules and forms calcifications in lobules, which are typically punctate. In this cluster, the fine linear branching calcification is highly suspicious for DCIS. The presence of the punctate calcifications should not rule out classifying this cluster as suspicious.

It is impossible to predict definitely the subtype of DCIS based on the shape and distribution of the calcifications; however, the coarse heterogeneous pattern seen in patient 1 is often seen in micropapillary type with necrosis, which was her histology. Patient 2 had a high–nuclear grade solid and cribriform pattern, with extension into lobules, which is commonly seen in the fine linear branching form of DCIS.

Notes

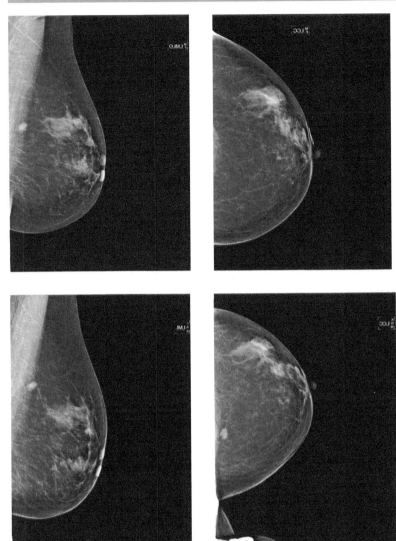

History: A 58-year-old woman presents for screening mammogram.

1. What is the differential diagnosis, based on the images presented? (Choose all that apply.)
   A. Normal left mammogram
   B. Focal asymmetric density in the posterior breast on the mediolateral oblique (MLO) view, possible lymph node
   C. Focal density on MLO view only, possible mass
   D. Without prior films, there is no way to give a diagnosis

2. What is the next step of the work-up?
   A. Do a 90-degree lateral mediolateral (ML) view.
   B. Do a rolled craniocaudal (CC) view.
   C. Do an ultrasound of the entire breast, looking for a mass.
   D. Do an MRI, looking for an enhancing lesion.

3. You do a 90-degree mediolateral (ML) view next. Why?
   A. To see if the image is a real lesion or is caused by overlapping normal structures
   B. To identify the location of the density in the medial or lateral breast
   C. To include more lateral breast tissue in the image
   D. To determine if the density is more likely a lymph node

4. What is "triangulation"?
   A. The process of eliminating an image you think is not a real lesion
   B. The process of comparing the MLO, ML, and CC views to determine the location of a mass in all three views
   C. Finding a mass in the lateral aspect of the breast not included on the CC view
   D. Using ultrasound to help find a mass seen only on one view

CASE 58

Mass Seen on One View

1. B and C
2. A
3. B
4. B

References

Sickles EA: Practical solutions to common mammographic problems: tailoring the examination. *AJR Am J Roentgenol* 1988;151:31-39.

Sickles EA: Breast imaging: from 1965 to the present. *Radiology* 2000;215:1-16.

Cross-Reference

Ikeda D: *Breast Imaging: THE REQUISITES*, 2nd ed, Philadelphia: Saunders, 2010, p 49.

Comment

This asymptomatic patient presented for a routine mammogram. Not shown are her prior mammograms, which are negative. The focal density in the upper posterior left breast is a new finding. However, even in the absence of old films, this focal asymmetric density must be viewed with suspicion. Even though it is seen on only one view, it is no less suspicious. Its location in the posterior breast means that it might not have been included on the CC view, even though the CC view appears adequate for interpretation.

The way to determine the location of the lesion is to find it on two orthogonal views. The true lateral view is orthogonal to the CC view. The location of the density on the true lateral view is helpful in locating the lesion in two ways: It gives the distance from the nipple in the vertical plane, and by comparing the two views, the MLO and the true lateral, you can determine the location of the lesion in the breast, either medial or lateral to the nipple. This is well illustrated in the article by Dr. Sickles in 1988. If the lesion is more cephalad on the ML view, compared to the MLO view (goes up), it is in the medial breast. If it is more caudal on the ML view compared to the MLO view, it is in the lateral breast. This process is termed *triangulation* and can be visually demonstrated by lining up three views of the same breast in the order ML, MLO, CC, with the nipples at the same level and pointing the same way. A line drawn between the lesion on the two views predicts the location in the third view.

In this patient, the lesion is in the upper breast on the MLO view (see the figures) and is located more cephalad in the breast on the ML view (see the figures). Thus, you can determine that it is a medial lesion and instruct the technologist to perform a CC view, exaggerated to the medial aspect. This specialized view is shown in the fourth figure. The lesion is seen, and it can now be determined to be a true mass, located in the upper inner aspect of the left breast, at about the 10 o'clock position. The distance from the nipple in the vertical plane can be determined from the ML view, and the distance from the nipple in the radial plane can be determined from the exaggerated medial CC (XCCM) view. The next step would be to perform an ultrasound of the left 10 o'clock location to find the mass, assess its characteristics, and target the lesion for biopsy. MRI is typically used after a diagnosis of cancer has been made, in order to evaluate extent of disease, because additional masses may be missed on the mammogram.

Notes

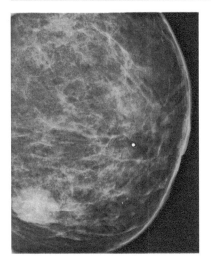
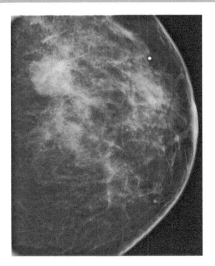

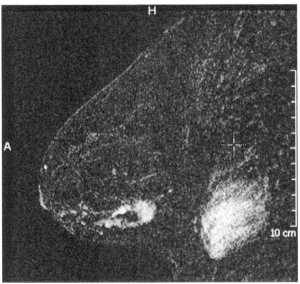
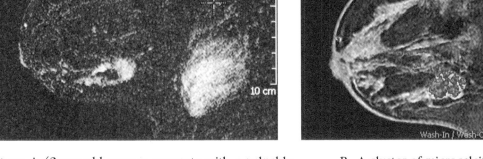

History: A 42-year-old woman presents with a palpable mass in her left breast.

1. What should be included in the differential diagnosis, based on the images provided? (Choose all that apply.)
   A. Malignant mass with ductal carcinoma in situ (DCIS) extending toward nipple
   B. Phyllodes tumor with adjacent DCIS
   C. Simple cyst and benign calcifications
   D. Malignant mass with benign calcifications

2. What is an extensive intraductal component?
   A. Malignancy that contains a large proportion of DCIS
   B. Purely intraductal carcinoma
   C. DCIS and atypical ductal hyperplasia
   D. A long segment of DCIS involving the entire quadrant of the breast

3. What mammographic features suggest an extensive intraductal component?
   A. A spiculated mass

   B. A cluster of microcalcifications less than 1 cm in diameter
   C. Architectural distortion
   D. Mass with microcalcifications in an area greater than 3 cm

4. Which of the following statements is *not* true about calcifications adjacent to a suspicious mass?
   A. Unless the calcifications are recognized and removed, the patient's risk of recurrence is higher.
   B. It is not important to remove calcifications because the patient will have radiation therapy, which will sterilize any remaining disease.
   C. The size of the tumor in the breast affects staging.
   D. It is important to recognize calcifications on the mammogram because DCIS can have a variable appearance on MRI.

Extensive Intraductal Component

1. A, B, and D
2. A
3. D
4. B

References

Stomper PC, Connolly JL: Mammographic features predicting an extensive intraductal component in early-stage infiltrating ductal carcinoma. *AJR Am J Roentgenol* 1992;158(2):269-272.

Van Goethem M, Schelfout K, Kersschot E, et al: MR mammography is useful in the preoperative locoregional staging of breast carcinomas with extensive intraductal component. *Eur J Radiol* 2007;62 (2):273-282.

Cross-Reference

Ikeda D: *Breast Imaging: THE REQUISITES*, 2nd ed, Philadelphia: Saunders, 2010, p 95.

Comment

An extensive intraductal component is a histologic feature that is associated with a higher recurrence rate after breast conservation therapy. In studies in which the tumor was excised, without regard to evidence of DCIS at the margins, 24% of patients had recurrence of their cancer after treatment compared with 6% of patients who had histologically benign margins. Radiation therapy at the accepted dose may be inadequate to treat the residual tumor. It is important to recognize when an extensive intraductal component may be present to guide the treating physician to excise all the malignant tissue before radiation.

Microcalcifications, in particular, when they extend from the tumor in linear distribution at least 3 cm, are the mammographic feature most commonly associated with an extensive intraductal component. Studies show that the proportion of infiltrating ductal carcinomas with an extensive intraductal component is approximately 25% to 35%, so evaluation of the mammogram with a suspicious mass for adjacent calcifications is prudent (see the figures).

MRI is also useful for evaluation of an extensive intraductal component. Linear enhancement, long spicules, a regional enhancing area, and nodules adjacent to a mass are suspicious MRI findings for an extensive intraductal component (see the figures). In one more recent study, MRI was shown to be superior to the mammogram in predicting an extensive intraductal component and assessing total tumor size.

This patient presented for baseline mammogram at age 42 with a palpable mass in the left breast. Microcalcifications were recognized in the same quadrant as the mass and extending toward the nipple in segmental distribution. She underwent image-guided biopsy of both the mass and the calcifications that were seen farthest away from the mass to establish the extent of disease. The mass was invasive ductal carcinoma, grade III, and the calcifications were DCIS, grade III.

If breast conservation therapy is desired in patients with an extensive intraductal component, bracketing the location of calcifications is necessary at the time of needle localization to include all of the suspected and known disease in the lumpectomy specimen. A mammogram after surgery is helpful to assess the complete excision of all suspicious calcifications before radiation therapy.

Note

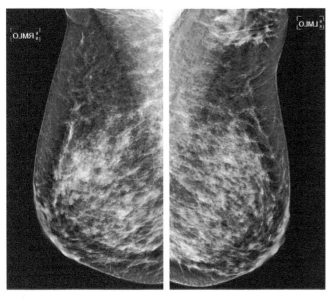

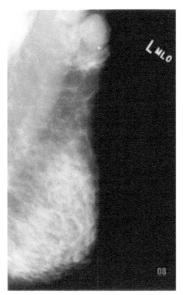

Three years previously.

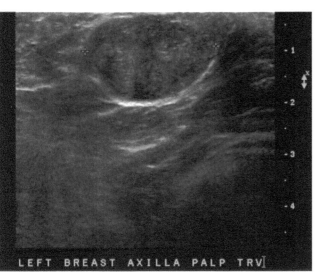

Three years previously.

History: A 43-year-old woman presents for routine screening mammogram. She had an excisional biopsy in her left axilla 3 years previously with benign findings.

1. What should be included in the differential diagnosis of the more recent mammogram? (Choose all that apply.)
   A. Ectopic breast tissue in the left axilla
   B. Spiculated suspicious mass in the left axilla
   C. Supernumerary breast in the left axilla
   D. Left axillary adenopathy

2. What is the clinical concern regarding ectopic gland tissue?
   A. Malignancy is more common in ectopic locations.
   B. Malignancy can occur in ectopic breast tissue.
   C. The concern is primarily cosmetic.
   D. Malignancy in the axilla is much more likely to become metastatic.

3. Which of the following statements is *not* true about the "milk line"?
   A. It is an area where primordial rests of breast tissue are present.
   B. It relates to animals, not humans.
   C. The axilla is the most common site of tissue development along the milk line, outside the normal breast location.
   D. Accessory nipples occur along this line.

4. What is the one best diagnosis of the mammogram and ultrasound from 3 years previously?
   A. Left axillary adenopathy
   B. Left axillary malignancy
   C. Left axillary fibroadenoma
   D. Left axillary complex cystic mass

CASE 60

Ectopic Tissue

1. A and C
2. B
3. B
4. C

References

Ciralik H, Bulbuloglu E, Arican O, et al: Fibroadenoma of the ectopic breast of the axilla—a case report. *Pol J Pathol* 2006;57(4):209-211.

Coras B, Landthaler M, Hofstaedter F, et al: Fibroadenoma of the axilla. *Dermatol Surg* 2005;31(9 Pt 1):1152-1154.

Sanguinetti A, Ragusa M, Calzolari F, et al: Invasive ductal carcinoma arising in ectopic breast tissue of the axilla: case report and review of the literature. *G Chir* 2010;31(8-9):383-386.

Cross-Reference

Ikeda D: *Breast Imaging: THE REQUISITES*, 2nd ed, Philadelphia: Saunders, 2010, pp 36-37.

Comment

Ectopic breast tissue refers to the presence of breast tissue outside the normal confines of the central breast cone and typically occurs along the "Hughes line," or "milk line," which extends from the axilla inferomedially into the abdomen. It is seen in approximately 2% to 6% of women. The ectopic tissue can be associated with an extra nipple (*polythelia*) and can form into a cone of breast tissue, as an accessory breast (*polymastia*). Although most common along the milk line, ectopic tissue can also occur anywhere in the body and can occur in men, although it is much more common in women. Along the milk line, ectopic tissue is most commonly seen in the axilla (see the figures).

The ectopic tissue arises from quiescent primordial rests of breast tissue. It may remain subclinical and then become manifest during pregnancy and lactation. Because the tissue is normal glandular tissue, albeit located in an aberrant spot, it can develop any change that can occur in the central breast tissue; breast cysts, fibroadenomas, and malignancy can develop.

Masses in the axilla that are of breast origin must be differentiated from axillary adenopathy. Ultrasound is useful in the evaluation of the axilla. Solid benign masses such as fibroadenoma in the axilla should have the same appearance as fibroadenoma anywhere in the breast (see the figures). Adenopathy may appear as a node with a central fatty hilum and a thickened eccentric cortex, or the node may be completely involved with tumor, and the fatty hilum is not seen. In this instance, the abnormal node can appear anechoic and cystic. Color flow Doppler of the axillary mass should always be performed so that adenopathy is not confused with a cyst in axillary ectopic gland tissue.

Notes

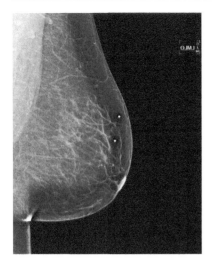

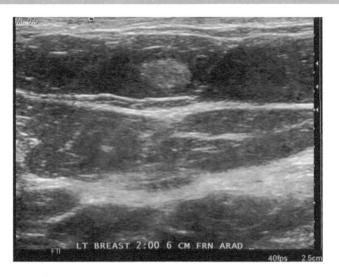

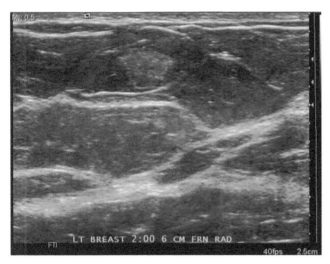

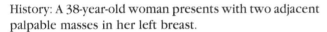

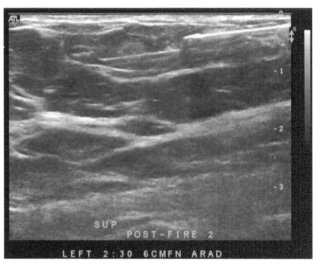

History: A 38-year-old woman presents with two adjacent palpable masses in her left breast.

1. What is the differential diagnosis? (Choose all that apply.)
   A. Hematoma
   B. Hemangioma
   C. Angiolipoma
   D. Fibroadenoma

2. How would you proceed with the work-up after mammography and ultrasound?
   A. Surgery is needed.
   B. Perform an MRI to check for abnormal blood supply.
   C. No further work-up is needed.
   D. Perform a clinical history.

3. After a 6-week delay, the masses are unchanged. Should biopsy be the next step?
   A. Yes, the patient must be seen by a surgeon because the lesions are palpable.
   B. Yes, image-guided needle biopsy should be performed using ultrasound guidance.
   C. Yes, a stereotactic biopsy should be performed.
   D. No, follow-up ultrasound in 3 months is recommended.

4. What is the ultrasound finding that is not typical of benign lesions?
   A. Echogenic
   B. Irregular contour
   C. Location in the subcutaneous tissue
   D. Heterogeneous texture

Angiolipoma

1. A, B, and C
2. D
3. B
4. B

References

Noel JC, Geertruyden JV, Engohan-Aloghe C: Angiolipoma of the breast in a male: a case report and review of the literature. *Int J Surg Pathol* 2009 Dec 24.

Stavros AT, Thickman D, Rapp CL, et al: Solid breast nodules: use of sonography to distinguish between benign and malignant lesions. *Radiology* 1995;196:123-134.

Weinstein SP, Conant EF, Acs G: Case 59: angiolipoma of the breast. *Radiology* 2003;227:773-775.

Cross-Reference

Ikeda D: *Breast Imaging: THE REQUISITES*, 2nd ed, Philadelphia: Saunders, 2010, p 139.

Comment

This patient presents with two adjacent palpable, superficial masses. On the mammogram, there is no evidence of a mass (see the figures). Ultrasound shows two adjacent masses in the subcutaneous tissues, corresponding to the palpable masses (see the figures). The margin of one of the masses is microlobulated, and the masses are almost purely echogenic. These features are indeterminate for the presence of malignancy, although they favor a benign diagnosis. The differential diagnosis includes angiolipoma, angiosarcoma, hemangioma, and hematoma.

The patient related no history of trauma. However, a common presentation after trauma is a palpable mass, a hematoma, that can have an identical appearance on mammography and ultrasound. Careful questioning of the patient for any history of recent trauma is helpful, as is examination of the breast for signs of bruising. If the clinical presentation is consistent with trauma, no biopsy is necessary. The patient can be asked to return for follow-up in 6 to 8 weeks, and if the mass resolves completely, no further evaluation is needed. Trauma can cause an occult breast malignancy to manifest as a palpable concern if the mass bleeds and enlarges.

This patient underwent a needle core biopsy using vacuum technique (see the figures), and the histology report was that of an angiolipoma. Excision of the remainder of the mass was advised to exclude angiosarcoma. The histology of the excised specimen was two cellular angiolipomas, and no malignant transformation was seen. This is a relatively unusual tumor of the breast; it is more typically seen in the back, neck, and shoulder.

Notes

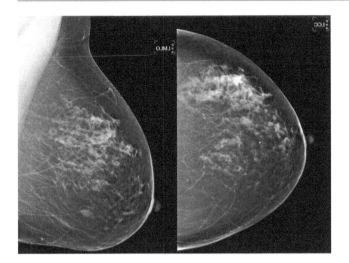
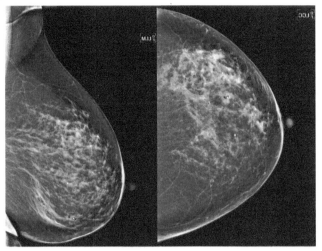

History: A 53-year-old woman has a developing mass, seen best on mediolateral oblique (MLO) view, in the left lower breast. A stereotactic biopsy was performed.

1. What should be included in the differential diagnosis for the left mammogram presented? (Choose all that apply.)
   A. Infiltrating lobular carcinoma
   B. Fibroadenoma
   C. Pseudoangiomatous stromal hyperplasia (PASH)
   D. Lymph node

2. What is PASH?
   A. A high-risk lesion
   B. A benign condition
   C. Always an incidental finding on a biopsy specimen of another finding
   D. A premalignant lesion

3. Which of the following is *not* in the management scheme of PASH, when found on histology of core needle biopsy?
   A. Surgical excision
   B. Return to screening
   C. Close follow-up
   D. Clinical follow-up

4. Is this patient at increased risk of future breast cancer?
   A. No, but short-interval follow-up is necessary.
   B. No, she is at no increased risk.
   C. Yes, her risk doubles.
   D. Yes, her risk is increased threefold.

Pseudoangiomatous Stromal Hyperplasia

1. A, B, and C
2. B
3. C
4. B

References

Polger MR, Denison CM, Lester S, et al: Pseudoangiomatous stromal hyperplasia: mammographic and sonographic appearances. *AJR Am J Roentgenol* 1996;166(2):349-352.

Salvador R, Lirola J, Dominguez R, et al: Pseudo-angiomatous stromal hyperplasia presenting as a breast mass: imaging findings in 3 patients. *Breast* 2004;13(5):431-435.

Cross-Reference

Ikeda D: *Breast Imaging: THE REQUISITES*, 2nd ed, Philadelphia: Saunders, 2010, pp 134, 231.

Comment

PASH is a benign, relatively rare condition. It was initially described in 1986 in premenopausal women or in post-menopausal women taking hormone supplements but more recently has been found in girls as young as 12 years old and in men. The histology is a proliferation of stromal and epithelial elements. These form slitlike spaces that appear similar to vascular channels, which give this lesion its name of *pseudoangiomatous*.

PASH can manifest radiographically as an incidental finding on a biopsy specimen of an adjacent lesion, such as a mass or calcifications; it can manifest as a palpable mass because the stromal overgrowth may coalesce similar to a tumor, such as a fibroadenoma; or it may manifest as a nonpalpable developing density on mammogram, not visible on ultrasound, as in this patient (see the figures). On mammography, PASH is commonly ill defined, as in this patient. It characteristically is not associated with calcification. If a mass is seen on mammography, ultrasound should be performed. Ultrasound features are similar to fibroadenoma or phyllodes tumor; cystic spaces may be present within an oval mass that is wider than tall. However, PASH may also have features overlapping with malignancy on ultrasound; it may be irregular and vertically oriented. In this patient, the focal density was seen best on MLO view and could not be identified on ultrasound.

When PASH is the predominant lesion determined after a needle core biopsy, correlation of clinical and ultrasound findings is crucial to ensure that the targeted area was sampled. Correlation can be obtained by placing a clip after the biopsy and repeating the mammogram and comparing with the initial study.

Management can be routine follow-up if the patient is asymptomatic. However, there are cases of very large (9 cm) palpable masses that are PASH, and these may be best treated with surgical excision, after needle core biopsy establishes the benign diagnosis of PASH. The lesions can recur and can be multiple.

Notes

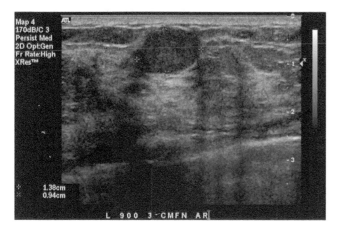

History: A 15-year-old girl presents with a solitary breast mass.

1. What is the differential diagnosis for this ultrasound image of the palpable mass? (Choose all that apply.)
   A. Simple cyst
   B. Complicated cyst
   C. Fibroadenoma
   D. Malignant tumor

2. How should imaging of this patient proceed?
   A. Mammogram as initial work-up, then ultrasound if needed
   B. Mammogram as initial work-up, then MRI to assess for additional masses
   C. Ultrasound
   D. MRI

3. What is the management for this lesion?
   A. Perform histology.
   B. Perform stereotactic biopsy.
   C. No management is needed. Have the patient return for routine mammogram at age 40 years.
   D. Follow with mammogram in 1 year.

4. What are the ultrasound features that predict benign histology?
   A. Taller-than-wide orientation
   B. Microlobulated contour
   C. Heterogeneous internal echotexture
   D. Oval or bilobed shape

CASE 63

Palpable Mass in a Teenager

1. B and C
2. C
3. A
4. D

References

Kronemer KA: Gray scale sonography of breast masses in adolescent girls. *J Ultrasound Med* 2001;20(8):881.

Stavros AT, Thickman D, Rapp CL, et al: Solid breast nodules: use of sonography to distinguish between benign and malignant lesions. *Radiology* 1995;196:123-134.

Cross-Reference

Ikeda D: *Breast Imaging: THE REQUISITES*, 2nd ed, Philadelphia: Saunders, 2010, p 117.

Comment

Ultrasound is the imaging method of choice in the young, since it uses no ionizing radiation. Ultrasound is used to determine if the palpable finding is cystic or solid. A solid mass may be hyperechoic, hypoechoic, or isoechoic to neighboring fat. When evaluating a solid mass, look for features that help characterize the lesion as benign or malignant. These characteristics include margin analysis, acoustic shadowing, and echotexture. Benign masses are oval, gently lobulated, parallel to the skin, and sharply circumscribed, with no acoustic shadowing.

In this patient, there is a hypoechoic mass with gentle lobulations and sharply circumscribed borders, corresponding to the palpable finding. It is most consistent with a fibroadenoma, although other etiologies cannot be excluded, such as papilloma, hamartoma, or hematoma (see the figure).

The fibroadenoma is a common benign mass of the breast occurring in 10% to 25% of women. The mass arises from the breast lobule and is most likely stimulated by estrogen. Fibroadenomas occur as multiple masses in approximately 20% of cases. Histologically, there is a fibrous stroma without cytologic atypia, and there is also an epithelial component. Morphologically, fibroadenomas are circumscribed round, oval, or bilobed, and they can occur anywhere in the breast.

In a study of 57 masses in adolescent girls (median age, 15.4 years), 36 masses were fibroadenoma. All masses were benign. Malignancy is extremely rare in this age group.

Because malignancy is unusual, there are options in the management of the solid mass in the breast of an adolescent. Traditionally, excisional biopsy was performed. It is now acceptable to follow the mass, once benign characteristics have been established with ultrasound evaluation. If there is growth, excision is recommended. If knowledge of the histology is desired but surgery is not, needle core biopsy gives a reliable histologic diagnosis. In this patient, excision was performed and the mass was a fibroadenoma.

Notes

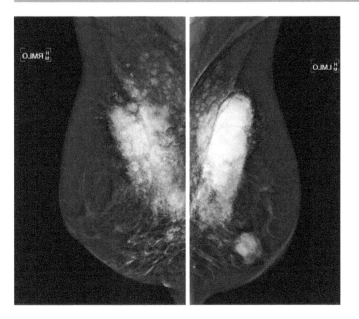
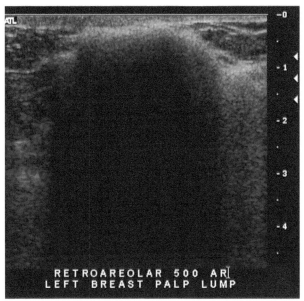

History: A 56-year-old woman presents for routine screening mammogram. Ultrasound image is also shown from a previous diagnostic examination performed because of a palpable lump.

1. What should be included in the differential diagnosis for the images shown? (Choose all that apply.)
   A. Patient had liquid silicone injected into the breasts
   B. Previous bilateral silicone implant rupture
   C. Previous bilateral saline implant rupture
   D. Silicone granulomas

2. Which breast evaluation modality is *least* affected by injected silicone?
   A. Mammography
   B. MRI
   C. Ultrasound
   D. Physical examination

3. What is the next step in management for this patient?
   A. MRI is necessary because of the limited mammogram.
   B. Routine screening mammogram should be performed.
   C. Ultrasound should be performed as a routine adjunct to mammogram.
   D. Breast-specific gamma imaging should be performed annually.

4. Which of the following is *not* a complication of free silicone?
   A. Delayed discovery of breast cancer
   B. Granuloma formation
   C. Increased risk of breast cancer
   D. Migration of silicone into the arm

CASE 64

Silicone Injections

1. A, B, and D
2. B
3. B
4. C

References

Caskey CI, Berg WA, Hamper UM, et al: Imaging spectrum of extracapsular silicone: correlation of US, MR imaging, mammographic, and histopathologic findings. *Radiographics* 1999;19 (Spec No): S39-S51.

Yang N, Muradali D: The augmented breast: a pictorial review of the abnormal and unusual. *AJR Am J Roentgenol* 2011;196(4): W451-W460.

Cross-Reference

Ikeda D: *Breast Imaging: THE REQUISITES*, 2nd ed, Philadelphia: Saunders, 2010, p 349.

Comment

Liquid silicone is used as a method for augmenting the size of the breasts. It was used in the United States until the 1970s, when its use was banned by the U.S. Food and Drug Administration (FDA). It is still used in Asia. When seen on the mammogram, liquid silicone has a characteristic appearance of dense material, typically in rounded masses, which often have a calcified rim. It can also cause a spiculated mass (see the figures). The rounded masses are granulomas, which is a natural response of the host to the foreign material.

On ultrasound, the appearance is also characteristic, with a highly echogenic surface and dense shadowing, with loss of information deep to the surface, caused by scatter of the sound beam (see the figures). This has been termed "snowstorm" appearance. Because of the dense shadowing and scatter of the beam, very little information about adjacent breast abnormalities can be gained when free silicone is present.

Silicone is inert and in a study published in 1994 was not found to cause connective tissue disease. However, it can have many adverse effects, including adenopathy, infection, granuloma formation, granulomatous hepatitis, and embolism. Patients with free silicone may present with a palpable mass, as this patient did in the past (see the figures). The silicone granulomas, or "siliconomas," are hard masses that may feel like a cancerous mass. Physical examination of the breast is limited when silicone has been injected into the breasts. MRI can be used to obtain more complete information in a patient with free silicone because the silicone is hyperintense on T2-weighted images. If water suppression is also used, the silicone should be the only hyperintense material on the image.

Notes

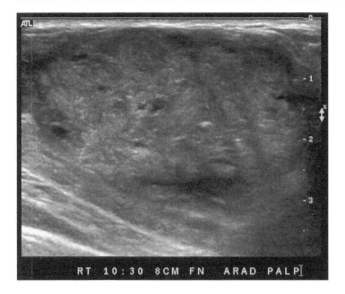

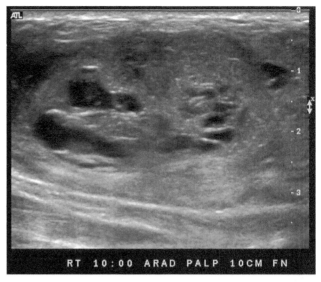

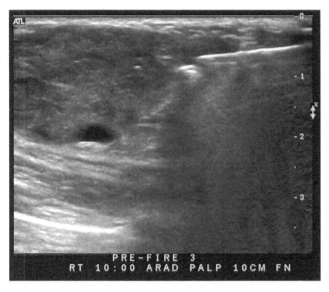

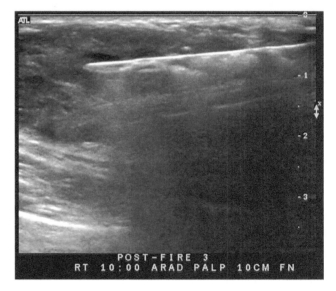

History: A 23-year-old woman noticed a mass in her right breast during pregnancy; she described the mass as growing during the course of the pregnancy. She presents 4 weeks after delivery for imaging evaluation and biopsy.

1. What should be included in the differential diagnosis for the mass in the right breast? (Choose all that apply.)
   A. Lactating adenoma
   B. Fibroadenoma
   C. Phyllodes tumor
   D. Highly suspicious for invasive ductal carcinoma

2. Which of the following is *not* a complication of ultrasound-guided core biopsy during pregnancy?
   A. Vasovagal reaction
   B. Milk fistula
   C. Hematoma
   D. Inadequate sampling

3. Should biopsy of a breast mass be postponed until after parturition?
   A. Yes, it is not safe to perform a biopsy of a breast mass during pregnancy.
   B. Yes, nearly all breast masses found during pregnancy are benign.
   C. No, biopsy should always be performed when a mass is found because there is always a chance of cancer.
   D. No, although benign-appearing masses can be followed, biopsy of suspicious or indeterminate masses should be performed when such masses are discovered.

4. What is the most common reason for a palpable solid mass during pregnancy?
   A. Galactocele
   B. Lactating adenoma
   C. Fibroadenoma
   D. Infiltrating ductal carcinoma

C A S E 6 5

Mass Developing during Pregnancy

1. A, B, and C
2. A
3. D
4. C

References

Darling ML, Smith DN, Rhei E, et al: Lactating adenoma: sonographic features. *Breast J* 2000;6(4):252-256.

Sabate JM, Clotet M, Torrubia S, et al: Radiologic evaluation of breast disorders related to pregnancy and lactation. *Radiographics* 2007;27 (Suppl 1):S101-S124.

Sumkin JH, Perrone AM, Harris KM, et al: Lactating adenoma: US features and literature review. *Radiology* 1998;206(1):271-274.

Cross-Reference

Ikeda D: *Breast Imaging: THE REQUISITES*, 2nd ed, Philadelphia: Saunders, 2010, p 376.

Comment

Benign masses are the most common palpable masses that develop during pregnancy. Pregnancy-associated breast cancer can occur and should always be considered. The incidence of breast cancer in pregnant women is 1:3000 to 1:10,000. Benign masses include fibroadenoma and lactating adenoma. Abscess and galactocele also manifest as palpable masses and should be considered. These lesions can appear as complex or complicated cysts and can be mistaken for solid masses. Ultrasound is the initial method of imaging used in pregnant women (and in women < 30 years old), although if a mass looks suspicious on ultrasound, mammography should be performed, even in a pregnant patient. Scatter radiation to the fetus is minimal (about 0.4 mrad to the fetus from two mammographic views), and shielding can be used to limit the scatter radiation.

This mass has many benign features (see the figures), including oval shape, wider-than-tall appearance, and thin smooth margin. However, the cystic spaces in the mass are unusual for a fibroadenoma or lactating adenoma; these can be seen in phyllodes tumor, which can be locally aggressive and needs excision. The patient in this case expressed concern because of the large size of the mass (approximately 7 cm), and core biopsy was performed. It is important to determine the histology of the mass because a phyllodes tumor needs to be widely excised, whereas a lactating adenoma or fibroadenoma can be excised without a wide margin or can be followed. Performing core needle biopsy in women who are lactating or pregnant can cause the complication of milk fistula. The present patient was postpartum and was not breastfeeding.

Ultrasound-guided core needle biopsy is an inexpensive diagnostic tool to obtain the histology of a breast mass. The technique involves cleansing and numbing the skin and subcutaneous tissues and inserting a needle into the mass under ultrasound direct visualization. This technique allows real-time monitoring of the needle in the breast, which is impossible when performing stereotactic or MRI-guided biopsies. The last two figures illustrate the placement of the needle, parallel to the skin and adjacent to the mass; the core needle is "fired" into the breast, using a spring device built into the handle of the needle. At least five samples are taken; more may be necessary to sample the lesion adequately. In this patient, the mass was a fibroadenoma, with lactational change, explaining the cystic spaces. There was no evidence of malignancy.

Notes

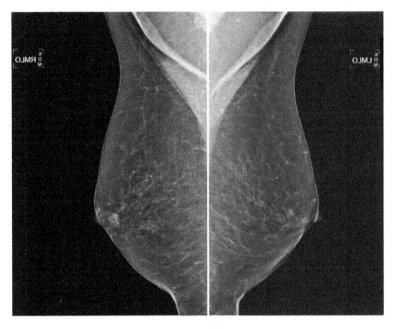

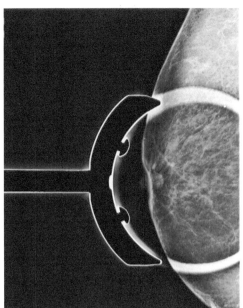

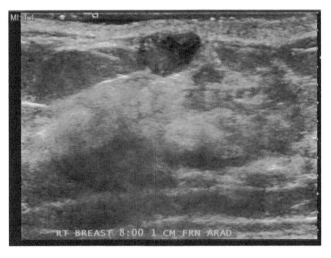

History: A 67-year-old woman presents for a screening mammogram. She has a family history of breast cancer in her sister at age 50, mother at age 65, and three maternal aunts.

1. What should be included in the differential diagnosis of the mammogram and ultrasound images shown? (Choose all that apply.)
   A. Subareolar complex cyst
   B. Papilloma
   C. Normal lymph node
   D. Malignant mass

2. What is the next step in management?
   A. Clinical examination—if this superficial mass is not palpable, it can be followed
   B. MRI to check for enhancement
   C. Biopsy
   D. PET/CT to check for enhancement

3. If the mass is a papilloma, what is the management?
   A. Routine mammogram in 1 year because papilloma is benign
   B. Referral to a surgeon for excision
   C. MRI to check for abnormal enhancement
   D. Short-interval follow-up with ultrasound

4. If the patient had bloody nipple discharge, does that change management?
   A. Yes, the patient would go directly to surgical consultation instead of imaging evaluation.
   B. Yes, the mass is more likely to be malignant if bloody discharge is present.
   C. No, management is the same.
   D. Yes, the patient would have a ductogram in her work-up.

CASE 66

Subareolar Cancer

1. A, B, and D
2. C
3. B
4. C

References

Chang JM, Moon WK, Cho N, et al: Management of ultrasonographically detected benign papillomas of the breast at core needle biopsy. *AJR Am J Roentgenol* 2011;196(3):723-729.

Liberman L, Tornos C, Huzjan R, et al: Is surgical excision warranted after benign, concordant diagnosis of papilloma at percutaneous breast biopsy? *AJR Am J Roentgenol* 2006;186(5):1328-1334.

Cross-Reference

Ikeda D: *Breast Imaging: THE REQUISITES*, 2nd ed, Philadelphia: Saunders, 2010, p 120.

Comment

This patient has a developing mass with benign features on mammography and ultrasound: relatively low density and round on mammography and sharply circumscribed, oval shape, and wider than tall on ultrasound (see the figures). Its subcutaneous location in the subareolar breast suggests a diagnosis of papilloma, complicated or complex cyst, or sebaceous cyst. However, any developing mass in a postmenopausal woman with a strong family history should be viewed with concern.

This woman underwent core needle biopsy, and the histology was consistent with malignant cells in a papillary lesion. The area of the mass was completely removed at core biopsy; when the patient had surgery, no malignancy was seen in the breast. It had been entirely removed at core biopsy. Her sentinel node was negative.

Clinical examination of the subareolar area is difficult because of the presence of the nipple, and masses in this location may escape clinical notice. This area should be carefully examined on mammography. The round shape and low density of this mass on mammography suggest a benign etiology; however, there is overlap in the appearance of benign and malignant processes in the breast on mammography and ultrasound, so care must be taken not to dismiss a potentially malignant developing mass. If the histopathology on core biopsy had been benign (e.g., a benign papilloma), surgical excision would still be recommended because there is a small but significant risk of malignant histology in papillomas (3% to 14% in several series).

Notes

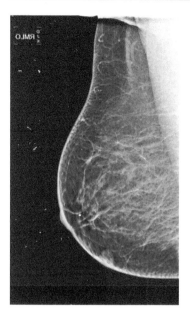
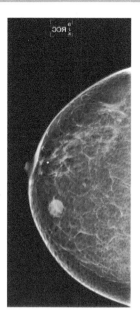
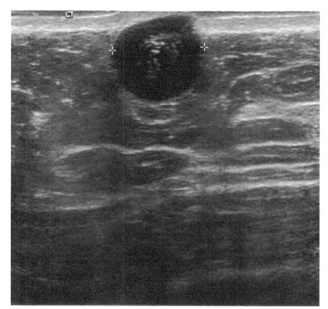

History: An asymptomatic 51-year-old woman presents for a screening mammogram.

1. What is the differential diagnosis for the round mass in the lower right breast on the mammogram? (Choose all that apply.)
   A. Skin mole
   B. Breast cyst
   C. Oil cyst
   D. Sebaceous cyst

2. If the patient presents with a palpable mass and this mammogram, what would the next step be?
   A. Spot compression views of the mass
   B. Placing a metal BB on the skin and repeating a view with the marker in tangent, to confirm a skin lesion
   C. Ultrasound of the palpable finding
   D. MRI of the right breast

3. What Breast Imaging Reporting and Data System (BI-RADS) score would you give when reporting this mammogram, if it is seen as a screening exam?
   A. BI-RADs 0—incomplete, needs further evaluation
   B. BI-RADs 2—benign
   C. BI-RADs 4—suspicious, biopsy should be considered
   D. BI-RADS 3—probably benign, recommend short-interval follow-up

4. Where in the right breast is the lesion located?
   A. Right breast at 2:00 o'clock position
   B. Right breast at 10:00 o'clock position
   C. Right breast at 8:00 o'clock position
   D. Right breast at 5:00 o'clock position

C A S E 6 7

Sebaceous Cyst

1. A, B, and D
2. C
3. B
4. D

References

Baker JA, Soo MS: Breast US: assessment of technical quality and image interpretation. *Radiology* 2002;223:229-238.

Stavros AT: *Breast Ultrasound*, Philadelphia: Lippincott Williams & Wilkins 2004, pp 325-333.

Cross-Reference

Ikeda D: *Breast Imaging: THE REQUISITES*, 2nd ed, Philadelphia: Saunders, 2010, p 141.

Comment

The mammographic views show a round mass that triangulates to the lower inner aspect of the breast (see the figures). On the craniocaudal (CC) view, the mass is in the medial breast. On the mediolateral oblique (MLO) view, the mass is seen in the skin, projecting in toward the breast tissue, rather than outward into the air. This is pathognomonic for a dermal mass. The three most likely dermal masses are sebaceous cyst, which is a retention cyst of a hair follicle in the dermis; an epidermal inclusion cyst, which arises as a result of traumatic skin disruption, such as biopsy; and a Montgomery gland cyst, which arises from the superficial Montgomery gland of the areola. Questioning (and/or examination) of the patient might reveal an inflamed skin lesion consistent with a dermal cyst; however, with the mammographic appearance seen in this case (see the figures), such examination is not necessary.

On the film-screen mammogram, rather than on the digital mammogram as in this case, the skin is not as well seen, and there may be some doubt about the location of the mass. In these cases, physical examination of the skin often is diagnostic of a skin mass. If you are unsure, ultrasound can be used to help make the diagnosis. Ultrasound reveals a well-defined oval mass contained within the dermal layer, or just deep to the dermal layer with a thin neck, which is the hair follicle extending through the echogenic skin layer to the skin surface. To image the follicle, a standoff pad and a high-frequency transducer may be necessary.

Once the etiology has been determined, no further evaluation is needed. Routine screening mammography is recommended.

Notes

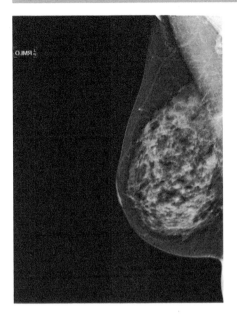

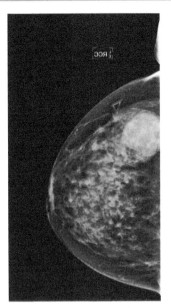

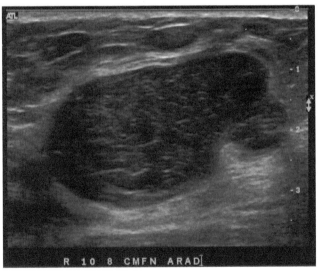

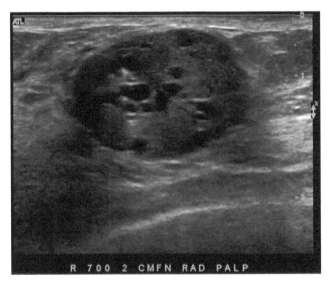

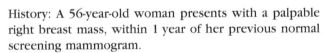

History: A 56-year-old woman presents with a palpable right breast mass, within 1 year of her previous normal screening mammogram.

1. What should be included in the differential diagnosis for the developing right breast mass? (Choose all that apply.)
   A. Breast cyst
   B. Radial scar
   C. Medullary cancer
   D. Phyllodes tumor

2. What is the next step in imaging?
   A. MRI to differentiate benign from malignant
   B. Ultrasound of the lesion
   C. Positron emission tomography (PET) scan to check for additional masses throughout the body
   D. Stereotactic biopsy

3. Ultrasound is performed, and the mass is solid, with benign features. What is the next step?
   A. Ultrasound-guided needle biopsy
   B. Following of benign-appearing masses; ultrasound examination in 6 months recommended
   C. MRI to assess enhancement characteristics to decide whether biopsy is needed
   D. Annual mammogram

4. The biopsy histology is benign phyllodes tumor. What is the next step?
   A. Follow-up of the benign lesion in 6 months with ultrasound
   B. Annual mammogram
   C. Surgical consultation
   D. MRI to determine if mass needs excision

Phyllodes Tumor

1. A, C, and D
2. B
3. A
4. C

References

Liberman L, Bonaccio E, Hamele-Bena D, et al: Benign and malignant phyllodes tumors: mammographic and sonographic findings. *Radiology* 1996;198(1):121-124.

Wurdinger S, Herzog AB, Fischer DR, et al: Differentiation of phyllodes breast tumors from fibroadenomas on MRI. *AJR Am J Roentgenol* 2005;185(5):1317-1321.

Cross-Reference

Ikeda D: *Breast Imaging: THE REQUISITES*, 2nd ed, Philadelphia: Saunders, 2010, p 120.

Comment

Phyllodes tumor is rare, constituting approximately 1% of breast masses, and can be either benign or malignant. Approximately 25% are malignant. The older term was *cystosarcoma phyllodes,* which implied malignancy, and this term is no longer used. Growth is characteristically rapid; benign phyllodes tumors can grow faster than infiltrating ductal carcinomas.

Histologically, there is stromal overgrowth, which is markedly hypercellular, and the stroma forms leaflike patterns that protrude into cystic spaces microscopically. The name *phyllodes* is derived from these leaflike patterns. The malignant form can metastasize hematogenously to the lungs and liver and can be fatal. The benign type can recur after excision but does not spread outside the breast.

The benign and malignant forms can be identical on imaging. Larger masses (> 3 cm) are statistically more likely to be malignant, according to one report. On mammography, phyllodes tumor is a circumscribed mass, with lobulated contours, and is relatively dense. On ultrasound, the mass is circumscribed, with a hypoechoic internal texture that can show through transmission. Cystic spaces are common, as seen in the last figure, from a different patient. The cystic spaces are characteristic of a phyllodes lesion. When cystic spaces are seen in a mass on ultrasound, phyllodes tumor should be considered, and biopsy should be performed.

Notes

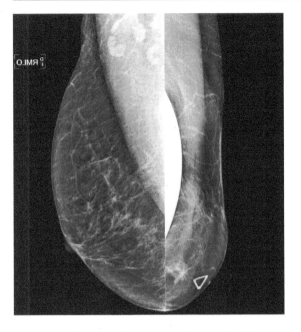

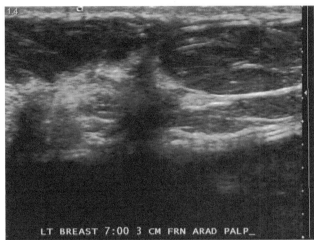

History: A 63-year-old woman who had left breast cancer diagnosed in 1998 and treated with mastectomy has a palpable finding on her mastectomy side. She has a silicone implant reconstruction.

1. What should be included in the differential diagnosis of the bilateral mammogram and ultrasound image shown? (Choose all that apply.)
   A. Fat necrosis on the mastectomy side
   B. Recurrent cancer on the mastectomy side
   C. Distortion from surgical biopsy
   D. Lipoma on the mastectomy side

2. What is the incidence of recurrent tumor on the ipsilateral side after mastectomy?
   A. Relatively common, about 50%
   B. Unusual, about 5% to 10%
   C. Relatively uncommon, about 25%
   D. Extremely rare, less than 1%

3. Is ipsilateral mammography required after mastectomy?
   A. Yes, because of the risk of recurrence, mammography should be performed annually.
   B. There is no requirement, but it is strongly recommended.
   C. No, ipsilateral mammogram is usually not performed after mastectomy.
   D. No, but ultrasound screening is widely accepted as a replacement for mammography in screening the mastectomy side.

4. Which of the following statements is true regarding recurrence after mastectomy?
   A. Recurrence is typically found on physical examination.
   B. Recurrence is so unusual that there is no clinical utility in screening clinical examination for recurrence.
   C. Recurrence usually takes the form of a metastatic axillary node.
   D. Postoperative radiation therapy to the mastectomy site does not affect local recurrence rate.

CASE 69

Recurrent Cancer after Mastectomy

1. A, B, and C
2. B
3. C
4. A

References

Fajardo LL, Roberts CC, Hunt KR: Mammographic surveillance of breast cancer patients: should the mastectomy site be imaged? *AJR Am J Roentgenol* 1993;161(5):953-955.

Kim SJ, Moon WK, Cho N, et al: The detection of recurrent breast cancer in patients with a history of breast cancer surgery: comparison of clinical breast examination, mammography and ultrasonography. *Acta Radiol* 2011;52(1):15-20.

Kim SJ, Park JM: Normal and abnormal US findings at the mastectomy site. *Radiographics* 2004;24(2):357-365.

Cross-Reference

Ikeda D: *Breast Imaging: THE REQUISITES*, 2nd ed, Philadelphia: Saunders, 2010, p 328.

Comment

Mastectomy is a surgical procedure used to treat breast cancer. Mastectomy is often performed when the tumor occupies a large portion of the breast. It is also preferred by some women to treat small cancers that could be treated with local excision and radiation. Recurrence can occur after mastectomy because of incomplete local removal of tumor or as an early sign of disseminated disease. Tumors that are more likely to recur include larger tumors, tumors of higher stage, and tumors with negative hormone receptors. Local recurrence decreases survival. Radiation therapy has been shown to reduce recurrence by two thirds. It is important to be vigilant about the possibility of recurrence after mastectomy because it has been reported in various studies to occur in approximately 5% to 10% of patients. Most recurrence (70%) occurs in the first 3 years after surgery.

Mammography has been shown to be of limited usefulness in screening for recurrence after mastectomy because the chest wall is not included in the image and that is the primary site of local recurrence. The sensitivity of clinical examination is greater than that of mammography, so patients who have undergone mastectomy should be clinically evaluated routinely for any sign of palpable mass in the chest wall, supraclavicular region, or axilla. If a palpable mass is found, mammography may be useful, as in this patient (see the figures). Ultrasound is very useful because it can evaluate the chest wall better than mammography. Recurrent tumors have the same appearance as primary tumors and can be circumscribed, irregular, or spiculated masses. They can also manifest as microcalcification with or without a mass. Treatment of recurrence includes surgical excision, radiation therapy, systemic hormone therapy, or systemic chemotherapy.

Notes

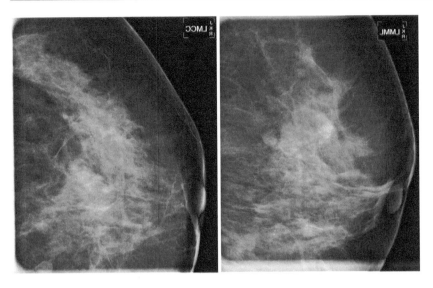

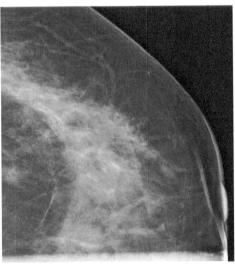
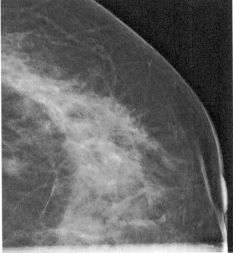

History: An asymptomatic patient who had developing microcalcifications on routine screening mammogram in her left breast had magnification views and returned for follow-up magnification views 2 years later.

1. What should be included in the differential diagnosis for the change between the two examinations shown? (Choose all that apply.)
   A. Fibrocystic change, with increasing calcifications
   B. Increasing calcifications, suspicious for DCIS
   C. Atypical ductal hyperplasia
   D. Invasive ductal carcinoma

2. What is the distribution of the calcifications in the second figure?
   A. Regional
   B. Diffuse
   C. Segmental
   D. Punctate

3. Why is it important to identify the extent of suspicious calcifications on the mammogram?
   A. It is important to establish all sites of disease before surgery.
   B. There is no cancer present where there are no calcifications.
   C. Biopsy is not needed if calcifications are seen in another quadrant.
   D. It is of academic interest and does not affect the surgical management.

4. What is the next step in management?
   A. Short-interval follow-up
   B. Stereotactic biopsy of one site in the center of the calcifications
   C. Biopsy of at least two areas of calcifications that are farthest apart
   D. MRI of the left breast

C A S E 7 0

Developing Calcifications and Ductal Carcinoma In Situ

1. B, C, and D
2. C
3. A
4. C

References

Majid AS, de Paredes ES, Doherty RD, et al: Missed breast carcinoma: pitfalls and pearls. *Radiographics* 2003;23(4):881-895.

Rosen EL, Baker JA, Soo MS: Malignant lesions initially subject to short-term mammographic follow-up. *Radiology* 2002;223(1):221-228.

Cross-Reference

Ikeda D: *Breast Imaging: THE REQUISITES*, 2nd ed, Philadelphia: Saunders, 2010, p 70.

Comment

DCIS develops in the duct and its branches. Distinguishing DCIS calcifications from benign calcifications can be difficult. The shape of each individual calcification is important. Benign calcifications are round (punctate) or cigar-shaped (secretory type). Suspicious calcifications are linear, branching, and pleomorphic (irregularly shaped particles that look like shards of broken glass).

In the patient in this case, the initial magnification views were interpreted as probably benign because the shape of the calcifications was thought to be punctate. However, the distribution of calcifications is also important, and clustered or grouped calcifications are suspicious. On the initial magnification views, this patient had calcifications that were mostly punctate but that were grouped together (see the figures).

This patient did not return for follow-up for 2 years. In the second set of magnification views, the calcifications have increased considerably, and now their suspicious appearance is more obvious (see the figures). The distribution is segmental, which indicates that the calcifications are filling a duct and its branches. One way to identify a segmental distribution is to look for a triangle-shaped area of calcifications, with the apex pointing toward the nipple (see the figures).

When calcifications are newly developing, care should be taken to identify the most aggressive-appearing feature seen. Biopsy should be performed if there are any suspicious features. The benefit of early diagnosis is clear: DCIS is a precursor to invasive ductal carcinoma. Cancer that is diagnosed by mammography as DCIS has a higher cure rate than invasive ductal carcinoma and is less likely to need aggressive local and general therapy.

Notes

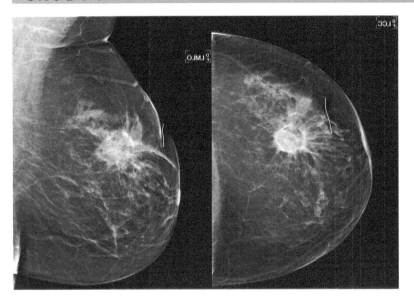

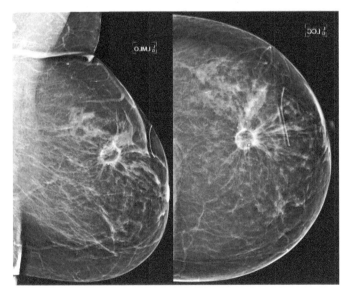

History: A 57-year-old woman had infiltrating ductal carcinoma, grade I, detected in her left breast in 2007. It was treated with lumpectomy and partial breast irradiation.

1. What should be included in the differential diagnosis for the mammographic images shown? (Choose all that apply.)
   A. Fat necrosis in the left breast
   B. Changes caused by partial breast irradiation
   C. Sequelae of lumpectomy without radiation
   D. Complicated cyst in the left breast

2. What mammographic findings are unique to accelerated partial breast irradiation (APBI) compared with external beam radiotherapy?
   A. The mammographic findings are similar.
   B. APBI causes much more distortion at the lumpectomy site.

C. Fat necrosis is much more common with APBI.
D. The changes associated with APBI are less focal.

3. Why may APBI be preferred instead of external beam radiotherapy?
   A. The long-term data show lower recurrence compared with external beam radiotherapy.
   B. Shorter duration of therapy improves patient compliance.
   C. Fewer side effects occur with APBI compared with traditional therapy.
   D. Larger tumors can be treated better with APBI.

4. What is the appropriate management in this case?
   A. Biopsy of the spiculated mass at the lumpectomy site
   B. Short-interval mammogram follow-up of the left breast in 6 months
   C. MRI of the left breast
   D. Mammogram in 1 year

Partial Breast Irradiation

1. A, B, and C
2. A
3. B
4. D

References

Ahmed HM, Dipiro PJ, Devlin PM, et al: Mammographic appearance following accelerated partial breast irradiation by using MammoSite brachytherapy. *Radiology* 2010;255(2):362-368.

Esserman LE, Da Costa D, d'Almeida M, et al: Imaging findings after breast brachytherapy. *AJR Am J Roentgenol* 2006;187(1):57-64.

Cross-Reference

Ikeda D: *Breast Imaging: THE REQUISITES*, 2nd ed, Philadelphia: Saunders, 2010, p 313.

Comment

Radiation therapy is administered to reduce the risk of recurrence in patients treated with lumpectomy. This treatment allows preservation of the breast. Traditionally, external beam radiation was used. More recently, brachytherapy has been used in a selected group of patients. *Brachytherapy* is the term given to the technique that inserts radioactive materials into the breast. Brachytherapy may take the form of multiple catheters or a balloon inserted into the lumpectomy cavity after excision of the malignant mass; this is termed *accelerated partial breast irradiation* (APBI).

Dosing may be twice a day for 5 to 7 days. In contrast, external beam radiation therapy is administered 5 days a week for 5 to 7 weeks. In brachytherapy, only the tumor site is treated. Several studies have shown that 90% of recurrence occurs at the lumpectomy site. APBI targets most potential recurrences, without exposing the entire breast, chest wall, and internal organs to radiation. However, recurrence or residual disease at a distance from the lumpectomy site would not be treated. Patient selection for APBI is important; patients with a relatively small, single tumor mass are appropriate candidates.

Mammographic findings after APBI are similar to the effects of external beam radiation, including skin thickening, diffuse and focal increased density, seroma, and fat necrosis (see the figures). However, with APBI, the changes of fibrosis and scarring may occur earlier than with external beam therapy and may be more severe, owing to the higher dose of APBI per treatment. In the patient in this case, the mammogram performed 6 months after surgery and APBI shows a focal mass, with a fluid-fluid level on mediolateral view, consistent with fat necrosis and scarring (see the figures). At 4 years after treatment, the mass has decreased in size, and the fibrosis has diminished. The patient did not develop calcifications after treatment. However, calcification is not unusual; it is seen in about 25% of patients after external beam treatment. This percentage may be higher with APBI.

Notes

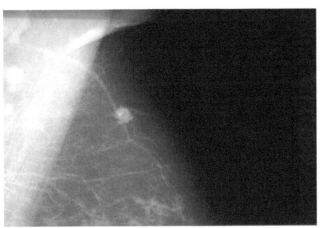

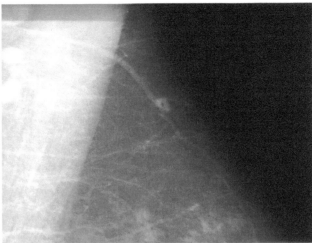

Prior examination

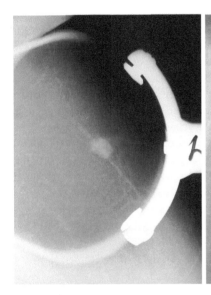

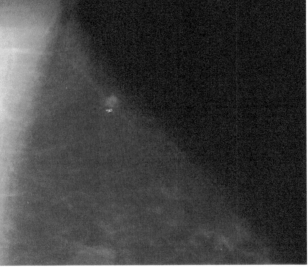

History: A 68-year-old woman underwent a screening mammogram. A mammogram from 2 years ago was available for comparison. She is called back for further evaluation of the left breast finding.

1. What should be included in the differential diagnosis? (Choose all that apply.)
   A. Metastatic lymph node
   B. Reactive lymph node
   C. Lymphoma
   D. Asymmetric glandular tissue

2. What imaging test should be performed next?
   A. Ultrasound
   B. MRI
   C. PET/CT
   D. No further imaging is needed

3. Which of the following is the *least* useful biopsy procedure for diagnosis?
   A. Fine-needle aspiration
   B. Core biopsy
   C. Vacuum-assisted core biopsy
   D. Surgical excision

4. Which of the following is *not* a reason for placing a clip after core biopsy?
   A. To document the location of the original finding
   B. To avoid additional unnecessary biopsies
   C. To guide radiation therapy
   D. To guide surgery

CASE 72

Lymphoma in Intramammary Node

1. A, B, and C
2. A
3. A
4. C

References

Cyrlak D, Carpenter PM: Breast imaging case of the day: intramammary and axillary lymph node metastases from infiltrating lobular carcinoma of the breast. *Radiographics* 1999;19 Spec No:S73-S79.

Lee CH, Giurescu ME, Philpotts LE, et al: Clinical importance of unilaterally enlarging lymph nodes on otherwise normal mammograms. *Radiology* 1997;203(2):329-334.

Lu H, Xu YL, Zhang SP, et al: Breast magnetic resonance imaging in patients with occult breast carcinoma: evaluation on feasibility and correlation with histopathological findings. *Chin Med J (Engl)* 2011;124(12):1790-1795.

Venizelos ID, Tatsiou ZA, Vakalopoulou S, et al: Primary non-Hodgkin's lymphoma arising in an intramammary lymph node. *Leuk Lymphoma* 2005;46(3):451-455.

Zack JR, Trevisan SG, Gupta M: Primary breast lymphoma originating in a benign intramammary lymph node. *AJR Am J Roentgenol* 2001;177 (1):177-178.

Cross-Reference

Ikeda D: *Breast Imaging: THE REQUISITES*, 2nd ed, Philadelphia: Saunders, 2010, p 395.

Comment

In this 68-year-old woman, a left intramammary node was noted to have enlarged on her screening mammogram when it was compared with the examination from 2 years earlier (see the figures). On the previous examination, the lymph node appeared oval, had a low density and symmetric cortex, and contained a fatty hilum. These are all features of a normal lymph node, so no further imaging was needed at that point. However, on the current mammogram, the same node appears larger and denser with irregular margins and loss of its fatty hilum. The previously normal architecture is no longer seen (see the figures).

This change in a solitary, unilateral node may be due to benign causes, such as granulomatous disease, collagen vascular disease, inflammation or infection, or hyperplasia, but metastatic disease and lymphoma must be considered first. Metastatic disease could develop in a node from a breast, lung, or melanoma primary.

After initial diagnostic mammography, ultrasound is the next step in evaluation, helping to characterize the lesion further and guide future biopsy. Core needle biopsy of the node gives the histology of the disease causing the enlargement, and it can help tailor the remaining work-up. The biopsy can be performed with or without vacuum assistance. Surgical excision is also helpful because it provides the entire node for histologic analysis; nevertheless, it constitutes a more invasive procedure. Fine-needle aspiration biopsy is not as useful in determining the exact etiology of the lesion because it may not provide sufficient information (only cells, not tissue). If the node contains metastatic breast cancer and no primary malignancy is seen on mammography, MRI is performed to evaluate for occult cancer because it has a higher sensitivity for invasive tumor than mammography and ultrasound.

This patient underwent an ultrasound-guided core needle biopsy that showed grade I follicular lymphoma. A clip was placed after the biopsy to document the location (see the figures).

Notes

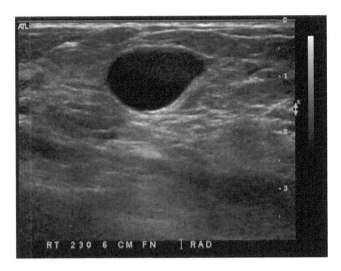 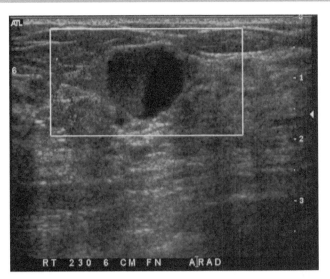

History: A 25-year-old woman presents with a palpable mass.

1. What is the differential diagnosis for the ultrasound images? (Choose all that apply.)
   A. Intracystic mass
   B. Simple cyst
   C. Cyst with two distinct fluid densities, with layering
   D. Debris within a complicated cyst

2. What is the first step in the imaging evaluation of a 25-year-old woman with a palpable breast lump?
   A. Bilateral mammogram with a marker over the area of concern
   B. Unilateral mammogram of the side of interest, with a marker over the area of concern
   C. MRI of the side of interest
   D. Ultrasound of the palpable concern

3. What is the definition of a simple cyst?
   A. A cyst that is anechoic, has imperceptible margins, and has enhanced through-transmission
   B. A cyst that is anechoic or has low-level echoes, has well-circumscribed margins, and has enhanced through-transmission
   C. Any cyst that is anechoic; margins can be irregular, lobulated, or circumscribed
   D. All anechoic structures in the breast

4. What is the echogenic intracystic fluid in this case?
   A. The echogenic fluid is debris.
   B. The echogenic fluid is an intracystic mass.
   C. The echogenic fluid contains fat.
   D. The echogenic fluid is milk of calcium.

CASE 73

Cyst with Layering Fluid

1. C and D
2. D
3. A
4. C

References

Berg WA, Sechtin AG, Marques H, Zhang Z: Cystic breast masses and the ACRIN 6666 experience. *Radiol Clin North Am* 2010;48 (5):931-987.

Daly CP, Bailey JE, Klein KA, Helvie MA: Complicated breast cysts on sonography: is aspiration necessary to exclude malignancy? *Acad Radiol* 2008;15(5):610-617.

Cross-Reference

Ikeda D: *Breast Imaging: THE REQUISITES*, 2nd ed, Philadelphia: Saunders, 2010, p 159.

Comment

This young patient presented with a palpable lump. Patients younger than 30 years should be evaluated with imaging that does not use ionizing radiation, and ultrasound is often diagnostic. MRI of the breast is not the first imaging method in the case of a palpable lump. The palpable finding may be a cyst, a solid mass, or normal glandular tissue. The radiologist should search for any suspicious features that might suggest malignancy, even in young women.

The simple cyst is completely anechoic, has a well-circumscribed, nearly imperceptible margin, and is enhanced through transmission. A complicated cyst may contain a fluid-debris level or fat-fluid level in the cyst, as in this case (see the figures). If the dependent layering fluid is more echogenic, this suggests debris, might indicate infection or inflammation, and is often seen in fibrocystic change. If the fluid-fluid level is not a straight level line, the presence of an intracystic mass must be excluded. The patient can be turned to a decubitus position while the cyst is observed under ultrasound, to watch the fluid level. It should change position within the cyst if it is layering fluid or debris; this change can take up to 10 minutes to occur. A mass will stay the same and will not change its position within the cyst when the patient's position is changed.

In this case, the echogenic fluid is nondependent, or floating (see the figures). This is consistent with fat. Fat may be seen in galactocele or in fat necrosis, but a cyst with a fat-fluid level is most commonly seen in fibrocystic change, as in this case. This type of cyst, with floating fat, is invariably benign, Breast Imaging Reporting and Data System (BI-RADS) 2, and aspiration is not necessary.

Notes

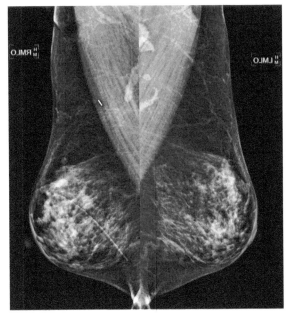

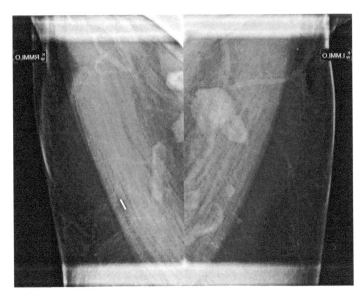

History: A 58-year-old woman presents for a routine screening mammogram. She is recalled for additional views to evaluate calcifications in the axillary nodes.

1. What should be included in the differential diagnosis for the mammographic views shown? (Choose all that apply.)
   A. Patient with history of granulomatous disease
   B. Patient who received gold therapy for rheumatoid arthritis
   C. Patient with history of prior bilateral saline implant rupture
   D. Patient with past history of bilateral silicone implant rupture

2. What is the next step in the work-up?
   A. Obtaining a thorough patient history
   B. Biopsy of an axillary node using ultrasound guidance

C. 6-Month follow-up
D. Annual mammogram

3. Can breast cancer manifest with calcifications in the axillary nodes?
   A. No, only ovarian cancer metastases can produce calcifications in axillary nodes.
   B. Yes, but only calcified ductal carcinoma in situ can produce calcifications.
   C. Yes, but the breast tumor must contain calcifications.
   D. Yes, infiltrating mammary carcinoma can cause metastases containing calcifications.

4. What is the management of a patient with history of gold therapy and with gold deposits in the axillary nodes?
   A. Biopsy of a node using ultrasound guidance
   B. Short-interval follow-up
   C. Annual mammography
   D. Comparison with prior films; this is mandatory

CASE 74

Gold Therapy
1. A, B, and D
2. A
3. D
4. C

References
Bruwer A, Nelson GW, Spark RP: Punctate intranodal gold deposits simulating microcalcifications on mammograms. *AJR Am J Roentgenol* 1987;163(1):87-88.

Cao MM, Hoyt AC, Bassett LW: Mammographic signs of systemic disease. *Radiographics* 2011;31(4):1085-1100.

Carter TR: Intramammary lymph node gold deposits simulating microcalcifications on mammogram. *Hum Pathol* 1988;19(8):992-994.

Cross-Reference
Ikeda D: *Breast Imaging: THE REQUISITES*, 2nd ed, Philadelphia: Saunders, 2010, p 396.

Comment
The axillary lymph nodes should be carefully assessed on each mammogram. Radiodense particles can deposit in the nodes from various sources, including calcifications from granulomatous disease, tattoo pigment, metal fragments from gunshot, metal fragments sheared off during needle localization, and gold therapy (also called *chrysotherapy*) for rheumatoid arthritis (see the figures). Artifacts on the skin can simulate radiodense materials in the nodes and are more common. Deodorant, lotion, and powder should be searched for, and if these materials are present, the skin should be cleaned and the images retaken.

Granulomatous disease typically has coarse calcifications, and gold therapy typically has very fine, almost imperceptible metal density particles, as in this patient (see the figures). These findings should be easily differentiated. Magnification views may be helpful to evaluate the material better. If the nodal material is due to a benign condition, the mammogram is benign (BI-RADS [Breast Imaging Reporting and Data System] 2), and routine screening mammogram is recommended.

Breast cancer and, rarely, ovarian cancer can cause calcifications in axillary lymph nodes and may be the first presentation of an occult cancer. This is a relatively rare presentation of breast cancer; one report found that 3% of breast cancers may cause microcalcifications in the axillary nodes. If there is no history of gold therapy, granulomatous disease, tattoo, needle localization, silicone implant, or gunshot wound, the material should be suspected to be malignant calcification, and biopsy of the node should be performed.

Notes

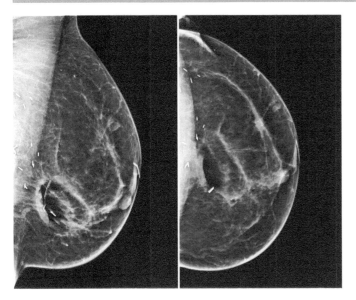

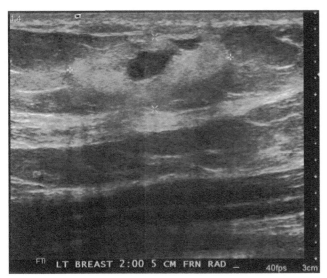

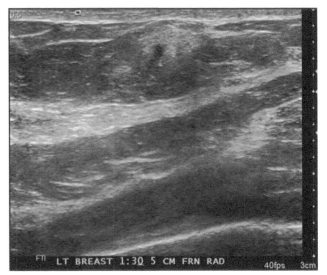

One month later.

History: A 60-year-old woman, who has a history of bilateral breast cancer, has a new area of pain and lump in her left breast. She had breast conservation therapy in the left breast 4 years earlier.

1. What should be included in the differential diagnosis of the mammogram and ultrasound images shown? (Choose all that apply.)
   A. Developing malignant mass
   B. Hematoma
   C. Simple cyst
   D. Fat necrosis

2. What is the next step in management?
   A. Biopsy must be performed because there is a chance of malignancy.
   B. This possible hematoma can be followed with ultrasound in about 1 month.

C. The patient can return for her regular mammogram in 1 year.
D. The patient can monitor the palpable finding and return only if it gets larger.

3. Which of the following is *not* an ultrasound appearance of a hematoma?
   A. Oval echogenic mass with cystic center
   B. Anechoic round mass with through-transmission and thin wall
   C. Hypoechoic, with thick and thin weblike echoes
   D. Oval, with fluid-debris level

4. What imaging study would *not* help differentiate hematoma from malignancy?
   A. MRI
   B. Color Doppler ultrasound
   C. Standard mammographic images
   D. Spot compression magnification views

Hematoma

1. A, B, and D
2. B
3. B
4. C

References

Pojchamarnwiputh S, Muttarak M, Na-Chiangmai W, et al: Benign breast lesions mimicking carcinoma at mammography. *Singapore Med J* 2007;48(10):958-968.

Stavros AT: *Breast Ultrasound*, Philadelphia: Lippincott Williams & Wilkins, 2004.

Cross-Reference

Ikeda D: *Breast Imaging: THE REQUISITES*, 2nd ed, Philadelphia: Saunders, 2010, p 139.

Comment

A developing mass in the breast of a patient who has been diagnosed with cancer in the past is suspicious. Additional views and ultrasound can help in differentiating malignancy from hematoma or fat necrosis. This patient (see the figures), who had undergone breast conservation therapy 4 years ago, presented with a new left breast mass and pain and had no recollection of a traumatic event. There was no bruising in the skin at the time she presented. It is helpful if the patient recalls a traumatic event and bruising because this can steer the diagnosis toward hematoma. However, many women do not recall the event and do not perceive the focal finding until the bruising has passed and the hematoma is felt as a lump.

Standard imaging of mammography and ultrasound can be helpful in making the diagnosis. Typically, the mammogram and ultrasound show features of fat and water density. The mass on mammography has fat lucency and may have high-density material (blood) appearing as a dense halo (see the figures). On ultrasound, there may be an echogenic mass (blood) with varying degrees of liquefaction, appearing as cystic areas (see the figures). The ultrasound appearance can be quite variable because acute hematoma is seen as a markedly hypoechoic mass, and then as clotting begins, varying degrees of echogenic material and clot can develop. The mass should not have increased blood flow on color Doppler because the echogenic material seen within is clot, not tumor.

The management of the finding can be close follow-up if there are features of a hematoma. If the ultrasound examination is repeated in 1 month, there should be a decrease in the size of the mass (see the figures). The time to full resolution varies, but it is helpful to follow the mass to complete resolution, if possible. Malignant masses are prone to bleeding if subjected to trauma, and this possibility must always be considered when following a hematoma, particularly in a high-risk patient. If the mass increases in size or does not change in 1 month, biopsy should be considered.

Notes

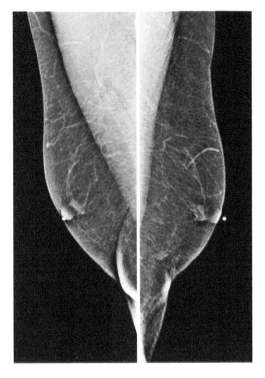

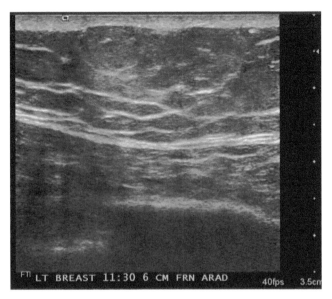

History: A 55-year-old man presents with a palpable mass in his left upper breast.

1. What is your differential diagnosis for palpable masses in the male breast? (Choose all that apply.)
   A. Breast cancer
   B. Lipoma
   C. Sebaceous cyst
   D. Fat necrosis
   E. Fibroadenoma

2. What is your interpretation of the findings presented on mammography and ultrasound?
   A. Normal mammogram, mass isoechoic to fat on ultrasound, likely lipoma
   B. Benign-appearing mass on mammography or ultrasound
   C. Left mammogram and ultrasound consistent with gynecomastia
   D. Malignant mass behind left nipple, not demonstrated on ultrasound

3. What is your recommendation and Breast Imaging Reporting and Data System (BI-RADS) code based on the imaging presented?
   A. Biopsy is needed, BI-RADS 4
   B. Incomplete exam, recommend MRI of breasts, BI-RADS 0
   C. Benign, BI-RADS 2
   D. Probably benign, recommend 6-month follow-up, BI-RADS 3

4. Why is it important to perform a mammogram in a man presenting with a breast mass?
   A. Men should be screened annually or semiannually for breast cancer with a mammogram.
   B. Mammography is the first tool to evaluate for breast cancer in the male or female patient who presents with a lump.
   C. Mammography is not necessary; the exam should begin with ultrasound of the area of concern.
   D. Mammography is not important. All men with a palpable area of concern only need surgical evaluation.

Palpable Mass in a Male Patient (Lipoma)

1. A, B, C, and D
2. A
3. C
4. B

References

Bancroft LW, Kransdorf MJ, Peterson JJ, O'Connor MI: Benign fatty tumors: classification, clinical course, imaging appearance, and treatment. *Skeletal Radiol* 2006;35(10):719-733.

Lanng C, Eriksen BO, Hoffman J: Lipoma of the breast: a diagnostic dilemma. *Breast* 2004;13(5):408-411.

Cross-Reference

Ikeda D: *Breast Imaging: THE REQUISITES*, 2nd ed, Philadelphia: Saunders, 2010, p 137.

Comment

Male patients can present with palpable masses in the breast. The findings fall into three broad categories: breast cancer, gynecomastia, and masses that could arise anywhere in the body, deriving from the skin, lymph system, or blood vessels. As in female patients, the most important consideration for the radiologist is to evaluate for the possibility of cancer. Thus, male patients who present with a palpable finding may first have a bilateral mammogram, followed by a directed ultrasound exam if needed. (Ultrasound might not be necessary when the mammogram demonstrates a characteristic appearance of gynecomastia.)

Lipomas are common masses in male and female patients. They arise from the subcutaneous fat, and they may be palpable owing to the superficial location. They can become large and may be cosmetically unappealing, but they are not otherwise clinically important. The lipoma is usually not recognized on a male mammogram (see the figures) because the normal male breast is composed predominantly of subcutaneous fat. In the female breast, the lipoma may be recognized on the mammogram if it is outlined by dense glandular tissue. On ultrasound, the lipoma typically is horizontally aligned and isoechoic or hyperechoic to the surrounding fat. The margins are smooth, and a thin, echogenic capsule may be seen (see the figures). The lipoma may be difficult to distinguish from the surrounding subcutaneous fat. The lipoma is soft, and it can compress on pressure of the transducer.

Notes

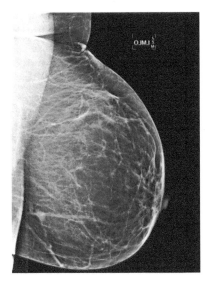
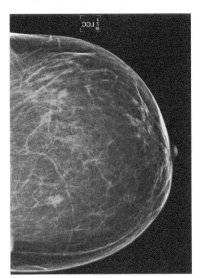

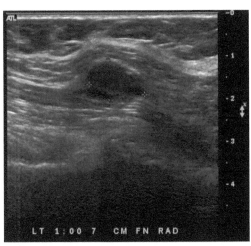
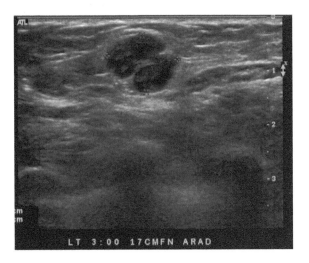

History: A 65-year-old woman who had a melanoma removed from her right leg 10 years ago undergoes a routine screening mammogram. The left breast only is shown.

1. What should be included in the differential diagnosis for the two developing masses in the left breast? (Choose all that apply.)
   A. Cysts in the breast
   B. Metastatic masses in the breast
   C. Primary carcinoma of the breast
   D. Breast abscess

2. Which of the following statements is true about hematogenous spread of tumor to the breast?
   A. There are almost always multiple masses in both breasts.
   B. Masses are most often spiculated.
   C. Masses are usually in a ductal distribution.
   D. Masses are typically hypervascular.

3. What is the most common cancer to spread to the breast?
   A. Breast cancer
   B. Lung cancer
   C. Medullary thyroid cancer
   D. Melanoma

4. Would you be more likely to recommend biopsy of a benign-appearing breast mass in a woman with known malignancy such as melanoma?
   A. No, you should treat each lesion on its own merits; if benign in appearance, it can be followed instead of performing biopsy.
   B. Yes, you should perform biopsy of a new mass in the breast regardless of appearance.
   C. Yes, you should perform biopsy of a new mass if its appearance is inconclusive in a patient with known cancer.
   D. A patient's cancer history bears no relationship to the decision to recommend biopsy.

Metastatic Melanoma

1. A, B, and C
2. D
3. A
4. C

References

Akçay MN: Metastatic disease in the breast. *Breast* 2002;11(6):526-528.
Yang WT, Metreweli C: Sonography of nonmammary malignancies of the breast. *AJR Am J Roentgenol* 1999;172(2):343-348.

Cross-Reference

Ikeda D: *Breast Imaging: THE REQUISITES*, 2nd ed, Philadelphia: Saunders, 2010, p 117.

Comment

Nonbreast primary tumors can spread hematogenously and can involve the breast. When single or multiple new masses are seen in a nonductal pattern in the breast in a patient with a known cancer, metastases should be considered. Metastatic involvement of the breast is rare, representing approximately 1% of all breast malignancies. The most common cause of metastatic involvement is from a contralateral breast cancer; melanoma is the most frequent nonbreast cancer to spread to the breast. Lymphoma, lung cancer, and ovarian cancer are the next most frequent cancers to metastasize to the breast. Sometimes metastases are the first indication that a cancer is present. This is more common in the case of enlarged axillary nodes seen on mammogram that herald a previously unknown malignancy.

Metastatic deposits in the breast are often multiple, as in this patient (see the figures), bilateral, and well defined. Microcalcification in the masses is rare, as are spiculated margins. The mammographic and ultrasound appearance overlaps with many benign masses, such as cysts and fibroadenomas. On mammography, the masses are round or oval, with circumscribed margins. On ultrasound, the masses usually are well defined, without shadowing, and without a thick echogenic halo because there is typically no desmoplastic reaction in the surrounding tissue. They are often hypoechoic or even appear anechoic. Color flow Doppler should show increased vascularity because the masses are spread hematogenously. It is important to recognize the possibility of metastases and to perform a biopsy of lesions with imaging guidance. Biopsy may avoid unnecessary breast surgery and lead to appropriate oncologic management.

This patient was diagnosed with melanoma 10 years previously and had no metastasis until the mammogram showed masses. The patient was initially recalled for additional views of the left breast and ultrasound evaluation. When she returned for the biopsy appointment 2 months after the mammogram, ultrasound revealed a new mass deep in the breast at the 1 o'clock position, near the pectoral muscle (see the figures), and another at 3 o'clock (see the figures), which had not been seen on the mammogram. Biopsy specimens of these two masses were obtained with core needle technique and ultrasound guidance, and a diagnosis of melanoma metastases was made.

Notes

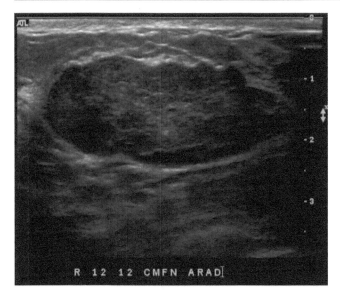

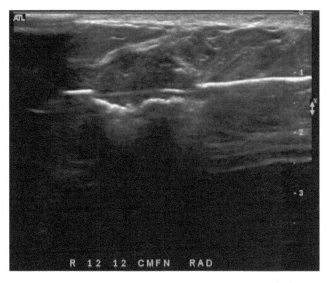

History: A 19-year-old woman who is 2 months postpartum presents for evaluation of a mass in the right upper breast.

1. What should be included in the differential diagnosis for this breast mass? (Choose all that apply.)
   A. Lactating adenoma
   B. Tubular adenoma
   C. Lipoma
   D. Malignancy

2. How do you evaluate a 19-year-old woman with a mass?
   A. Mammogram must always be performed in the setting of a palpable mass.
   B. A patient of this age should always have surgical evaluation first.
   C. Ultrasound of the palpable mass should be performed.
   D. MRI of both breasts should be performed.

3. Is the mass related to the patient's recent pregnancy?
   A. Yes, the mass likely developed during pregnancy.
   B. No, tubular adenomas are related to radial scars, not pregnancy.
   C. No, pregnancy and breast masses are not related.
   D. Yes, all breast masses in young women develop during pregnancy.

4. Are fibroadenomas, tubular adenomas, and lactating adenomas the same pathology?
   A. No, they are not related; the names are similar, but the pathology is very different.
   B. Yes, the masses have the same etiology, occurring at different times during the reproductive years.
   C. No, they are not the same pathology, but they are related.
   D. Yes, they are the same pathology, differing only in size.

Tubular Adenoma

1. A, B, and D
2. C
3. A
4. C

References

Soo MS, Dash N, Bentley R, et al: Tubular adenomas of the breast: imaging findings with histologic correlation. *AJR Am J Roentgenol* 2000;174(3):757-761.

Stavros AT: *Breast Ultrasound*, Philadelphia: Lippincott Williams & Wilkins, 2004, pp 554-557.

Cross-Reference

Ikeda D: *Breast Imaging: THE REQUISITES*, 2nd ed, Philadelphia: Saunders, 2010, pp 127, 379.

Comment

Tubular adenoma is a relatively rare, benign mass that develops during the reproductive years. This mass is related to lactating adenoma, which is more common and typically develops during pregnancy and lactation. These two adenomas have similar pathologic features, consisting mainly of epithelial cells, with very little stromal component. Fibroadenoma, much more common, has a greater degree of stromal cells.

The ultrasound and mammographic appearance of tubular adenoma is similar to fibroadenoma: oval shape, wider than tall, and possibly enhanced through-transmission. The mass surface may be smooth or microlobulated (see the figures). The microlobulated surface is a feature that can be seen in malignancy, making the lesion a BI-RADS (Breast Imaging Reporting and Data System) 4 when this feature is present. Calcifications can occur within the mass, although in one series, calcifications were seen only in tubular adenomas of older women.

Histologic diagnosis is indicated in this patient owing to the ultrasound features. Patients may choose a surgical resection, especially when the mass is large and palpable. However, they may choose follow-up, rather than excision, if the histology is known. Ultrasound-guided core needle biopsy can provide the histologic diagnosis, and a patient can choose follow-up or excision at her leisure.

This patient chose a needle biopsy, which was performed with a vacuum-assisted device (see the figures). Histology was tubular adenoma.

Notes

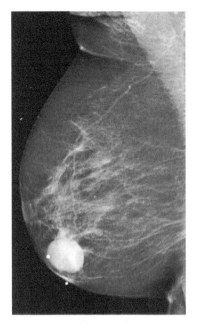
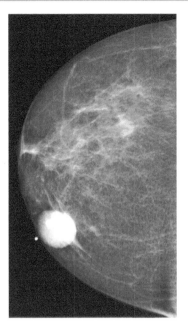

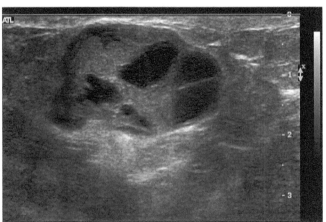

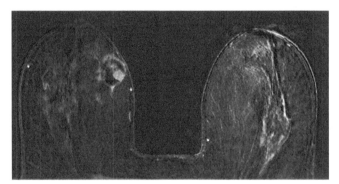

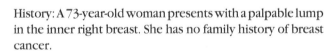

MR Subtraction view after contrast enhancement.

History: A 73-year-old woman presents with a palpable lump in the inner right breast. She has no family history of breast cancer.

1. What is the differential diagnosis? (Choose all that apply.)
   A. Cyst
   B. Ductal carcinoma in situ
   C. Intracystic papilloma
   D. Papillary carcinoma

2. Which of the following statements regarding papillary carcinomas is true?
   A. Papillary carcinomas are common.
   B. Papillary carcinomas are more common in premenopausal women.
   C. Treatment consists of radiation and hormonal treatment.
   D. The overall prognosis of papillary carcinomas is excellent.

3. Which of the following statements regarding imaging of papillary carcinomas is true?
   A. The presence of multiple masses excludes the diagnosis of papillary carcinoma.
   B. Small lesions manifest as architectural distortion or nipple retraction or both.
   C. Papillary carcinomas may manifest as complex cystic lesions or solid masses.
   D. On MRI, the fluid component is dark on T1-weighted images and bright on T2-weighted images.

4. Which of the following statements is *false*?
   A. Diagnosis of papillary carcinoma is made by biopsy.
   B. Histologically, papillary carcinomas are a heterogeneous group of lesions.
   C. Papillary carcinomas arise from benign papillomas.
   D. Distinction between benign papillary lesions and papillary carcinoma is important.

Papillary Carcinoma

1. C and D
2. D
3. C
4. C

References
Bhosale SJ, Kshirsagar AY, Sulhyan SR, et al: Invasive papillary breast carcinoma. *Case Rep Oncol* 2010;3(3):410-415.

Pal SK, Lau SK, Kruper L, et al: Papillary carcinoma of the breast: an overview. *Breast Cancer Res Treat* 2010;122(3):637-645.

Rodriguez MC, Secades AL, Angulo JM: Best cases from the AFIP: intra-cystic papillary carcinoma of the breast. *Radiographics* 2010;30 (7):2021-2027.

Cross-Reference
Ikeda D: *Breast Imaging: THE REQUISITES*, 2nd ed, Philadelphia: Saunders, 2010, p 116.

Comment

Papillary carcinomas are rare, accounting for approximately 1% of all newly diagnosed breast cancers. They are more common in older patients (average age of onset is approximately 70 years) and frequently manifest as a solitary palpable mass in the subareolar location or multiple peripheral masses; they may also manifest as bloody nipple discharge or be found incidentally on routine imaging. Retraction of the nipple or skin may be an associated clinical finding.

Mammographic findings are usually nonspecific. Lesions commonly appear as a dense, round or lobulated mass, with architectural distortion or nipple retraction as they become larger (see the figures). Less commonly, multiple or bilateral masses may be seen.

On ultrasound, lesions appear as complex cystic masses, with solid mural nodules with or without septa (see the figures). The solid component is often highly vascular. They may also appear as entirely solid masses.

MRI usually shows a well-circumscribed, heterogeneous round or oval mass, with cystic component and mural solid nodules (see the figures). The solid component has intermediate signal intensity, whereas the cystic areas may have a different appearance depending on the fluid composition (serous content appears hypointense on T1-weighted images and hyperintense on T2-weighted images; hemorrhagic content appears hyperintense on both T1-weighted and T2-weighted images). With addition of contrast agent, there is marked enhancement of the walls, septa, and solid nodules.

Biopsy should be performed to obtain a definitive diagnosis. Ultrasound-guided core needle biopsy establishes the initial diagnosis, as it can accurately target the solid components. Histologically, papillary carcinomas are a morphologically heterogeneous group of lesions, having in common a growth pattern characterized by arborescent fibrovascular stalks lined by epithelial cells. The mass is surrounded by thick stromal fibrosis. Papillary carcinomas can be distinguished from benign papillary lesions by the absence of myoepithelial cells in the malignant form. Distinction between benign papillary lesions and papillary carcinoma is important because it has an impact on treatment.

Treatment of papillary carcinoma, as in any type of breast cancer, includes surgery (lumpectomy or mastectomy) in association with radiation and hormonal treatment for hormone-sensitive tumors, chemotherapy, or both chemotherapy and radiation. The overall prognosis of papillary carcinoma is excellent because it tends to be low grade and slow growing. The survival rate approaches 100% at 10 years. Lymph node metastases occur less commonly than in invasive ductal carcinomas not otherwise specified.

Notes

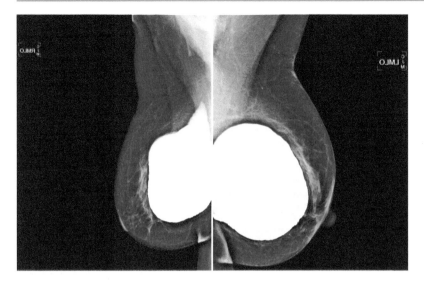

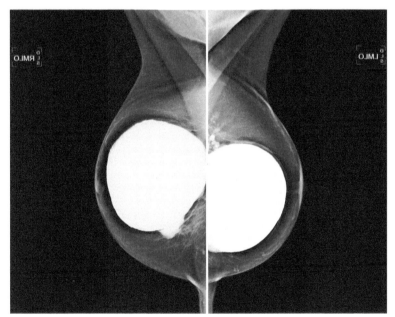

History: A 60-year-old asymptomatic woman with silicone implants placed 20 years ago undergoes mammography.

1. What should be included in the differential diagnosis for the images shown in the first figure? (Choose all that apply.)
   A. Saline implants with right saline implant rupture
   B. Mass suspicious for cancer, developing at the chest wall on the right
   C. Right silicone implant rupture
   D. Bilateral silicone implant rupture

2. What is the location of the implants, and what type are they?
   A. Subglandular silicone
   B. Subglandular saline
   C. Subpectoral silicone
   D. Subpectoral saline

3. What is the next step in imaging for this patient?
   A. MRI is needed to evaluate integrity of the right implant.
   B. Ultrasound is needed to evaluate possible right implant rupture.
   C. No further work-up is needed.
   D. Additional mammographic views are needed.

4. What is the management of this problem?
   A. No management is needed.
   B. Recommend that the patient discuss implant rupture with her clinician.
   C. The patient must be referred to a surgeon for implant removal.
   D. Silicone granulomas must be surgically removed because of autoimmune sequelae.

Mammography of Silicone Implant Leak

1. C
2. A
3. C
4. B

Reference

Berg WA, Caskey CI, Hamper UM, et al: Diagnosing breast implant rupture with MR imaging, US, and mammography. *Radiographics* 1993;13(6):1323-1336.

Cross-Reference

Ikeda D: *Breast Imaging: THE REQUISITES*, 2nd ed, Philadelphia: Saunders, 2010, p 343.

Comment

Asymptomatic silicone implant rupture is seen in approximately 5% of implants on screening mammography. Several factors predispose to implant rupture: subglandular location (as in this patient), implant age, and closed capsulotomy (a procedure in which pressure is applied to the implant to break the fibrous capsule and keep the implant from feeling hard).

When interpreting a mammogram of a woman with implants, it is important to distinguish the type of implant. Implant type is distinguished by assessing the density of the fluid—silicone is denser than saline—and checking for the presence of a valve—saline implants have a valve, but silicone implants do not. It is important to know the type of implant because when saline implants rupture, they collapse, and the saline is reabsorbed by the body. Only the implant shell remains, flattened against the posterior breast. For this reason, MRI is not used to evaluate for saline implant rupture: It is not a diagnostic dilemma; the rupture is clinically obvious. When silicone implants rupture, silicone gel leaks out of the implant shell, but the bulk of the silicone remains in the shell. The silicone leaks into the capsule (intracapsular rupture) and then may leak into the breast if there is also a rupture of the fibrous capsule around the implant (extracapsular rupture) (see the figures).

The second figure shows a different patient, also asymptomatic, with bilateral extracapsular silicone implant rupture. Silicone that has leaked outside the capsule can form into silicone granulomas, which can be found in the breast and axilla and in the rest of the body; silicone also can be taken up by the lymph nodes. A patient may be asymptomatic, similar to both of the patients discussed in this case; symptoms may be minimal; or the patient may experience pain and lumps. The American College of Rheumatology issued a report in 1995 stating that silicone implants do not expose patients to additional risk for connective tissue disease.

Notes

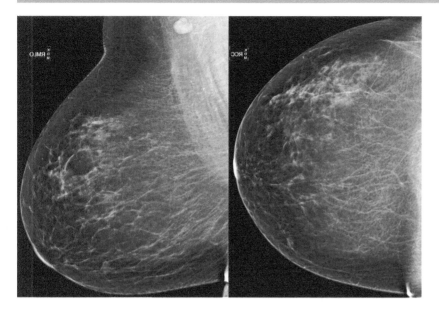

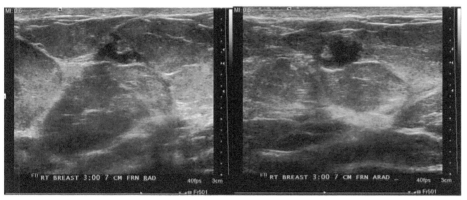

History: A 63-year-old woman for routine mammogram. Two years previously, she was diagnosed with ductal carcinoma in situ in the left breast, which was treated with breast conservation therapy. A new mass was noted to develop in the right breast.

1. What should be included in the differential diagnosis, based on the right mammogram and ultrasound images shown? (Choose all that apply.)
    A. Simple cyst in the right breast
    B. Right breast malignancy
    C. Papilloma in the right breast
    D. Complex cystic mass in the right breast

2. Which of the following statements is true about color Doppler imaging?
    A. If there is no flow, you can be confident there is no malignancy.
    B. Flow seen at the edge of the mass excludes a benign cyst.
    C. Flow seen within an intracystic mass raises the suspicion for malignancy.
    D. If the lesion is round and anechoic, color Doppler is not needed.

3. What is the next step in management?
    A. Short-interval follow-up for this likely benign mass
    B. Return to routine mammogram for this likely benign lesion
    C. Biopsy using ultrasound guidance
    D. MRI to check for abnormal enhancement

4. If the tissue diagnosis from the core needle biopsy is "benign breast tissue," what is the next step?
    A. Consider the biopsy nondiagnostic and repeat.
    B. Consider the biopsy result definitive, and recommend mammogram in 1 year.
    C. Consider the biopsy result unsatisfactory, and recommend short-interval follow-up to check for growth.
    D. Consider the biopsy diagnostic, and recommend that she be followed by her surgeon.

Cystic-Appearing Cancer

1. B, C, and D
2. C
3. C
4. A

References

Berg WA, Campassi C, Ioffe OB: Cystic lesions of the breast: sonographic-pathologic correlation. *Radiology* 2003;227(1):183-191.

Doshi DJ, March DE, Crisi GM, et al: Complex cystic breast masses: diagnostic approach and imaging-pathologic correlation. *Radiographics* 2007;27(Suppl 1):S53-S64.

Huff JG: The sonographic findings and differing clinical implications of simple, complicated, and complex breast cysts. *J Natl Compr Canc Netw* 2009;7(10):1101-1105.

Rinaldi P, Ierardi C, Costantini M, et al: Cystic breast lesions: sonographic findings and clinical management. *J Ultrasound Med* 2010;29(11):1617-1626.

Cross-Reference

Ikeda D: *Breast Imaging: THE REQUISITES*, 2nd ed, Philadelphia: Saunders, 2010, p 159.

Comment

A complex cystic mass is a mass that contains fluid but also has a thick wall, intracystic masses, thick internal septations, or mural projections and requires biopsy. These masses may represent malignancy, intracystic papilloma, necrotic tumor, hematoma, or abscess.

This patient had a new mass develop in her right breast, seen on mammography (see the figures). On the mammogram the mass has an appearance more suggestive of a benign process, such as a cyst. It has low density and relatively sharp margins on the standard views. However, this postmenopausal woman who has survived breast cancer in the contralateral breast is at increased risk for a new cancer. Spot compression views and ultrasound are needed for further evaluation of the developing mass. On ultrasound, the mass appears cystic, with internal masses. The walls are not thick, but the shape of the mass is irregular, not round or oval (see the figures). These are suspicious characteristics, and biopsy is recommended.

It is important to differentiate a complex cystic mass from a complicated cyst. A complicated cyst is oval or round, has a thin wall, and has diffuse low-level internal echoes or internal debris. A complex cystic mass has a thick wall or an internal mass, or both, such as in this patient (see the figures). In one series, 35% of cystic masses with a thick wall or thick septations were malignant. High-grade infiltrating ductal carcinoma may have circumscribed borders. This patient had infiltrating ductal carcinoma, high grade on core biopsy.

Core biopsy of the complex cystic mass is preferred rather than aspiration. The cyst fluid may be necrotic or acellular, which may result in a false-negative result. If a nonspecific benign result is received after needle biopsy of a suspicious lesion, the biopsy should be repeated. The nonspecific benign diagnosis is nonconcordant and does not explain the reason for the intracystic masses or thick wall of the complex cystic mass. Lesions with a specific benign diagnosis such as papilloma or atypical hyperplasia should be excised. Clips should be placed at the time of needle biopsy because the lesion may be poorly seen after biopsy, particularly if small.

Notes

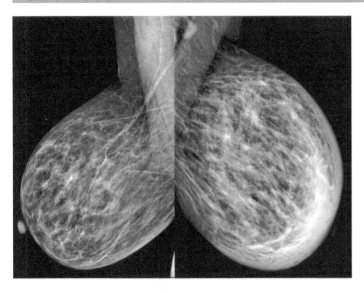

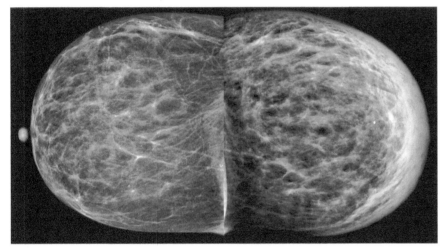

History: A 73-year-old woman presents with recent left breast enlargement. Her medical history includes long-term hypertension and multiple previous hospitalizations for shortness of breath and edema of the legs.

1. What should be included in the differential diagnosis? (Choose all that apply.)
   A. DCIS
   B. Mastitis
   C. Inflammatory breast cancer
   D. Congestive heart failure (CHF)

2. Considering the differential diagnosis, which of the following does *not* constitute a reasonable alternative in management?
   A. Breast biopsy
   B. Treatment with antibiotics and short-term follow-up
   C. Mastectomy
   D. Treatment with diuretics and cardiotherapeutic agents and short-term follow-up

3. Other conditions associated with unilateral breast edema include all of the following *except:*
   A. Changes after lumpectomy or radiation
   B. Lymphoma and leukemia
   C. Arteriovenous hemodialysis complications
   D. Diabetic mastopathy

4. Which of the following statements regarding breast edema secondary to CHF is true?
   A. Unilateral breast edema is a common manifestation of CHF.
   B. The edema is secondary to decreased hydrostatic pressure.
   C. Pitting edema can help distinguish between CHF and malignancy.
   D. A known clinical history of CHF excludes other etiologies of unilateral breast edema.

Unilateral Breast Edema

1. B, C, and D
2. C
3. D
4. C

References

Cao MM, Hoyt AC, Bassett LW: Mammographic signs of systemic disease. *Radiographics* 2011;31(4):1085-1100.

Kwak JY, Kim EK, Chung SY, et al: Unilateral breast edema: spectrum of etiologies and imaging appearances. *Yonsei Med J* 2005;46(1):1-7.

Oraedu CO, Pinnapureddy P, Alrawi S, et al: Congestive heart failure mimicking inflammatory breast carcinoma: a case report and review of the literature. *Breast J* 2001;7(2):117-119.

Cross-Reference

Ikeda D: *Breast Imaging: THE REQUISITES*, 2nd ed, Philadelphia: Saunders, 2010, p 389.

Comment

Unilateral breast edema raises concern for inflammatory breast carcinoma. However, edema can have different etiologies, including benign and malignant conditions. Conditions associated with unilateral breast edema include inflammatory breast carcinoma, mastitis, changes following surgical and radiation treatments, lymphatic obstruction, central venous obstruction, arteriovenous hemodialysis complications, granulomatous diseases, nephrotic syndrome, scleroderma, CHF, some skin conditions, lymphoma, leukemia, and metastasis.

Knowledge of these entities, in conjunction with a thorough clinical history including preexisting medical conditions and previous procedures, is important in developing an accurate diagnosis, affecting the patient's management. If inflammatory breast cancer is suspected, biopsy should be performed to obtain a definitive diagnosis; biopsy specimens of the skin and of any identifiable discrete mass should be obtained.

Clinically, breast edema, thickening, and associated enlargement are common to all of the above-mentioned etiologies. Nevertheless, additional distinctive features may be helpful in distinguishing some of these conditions. Inflammatory breast cancer also manifests with erythema that may be associated with sensation of heat in the affected breast; mastitis is accompanied by erythema, breast pain, and fever that regress after antibiotic treatment; CHF has pitting edema on clinical examination, with absence of a discrete palpable mass, and signs and symptoms resolve after standard treatment. Other entities can be suspected based on the clinical history (e.g., previous lumpectomy with axillary dissection or sentinel node biopsy, radiation to the breast, hemodialysis with upper extremity arteriovenous fistula).

The appearance of breast edema on mammography is characterized by skin thickening, increased parenchymal density, and prominent interstitial markings (trabecular thickening), regardless of the etiology (see the figures). The presence of a discrete mass or microcalcifications, or both, may help to diagnose breast malignancy.

On ultrasound, there is skin thickening, with associated lymphatic engorgement. The presence of a discrete mass may be helpful in diagnosing breast malignancy and can be targeted for biopsy.

On MRI, breast edema manifests as skin thickening and prominent interstitial markings, which appear hyperintense on T2-weighted images. If breast edema is the only finding, no enhancement is seen after injection of contrast material.

In the presented case, the edema of the left breast was secondary to CHF, which is a common clinical condition in the general population. When CHF causes breast edema, usually both breasts are affected because of increased hydrostatic pressure and subsequent lymphatic obstruction. Unilateral breast edema secondary to CHF is rare, and it may be due to lateralization to the dependent breast if the patient lies on one side for extended periods.

Notes

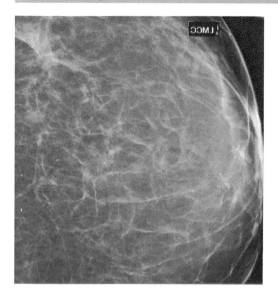
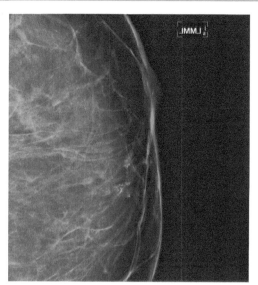

History: A 68-year-old woman presents with a chronic scaly red patch on her left nipple. Magnification views of the left subareolar area are shown.

1. What is the differential diagnosis and Breast Imaging Reporting and Data System (BI-RADS) category for these special views? (Choose all that apply.)
   A. Benign-appearing calcifications in the subareolar breast, BI-RADS 2
   B. Indeterminate calcifications in subareolar ducts, BI-RADS 3
   C. Microcalcifications in subareolar ducts, suspicious for ductal carcinoma in situ (DCIS), BI-RADS 4
   D. Normal, BI-RADS 1

2. What significance is the clinical finding of the scaly red patch on the nipple?
   A. This is not related to the mammographic concern.
   B. The area of concern is likely eczema, not related to breast disease.
   C. This might represent Paget's disease and may be related to the calcifications on the mammogram.
   D. This might represent Paget's disease, but it is not related to the calcifications on the mammogram.

3. What is the next step in diagnosis?
   A. Send the patient to a surgeon for a biopsy of the nipple abnormality.
   B. Schedule a 6-month follow-up of indeterminate calcifications.
   C. Perform an image-guided biopsy of the microcalcifications.
   D. The radiologist should perform a skin biopsy.

4. How often is there a mammographic abnormality in the setting of red, scaly nipple abnormality?
   A. Nearly always, 90%
   B. Rarely,10%
   C. About half of the time
   D. About 75% of the time

C A S E 8 3

Paget's Disease

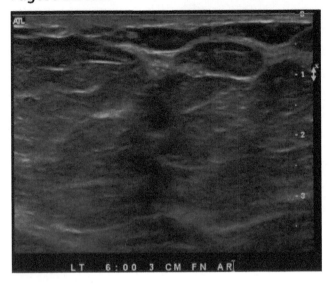

1. C
2. C
3. C
4. C

References

Ikeda DM, Helvie MA, Frank TS, et al: Paget disease of the nipple: radiologic-pathologic correlation. *Radiology* 1993;189(1):89-94.

Valdes EK, Feldman SM: Paget's disease of the breast. *Breast J* 2006;12 (1):83.

Cross-Reference

Ikeda D: *Breast Imaging: THE REQUISITES*, 2nd ed, Philadelphia: Saunders, 2010, p 397.

Comment

This patient presents with a suspicious clinical finding. When a red scaly patch is seen on or adjacent to the nipple-areolar complex, Paget's disease should be suspected. Skin biopsy will be needed, but the first step is to evaluate the mammogram for any evidence of intraductal or invasive malignancy. In this case (see the figures), there are casting-type calcifications filling the subareolar ducts, highly suspicious for ductal carcinoma in situ (DCIS). Note the calcifications within the nipple in the second figure.

The extent of disease should be established before the patient goes to surgery. Abnormal mammographic findings require a biopsy. Calcifications may be targeted for stereotactic biopsy; however, stereotactic biopsy can be difficult in the immediate subareolar area, and ultrasound can be used to try to image the calcifications in the distended ducts (see the figures). In this patient, ultrasound-guided biopsy was performed. The biopsy result was DCIS, grade III. On skin biopsy performed by the surgeon, the nipple area contained the same cells as were present in the breast biopsy, which is typical for Paget's disease.

Paget's disease is an uncommon form of breast cancer, accounting for less than 5% of all breast cancers. More than 97% of patients with pagetoid changes of the nipple have underlying breast cancer. The mammogram might not demonstrate the underlying malignancy, however. Only about 50% have a mammographic abnormality, including nipple, areolar, or subareolar distortion, nipple retraction, masses, or calcifications. The breast abnormality may be subareolar, as in this case (see the figures), or may be distant from the nipple. The disease may be multicentric or multifocal. MRI can be used to evaluate extent of disease, prior to definitive treatment.

Notes

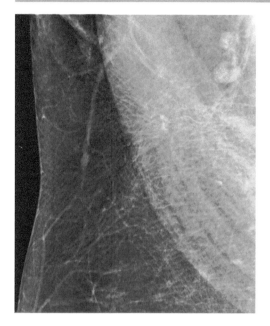 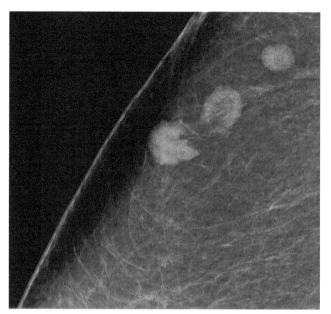

History: Two different patients present for routine screening mammograms. Portions of the view showing axillary nodes are provided.

1. What should be included in the differential diagnosis for this mammographic appearance? (Choose all that apply.)
   A. Hypercalcemia
   B. Gold deposits
   C. Granulomatous disease
   D. Metastatic disease
   E. Silicone

2. If the patient has a history of gold therapy for rheumatoid arthritis, what is the Breast Imaging Reporting and Data System (BI-RADS) category for this finding?
   A. BI-RADS 0—incomplete; further evaluation with magnification views is needed
   B. BI-RADS 4—biopsy of a node to confirm gold deposits
   C. BI-RADS 3—short-interval follow-up
   D. BI-RADS 2—benign

3. If this is a new finding in a patient with a history of ipsilateral breast cancer, what is the BI-RADS category for this finding?
   A. BI-RADS 4—biopsy should be considered
   B. BI-RADS 2—benign
   C. BI-RADS 3—short-interval follow-up
   D. BI-RADS 1—normal

4. If you elected to perform a biopsy of an axillary lymph node, can this procedure be accomplished with needle biopsy with image guidance?
   A. No, the node must be excised surgically.
   B. No, calcifications require stereotactic biopsy, which is not an option in the axilla.
   C. Yes, ultrasound-guided core needle biopsy is an option.
   D. No, the axillary nodes are seen best with MRI, and the axilla is not accessible for MRI-guided biopsy.

C A S E 8 4

Calcifications in Axillary Lymph Nodes

1. B, C, D, and E
2. D
3. A
4. C

References

Bruwer A, Nelson GW, Spark RP: Punctate intranodal gold deposits simulating microcalcifications on mammograms. *Radiology* 1987;163(1):87-88.

Dunnington GL, Pearce J, Sherrod A, et al: Breast carcinoma presenting as mammographic microcalcifications in axillary lymph nodes. *Breast Dis* 1995;8:193-198.

Singer C, Blankstein E, Koenigsberg T, et al: Mammographic appearance of axillary lymph node calcification in patients with metastatic ovarian carcinoma. *AJR Am J Roentgenol* 2001;176(6):1437-1440.

Cross-Reference

Ikeda D: *Breast Imaging: THE REQUISITES*, 2nd ed, Philadelphia: Saunders, 2010, p 396.

Comment

Calcifications or dense particulate matter may be seen in axillary lymph nodes, often in the setting of an asymptomatic woman undergoing a screening mammogram. If the material is calcium density, the differential diagnosis includes granulomatous disease, such as sarcoidosis and metastatic disease from breast cancer or ovarian cancer (psammomatous calcifications). In cases of metastatic disease, the lymph nodes have other features of malignancy in addition to calcifications, including loss of hilum and increased density. Axillary lymph node calcifications are identified in 3% of patients with breast cancer.

If the particulate matter in the nodes is of metal density, gold therapy (chrysotherapy) is often the reason. Other possibilities are silicone material in the nodes in patients who have had silicone implants or injections and tattoo pigment.

In the cases presented here, the woman in the first figure had a history of gold therapy for rheumatoid arthritis. The patient in the second figure underwent an ultrasound-guided core needle biopsy of an axillary node because of a concern that it might represent metastatic disease from ovarian cancer. The histology of the core biopsy was consistent with sarcoid, a granulomatous disease.

Notes

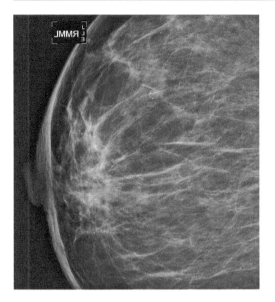

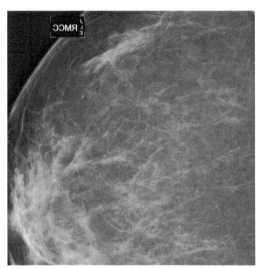

History: A woman with a personal history of left breast cancer presents for routine mammogram. New calcifications were seen in the right breast.

1. What should be included in the differential diagnosis for the magnification views shown? (Choose all that apply.)
   A. Benign calcifications
   B. Suspicious microcalcifications
   C. Milk of calcium
   D. Indeterminate calcifications

2. Why would ultrasound be utilized to evaluate calcifications?
   A. It is not useful; mammography is the only way to evaluate calcifications.
   B. Ultrasound is used to evaluate for a mass at the site of calcifications.
   C. It may be used to identify a mass but would not be used to target the biopsy.
   D. It is not helpful; MRI is better than ultrasound in evaluating extent of DCIS.

3. If ultrasound is performed and shows a mass associated with calcifications, what is the next step in management?
   A. Referral of the patient to a surgeon for excision
   B. Stereotactic biopsy
   C. Ultrasound-guided core biopsy
   D. Short-interval follow-up in 6 months

4. Which of the following is *not* an advantage of ultrasound-guided biopsy compared with stereotactic biopsy?
   A. Real-time imaging during the sampling
   B. Lack of ionizing radiation
   C. Patient comfort
   D. Improved samples from a larger bore needle

CASE 85

Use of Ultrasound to Evaluate Suspicious Microcalcifications

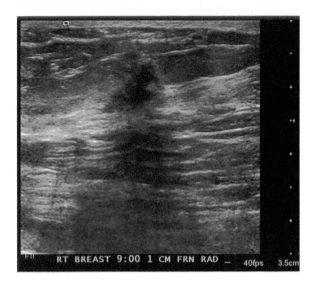

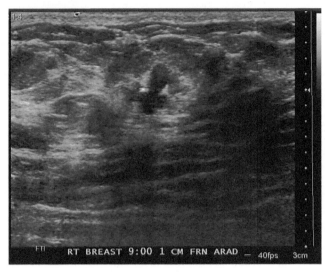

1. B and D
2. B
3. C
4. D

References

Cho N, Moon WK, Cha JH, et al: Ultrasound-guided vacuum-assisted biopsy of microcalcifications detected at screening mammography. *Acta Radiol* 2009;50(6):602-609.

Moon WK, Im JG, Koh YH, et al: US of mammographically detected clustered microcalcifications. *Radiology* 2000;217(3):849-854.

Soo MS, Baker JA, Rosen EL: Sonographic detection and sonographically guided biopsy of breast microcalcifications. *AJR Am J Roentgenol* 2003;180(4):941-948.

Cross-Reference

Ikeda D: *Breast Imaging: THE REQUISITES*, 2nd ed, Philadelphia: Saunders, 2010, p 212.

Comment

Newly developing microcalcifications detected on routine mammography may indicate malignant disease. The likelihood of calcifications representing malignancy is greater in elderly patients and in women with increased risk (see the figures). Biopsy is necessary unless the developing calcifications are characteristic of a benign type, such as milk of calcium, or lucent-centered calcifications. Stereotactic biopsy is often the method of choice for biopsy of calcifications. However, there are advantages to using ultrasound guidance, and if the finding can be seen on ultrasound, the biopsy can be performed using ultrasound guidance. Advantages of ultrasound-guided biopsy over stereotactic biopsy include real-time assessment of needle location during the sampling, patient comfort, quicker biopsy time, and lack of radiation exposure.

Several studies have shown that calcifications may not be seen on ultrasound, but if they are identified, there is a higher likelihood of malignancy. The calcifications may be in a mass, as in the patient in this case (see the figures) or in a duct. The presence of a hypoechoic mass heightens the visibility of tiny hyperechoic calcifications. Calcifications associated with a mass seen on ultrasound are more likely to be malignant (69% positive predictive value in one series).

Seeing a mass associated with microcalcifications on ultrasound and using ultrasound guidance to sample the mass, rather than just the calcifications on mammogram, increases the chances of sampling the invasive component of the disease. It is helpful to perform a specimen radiograph of the biopsied cores of tissue to check for calcifications.

In one study of 75 patients with microcalcifications seen on mammogram, 71% had calcifications retrieved on ultrasound-guided biopsy. The retrieval chance was higher when there was a mass or dilated duct associated with the calcifications (85% vs. 41% retrieval of calcifications not associated with a mass or dilated duct).

Notes

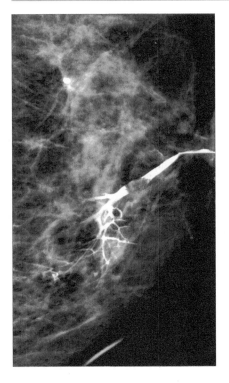 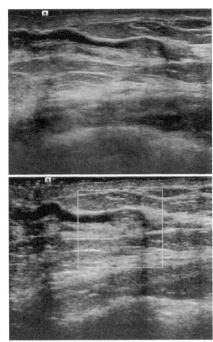 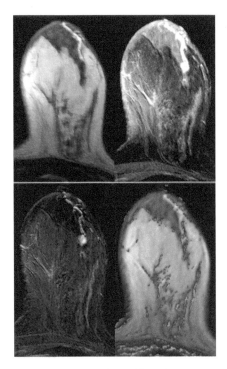

History: A 43-year-old woman presents with intermittent bloody discharge from the left nipple. The mammogram was negative (not shown). Ductography, ultrasound, and MRI were performed for further evaluation.

1. What should be included in the differential diagnosis? (Choose all that apply.)
   A. Ductal ectasia
   B. Ductal carcinoma in situ (DCIS)
   C. Intraductal papilloma
   D. Papillary carcinoma

2. Which of the following statements regarding nipple discharge is true?
   A. Bilateral nipple discharge and discharge from multiple openings should be evaluated with imaging.
   B. It is more common in postmenopausal women.
   C. Spontaneous bloody nipple discharge may be a sign of malignancy.
   D. Nipple discharge is a manifestation of breast pathology only.

3. Regarding imaging appearance of papillary lesions, which of the following statements is *false*?
   A. They may appear on the mammogram as microcalcifications.
   B. Ductogram usually shows involvement of multiple ductal systems.
   C. Intraductal papilloma appears on ultrasound as a solid mass with internal vascularity inside a duct.
   D. On MRI, papillomas appear as enhancing masses with or without a dilated duct.

4. Which of the following statements is *false*?
   A. Intraductal papillomas are considered high-risk lesions.
   B. Management of intraductal papillomas is controversial.
   C. A benign papilloma may evolve to a papillary carcinoma.
   D. Distinction between benign papillary lesions and papillary carcinoma is important.

Intraductal Papilloma

1. B, C, and D
2. C
3. B
4. C

References

Brookes MJ, Bourke AG: Radiological appearances of papillary breast lesions. *Clin Radiol* 2008;63(11):1265-1273.

Ibarra JA: Papillary lesions of the breast. *Breast J* 2006;12(3):237-251.

Kurz KD, Roy S, Saleh A, et al: MRI features of intraductal papilloma of the breast: sheep in wolf's clothing? *Acta Radiol* 2011;52 (3):264-272.

Cross-Reference

Ikeda D: *Breast Imaging: THE REQUISITES*, 2nd ed, Philadelphia: Saunders, 2010, p 383.

Comment

Papillary lesions are rare tumors, accounting for 0.7% to 4% of solid breast lesions. They include various pathologic processes, ranging from benign papillomas to papillary carcinomas. Benign papillary lesions are the most common intraductal mass. Histologically, they are benign ductal neoplasms with a papillary fibrovascular core covered with ductal epithelium and myoepithelial cells (the presence of myoepithelial cells differentiates benign papillomas from papillary carcinoma). Papillomas can be solitary or multiple, often arising in contiguous areas of a duct system. Solitary papillomas usually arise in a large duct near the nipple (central), whereas multiple papillomas most commonly occur in smaller, more peripheral ducts.

Many patients with solitary central papillomas present with nipple discharge. Bloody nipple discharge may occur if the papilloma twists on its fibrovascular stalk and becomes ischemic and necrotic, whereas clear (serous) nipple discharge may occur owing to secretions produced by the papilloma. Unilateral, bloody or serous nipple discharge from a single duct raises the level of concern because it may also be a manifestation of carcinoma. Bilateral or multiple duct, milky or green to brown discharges are not clinically significant, and they are usually associated with other conditions, such as fibrocystic change, hormonal imbalance, pregnancy and lactation, prolactinoma, and medication. In these cases, further evaluation with imaging is unnecessary. Nipple discharge generally may be present at any age.

Intraductal papillomas may be difficult to recognize with mammography. When visible, they may appear as round, often well-circumscribed subareolar masses with or without calcifications or as a small cluster of calcifications without a mammographically evident mass. Ductography can be helpful in localizing a papilloma within the discharging duct, which appears as an intraductal filling defect, sometimes with irregular borders (see the figures). On ultrasound, intraductal papillomas appear as a solid mass or masses with internal vascularity inside a duct, which may be focally dilated (see the figures).

MRI usually gives a more global picture and may reveal additional lesions in women with nipple discharge. On MRI, papillomas appear as enhancing masses with or without an accompanying dilated duct. The duct contents may have a different appearance depending on the fluid composition; serous content appears hypointense on T1-weighted images and hyperintense on T2-weighted images, whereas hemorrhagic content appears hyperintense on both T1-weighted and T2-weighted images.

Papillary lesions are considered high-risk lesions because some of them may be malignant, and many of them may contain atypical ductal hyperplasia or DCIS. In addition, DCIS and infiltrating ductal carcinoma may manifest as an intraductal mass. A benign papilloma does not evolve to a papillary carcinoma.

Histologic diagnosis is needed to exclude intraductal cancer. Recommendations on management vary. Although some clinicians advocate needle biopsy for initial diagnosis followed by excision, others recommend surgical excision only. If needle biopsy has been performed, some institutions excise all papillomas, whereas others excise only the ones with atypia. The patient in this case had a vacuum-assisted, ultrasound-guided core biopsy, which revealed an intraductal papilloma, with no atypia.

Notes

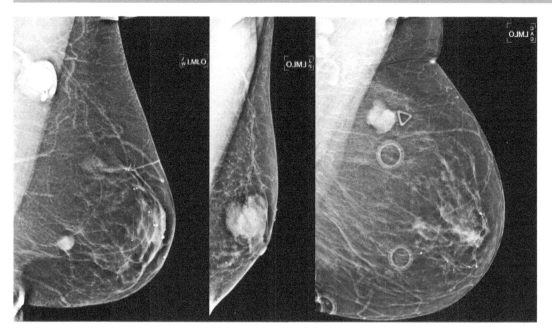

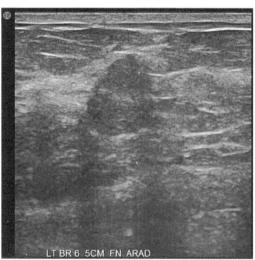

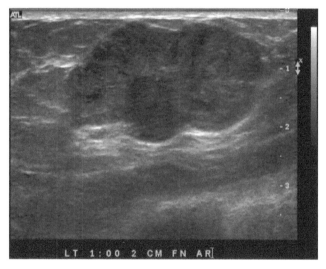

History: Three different patients present with a left breast palpable mass. The left mediolateral oblique (MLO) view and ultrasound images have been provided.

1. What should be included in the differential diagnosis of the palpable finding? (Choose all that apply.)
   A. Simple breast cyst
   B. Fibroadenoma
   C. Invasive ductal carcinoma (IDC), mucinous type
   D. Invasive ductal carcinoma, medullary type

2. What is the next step in management?
   A. MRI to differentiate benign from malignant
   B. Ultrasound-guided needle biopsy
   C. Fine-needle aspiration biopsy
   D. Short-interval follow-up ultrasound

3. What is mucinous carcinoma?
   A. A special type of invasive lobular carcinoma
   B. A tumor characterized by extracellular mucin
   C. Another name for medullary carcinoma
   D. A common subtype of IDC

4. What imaging characteristics are *not* seen with mucinous carcinoma?
   A. A dense mass on mammogram and isoechoic mass on ultrasound
   B. High signal intensity on T2-weighted MRI
   C. Markedly spiculated mass on mammography and dense shadowing on ultrasound
   D. Well-defined mass on mammography and cystic spaces seen on ultrasound

Mucinous Carcinoma

1. B, C, and D
2. B
3. B
4. C

References

Bode MK, Rissanen T: Imaging findings and accuracy of core needle biopsy in mucinous carcinoma of the breast. *Acta Radiol* 2011;52 (2):128-133.

Cardenosa G, Doudna C, Eklund GW: Mucinous (colloid) breast cancer clinical and mammographic findings in 10 patients. *AJR Am J Roentgenol* 1994;162(5):1077-1079.

Conant EF, Dillon RL, Palazzo J, et al: Imaging findings in mucin-containing carcinomas of the breast: correlation with pathologic features. *AJR Am J Roentgenol* 1994;163(4):821-824.

Cross-Reference

Ikeda D: *Breast Imaging: THE REQUISITES*, 2nd ed, Philadelphia: Saunders, 2010, p 114.

Comment

Mucinous carcinoma is a special type of IDC. The other special types are medullary, invasive papillary, and tubular carcinoma. The special types, as differentiated from IDC not otherwise specified (NOS), indicate a more differentiated cell type, with a better prognosis. Mucinous carcinoma manifests as a pure or mixed form. In the pure form, there are larger amounts of mucin (50% to 75%), and the lesion appears more well defined on mammography. The density of the tumor on mammography has been reported as denser than water, as in the patients in this case (see the figures), but also reported to be lower in density. In the pure form, the borders are smooth and lobulated. With the mixed form, the borders become more ill defined.

The pure form of mucinous carcinoma occurs more commonly in older women, average age 63, and is less likely to be palpable or, if palpable, is relatively soft. The pure form has positive axillary nodes in only 6%, and prognosis is better than in IDC NOS. However, in the mixed form, the tumor behavior is closer to IDC NOS, with a higher percentage of patients presenting with a hard palpable mass, positive nodes in 36%, and a worse prognosis.

The ultrasound appearance varies. Smaller masses (see the figures) are often isoechoic to fat and difficult to identify, and their appearance overlaps with fibroadenoma. However, in contrast to fibroadenomas, the tumors tend to be taller than wide, with a microlobulated surface (see the figures). They do not cause shadowing and may have enhanced through-transmission (see the figures). They may also contain cystic spaces.

On MRI, the mucinous carcinoma is bright on T2-weighted images and may have nonenhancing internal septa. These septa should be thicker than in fibroadenoma, but differentiating mucinous carcinoma from fibroadenoma on MRI may be difficult, particularly with the pure form of mucinous carcinoma. After contrast agent administration, the initial enhancement curve may be slow, intermediate, or rapid and then may be persistent or plateau, also overlapping with benign tumors.

Notes

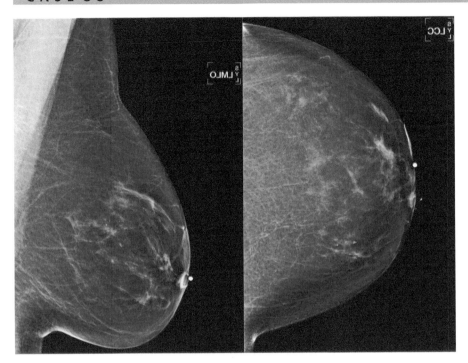

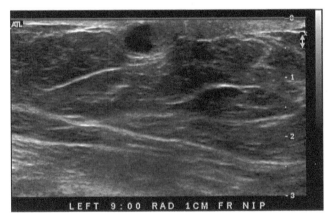

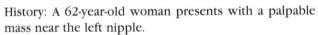

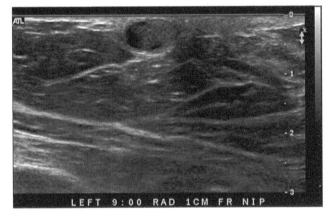

History: A 62-year-old woman presents with a palpable mass near the left nipple.

1. What should be included in the differential diagnosis based on the mammogram and ultrasound images shown? (Choose all that apply.)
   A. Sebaceous cyst
   B. Benign papilloma
   C. Lipoma
   D. Infiltrating ductal carcinoma

2. Is the ultrasound appearance diagnostic of a benign mass?
   A. No, because there is irregular solid material within the mass
   B. Yes, because the mass is oval and wider than tall
   C. Yes, because the location suggests it is in the dermal layer
   D. Yes, because the borders are smooth and well defined

3. What is the next step in management?
   A. Core biopsy
   B. Fine-needle aspiration biopsy
   C. Short-interval follow-up because this may be a sebaceous cyst
   D. MRI of both breasts to evaluate for abnormal enhancement

4. If pathology is benign papilloma on core biopsy, what is the next step?
   A. Short-interval follow-up
   B. Annual mammography
   C. Surgical consultation for excision
   D. MRI to evaluate enhancement of the mass

Palpable Subcutaneous Mass

1. A, B, and D
2. A
3. A
4. C

References

Berg WA, Campassi CI, Ioffe OB: Cystic lesions of the breast: sonographic-pathologic correlation. *Radiology* 2003;227(1):183-191.

Rinaldi P, Ierardi C, Costantini M, et al: Cystic breast lesions: sonographic findings and clinical management. *J Ultrasound Med* 2010;29(11):1617-1626.

Cross-Reference

Ikeda D: *Breast Imaging: THE REQUISITES*, 2nd ed, Philadelphia: Saunders, 2010, pp 120, 383.

Comment

This 62-year-old woman presented with a palpable mass near the nipple. Mammography was performed first (see the figures). Ultrasound was then performed, and the images showed an oval, sharply circumscribed, complex cystic mass, located in the superficial breast adjacent to the nipple. All of the ultrasound features are benign except for the echogenic, irregular material within the mass (see the figures).

The BI-RADS (Breast Imaging Reporting and Data System) code and the decision to perform a biopsy of a mass should be based on the worst characteristic, which is the irregular material within the cystic mass in this patient. This mass is termed a *complex cystic mass,* which has an increased chance of being malignant compared with a *complicated cyst* or *simple cyst.* (A complicated cyst contains internal echoes on ultrasound.) Ultrasound features of a complex cystic mass are thick, irregular septations; thick, irregular wall; indistinct or angular margins; intracystic mass; and associated solid component. In one series, 18 of 79 complex cystic lesions were malignant.

Core biopsy of this mass was performed, and histology showed intraductal papilloma. The mass was excised, and the surgical histopathology was infiltrating ductal carcinoma, grade II/III, micropapillary type, with ductal carcinoma in situ at the surgical margin.

This case illustrates that biopsy should be performed on cystic lesions that contain intracystic masses. If a papilloma is diagnosed at core biopsy, surgical excision should be considered. There is a 12% to 14% risk of "upgrading" the benign papillary lesion to carcinoma on excision.

This case also illustrates that palpable masses that are negative on mammography should be evaluated further with ultrasound. This is true particularly for a mass felt near the nipple, where a mass may be overlooked or obscured by the nipple and subareolar ducts.

Notes

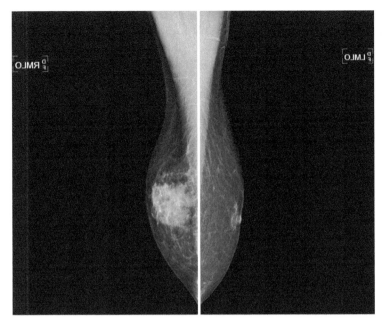

History: A 70-year-old man presents with a tender palpable right breast mass.

1. What is the differential diagnosis in this patient? (Choose all that apply.)
   A. Normal male breast tissue
   B. Right breast cancer
   C. Asymmetric gynecomastia
   D. Right breast lipoma

2. What imaging studies are needed to evaluate a palpable mass in a male?
   A. Unilateral mammogram and ultrasound of the area of concern
   B. Bilateral mammogram; add ultrasound if needed
   C. Both mammography and MRI
   D. Ultrasound only is sufficient.

3. What is the etiology of gynecomastia?
   A. Altered hormone levels, liver disease, renal disease, hyperthyroidism, medication
   B. Family history of breast cancer
   C. Overweight
   D. Multiple lipomas on the trunk, arms, and legs

4. What is the usual presentation?
   A. Tender mass behind the nipple
   B. Bilateral masses in the upper outer quadrant of the breast
   C. Axillary adenopathy and a palpable breast mass
   D. Nipple discharge

Male Gynecomastia

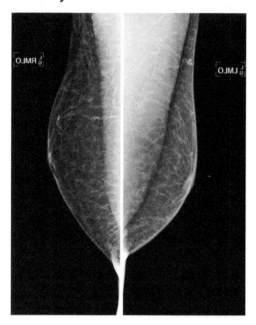

1. B and C
2. B
3. A
4. A

References

Appelbaum AH, Evans GFF, Levy KR, et al: Mammographic appearances of male breast disease. *Radiographics* 1999;19:559-568.

Braunstein GD: Gynecomastia. *N Engl J Med* 1993;328(7):490-495.

Chen L: Imaging characteristics of malignant lesions of the male breast. *Radiographics* 2006;26(4):993-1006.

Cross-Reference

Ikeda D: *Breast Imaging: THE REQUISITES*, 2nd ed, Philadelphia: Saunders, 2010, pp 370-374.

Comment

This patient is a 70-year-old man being treated for prostate cancer. Gynecomastia is a common condition in men, and it is the most common reason for men to present for a mammogram. It is an overgrowth of ductal epithelium and stromal elements; it may be tender on exam and may be detected by the patient or the referring physician. The differential diagnosis for a palpable mass in a man includes breast cancer, lipoma, epithelial inclusion cyst, fat necrosis, lymph node, and hematoma.

Gynecomastia develops from high exogenous or endogenous estrogen levels or a decrease in testosterone. It is also related to endocrine disorders; liver, kidney, or lung disease; and many medications. Men who present with a mass should initially have a bilateral mammogram.

The mammogram in gynecomastia classically shows a fan-shaped area of density behind the nipple. The edges of the mass fade into the surrounding fat (see the figures). There is also a nodular form in which the edges may be well circumscribed. The focal asymmetry seen can extend into the upper outer quadrant of the breast and is often asymmetric. It can also occur at some distance from the nipple. It can be unilateral or bilateral. Note in the first figure, the left breast also has a density behind the nipple, although smaller than on the right. Compare to the second figure, of a normal male breast.

Ultrasound of the palpable finding may be important because gynecomastia can obscure a small cancer on the mammogram. On ultrasound, the entire area of gynecomastia should be evaluated for a hypoechoic mass. Gynecomastia should not contain a mass. If the density is well evaluated by mammography alone, and there is no suggestion of mass within the glandular density, ultrasound is not necessary.

Solid masses or complex cysts seen on ultrasound are suspicious for malignancy. Hyperechoic masses contiguous with the skin are typical for epidermal inclusion cysts. Fat necrosis has a varying appearance but is usually hyperechoic and can shadow. Lipomas are typically hyperechoic, located in the subdermal layer, oval, and wider than tall. This is an example of bilateral, asymmetric gynecomastia. This concern is managed clinically. Surgery is not necessary.

In the second figure, a mammogram is shown of a symptomatic 45-year-old patient who felt palpable fullness on both sides. This is the mammogram of a normal male breast, with no ductal proliferation or masses. This is referred to as *pseudogynecomastia*.

Notes

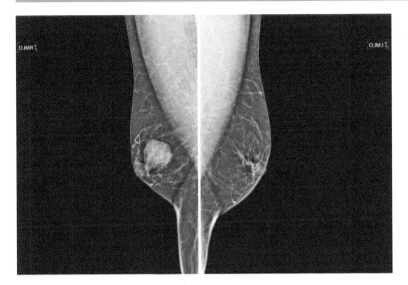

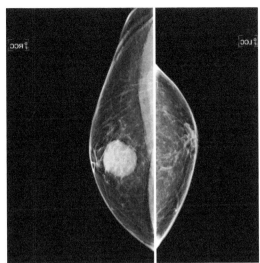

History: A 60-year-old man presents with a palpable mass in his right breast.

1. What is the differential diagnosis in this patient, based on the mammogram? (Choose all that apply.)
   A. Lipoma
   B. Sebaceous cyst
   C. Breast malignancy
   D. Gynecomastia

2. What is the next step in the work-up?
   A. MRI is performed to differentiate benign from malignant.
   B. Ultrasound
   C. Recommend a short-interval follow-up because this is possibly an infectious mass.
   D. No work-up is needed for this benign mass.

3. How common is male breast cancer?
   A. Men comprise approximately 10% of the breast cancer population.
   B. Men comprise approximately 25% of the breast cancer population.
   C. Men comprise approximately 5% of the breast cancer population.
   D. Men comprise approximately 1% of the breast cancer population.

4. What masses do *not* occur in the male breast?
   A. Lipoma
   B. Abscess
   C. Sebaceous cyst
   D. Fibroadenoma

C A S E 9 0

Male Breast Cancer

1. C and D
2. B
3. D
4. D

References

Appelbaum AH, Evans GFF, Levy KR, et al: Mammographic appearances of male breast disease. *Radiographics* 1999;19:559-568.

Fentiman IS, Fourquet A, Hortobagyi GN: Male breast cancer. *Lancet* 2006;367(9510):595-604.

Cross-Reference

Ikeda D: *Breast Imaging: THE REQUISITES*, 2nd ed, Philadelphia: Saunders, 2010, pp 370-376.

Comment

A mass in the male breast is most commonly benign. Gynecomastia is the most common finding and is typically a fan-shaped density centered on the nipple, although it can be remote from the nipple. Other masses include sebaceous cyst, lipoma, and abscess. Malignancy is relatively uncommon, but, as with palpable masses in women, it deserves serious consideration whenever a man presents with a palpable mass.

The work-up begins with a bilateral, four-view standard mammogram, with a marker placed over the area of clinical concern (see the figures). Ultrasound is a very useful imaging tool in the male patient, because it can help determine if the mass is in the skin, as in sebaceous cyst, an echogenic lipoma (typically the mammogram is normal, and the lipoma is not seen against the background of normal fatty breast), or an abscess (usually seen in the setting of an inflamed, tender breast). Breast cancer in men has an appearance similar to ductal carcinoma in women: a circumscribed mass that can rarely include the presence of calcifications (see the figures). Ductal carcinoma in situ (DCIS) can also occur; it accounts for approximately 10% of male breast cancer, with calcifications seen on the mammogram. Most tumors are of ductal origin. Presentation is usually more advanced than the presentation of breast cancer in women, with more than 40% presenting in stage III or IV. This late presentation is related to the lack of screening. Men are not screened with imaging for breast cancer, so detection is delayed until a mass is felt.

Risk factors include increased estrogen levels (Klinefelter's syndrome, gonadal dysfunction, cirrhosis, obesity), radiation exposure, and family history, particularly with *BRCA2* mutation. Male breast cancer is not related to gynecomastia. Peak age of incidence is 71 years, and in the majority of men, breast cancer is diagnosed after age 60 years.

Notes

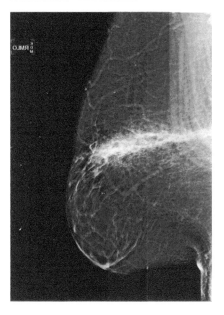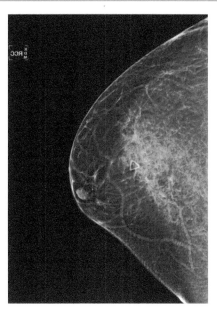

History: A 70-year-old woman presents with a palpable concern in her right breast. She reveals a recent history of a motor vehicle accident in which she was in the passenger seat.

1. What is the differential diagnosis for the mammographic findings in the right breast? (Choose all that apply.)
   A. Band of increased density, highly suspicious for malignancy
   B. Band of increased density, consistent with trauma from seat belt in motor vehicle accident
   C. Increased density in segmental distribution, suggesting malignant spread along ducts
   D. Band of increased density, consistent with surgical scar

2. What is the next step in the work-up?
   A. Nothing, the mammogram is diagnostic.
   B. MRI should be performed to differentiate malignancy from trauma.
   C. Ultrasound of the palpable finding should be performed.

3. What is the etiology of this finding on the mammogram?
   A. The seat belt forcibly compresses the breast tissue, causing trauma in the form of bleeding, which can lead to fat necrosis.
   B. The breast hits the steering wheel, causing trauma.
   C. There is increased density caused by fibrocystic change.
   D. Increased density is a result of malignancy in a regional distribution.

4. What follow-up should be recommended for traumatic injury to the breast?
   A. The patient should be followed every 6 months with mammograms and ultrasound.
   B. Biopsy is needed for the palpable mass.
   C. The patient should be referred to a surgeon.
   D. Annual mammogram is sufficient.

Seat Belt Trauma

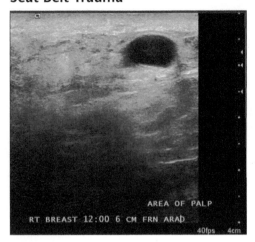

1. B and D
2. C
3. A
4. D

References
DiPiro P, Meyer J, Frenna T, Denison C: Seat belt injuries of the breast: findings on mammography and sonography. *AJR Am J Roentgenol* 1995;164:317-320.

Majeski J: Shoulder restraint injury of the female breast. *Int Surg* 2007;92:99-102.

Cross-Reference
Ikeda D: *Breast Imaging: THE REQUISITES*, 2nd ed, Philadelphia: Saunders, 2010, p 75.

Comment

The three-point seat belt is commonly used in automobiles. When a collision occurs, the breast can be forcibly compressed between the belt and the rib cage. The diagonal shoulder portion of the seat belt can cause a bandlike injury to the breast, usually to the left breast in the driver and to the right breast in the passenger. Fractures of the clavicle, ribs, and sternum can also occur, depending on the severity of the collision.

Mild injury results in bruising, skin blistering, breast swelling, tenderness, and friction burns over the contact area. More severe crush injury includes hematoma formation, fat necrosis, and skin laceration. Even more severe injury can result in laceration or even transection of the breast, with severe bleeding.

The mammographic appearance of the injury is typically a band of increased density that follows the path of the seat belt, diagonally across the breast. The increased density reflects edema and hematoma formation, and it is easier to see the injury if the breast tissue is predominantly fatty, as in this patient (see the figures). Fat necrosis can develop, typically seen as lucent round masses (oil cysts), often with rim-type calcification. The hematoma and fat necrosis can be palpable and tender.

In this patient (see the figures), the breast is predominantly fatty, and there is a discrete linear band of increased density in the upper breast. The palpable finding on the patient's self-exam has been marked with a marker, and ultrasound of the area (see the figures) demonstrates an anechoic mass, consistent with oil cyst, and surrounding echogenic edema. These mammographic and ultrasound findings indicate seat belt trauma. No further follow-up is necessary in this patient. Routine annual mammograms can be recommended.

Notes

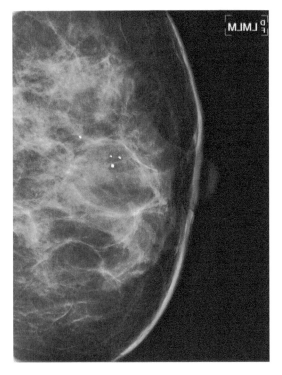
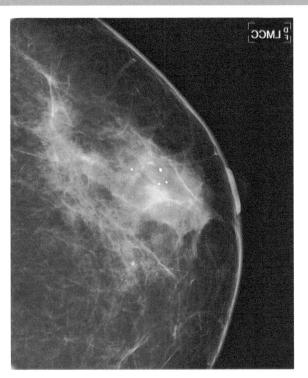

History: A 48-year-old woman whose mother was recently diagnosed with breast cancer at age 72 undergoes a routine screening mammogram. Microcalcifications are seen in the left breast.

1. What should be included in the differential diagnosis of the microcalcifications seen? (Choose all that apply.)
   A. Ductal carcinoma in situ (DCIS)
   B. Atypical ductal hyperplasia (ADH)
   C. Fibrocystic change
   D. Dermal calcifications in the lower left breast

2. What is the next step in management?
   A. MRI to check for abnormal enhancement
   B. Follow-up magnification views in 6 months
   C. Stereotactic needle biopsy
   D. Return to screening

3. When is a biopsy result discordant?
   A. When ADH is upgraded to DCIS on surgical excision
   B. When there are no calcifications on the specimen radiograph
   C. When the biopsy results match the expected outcome based on imaging
   D. When the patient has an infection as a result of the biopsy

4. Which of the following is a high-risk lesion?
   A. DCIS
   B. ADH
   C. Focal fibrosis
   D. Extensive intraductal component

CASE 92

Atypical Ductal Hyperplasia

1. A, B, and C
2. C
3. B
4. B

References

Eby PR, Ochsner JE, DeMartini WB, et al: Is surgical excision necessary for focal atypical ductal hyperplasia found at stereotactic vacuum-assisted breast biopsy? *Ann Surg Oncol* 2008;15(11):3232-3238.

Kohr JR, Eby PR, Allison KH, et al: Risk of upgrade of atypical ductal hyperplasia after stereotactic breast biopsy: effects of number of foci and complete removal of calcifications. *Radiology* 2010;255 (3):723-730.

Liberman L, Smolkin JH, Dershaw DD, et al: Calcification retrieval at stereotactic, 11-gauge, directional, vacuum-assisted breast biopsy. *Radiology* 1998;208(1):251-260.

Cross-Reference

Ikeda D: *Breast Imaging: THE REQUISITES*, 2nd ed, Philadelphia: Saunders, 2010, p 230.

Comment

ADH is a condition in the spectrum of epithelial proliferative disease that leads to DCIS and invasive ductal carcinoma. The presence of ADH increases a woman's risk of breast cancer to four to five times that of the general population. Histologically, ADH may contain all of the features of low-grade DCIS but to a limited degree. ADH is found on mammography by calcifications (see the figures). A focal density may be seen, and rarely ADH develops at the edge of a radial scar or focal area of sclerosing adenosis, seen on mammogram as spiculation. ADH may differ from DCIS only by degree of abnormality.

A core biopsy is a sampling procedure only. When ADH is found on core biopsy, as in the present patient, excision should be performed. The potential exists for inadequate sampling with core needle technique, and DCIS or invasive carcinoma may be adjacent to the ADH sampled. When ADH is excised, and the excision specimen shows malignancy, this is termed *upgrading*. The rate of upgrade from core biopsy to excision of ADH to DCIS is approximately 20%. When the degree of ADH is greater in the tissue specimens, the upgrade rate to DCIS is higher. In one recent study, if at least three foci of ADH were present in the needle biopsy samples, the rate of upgrade to DCIS was 28%.

ADH cannot be a Breast Imaging Reporting and Data System (BI-RADS) 3 lesion because this requires a 2% or less chance of malignancy. It is a BI-RADS 4 lesion, and excision is recommended. This patient had ADH on 10-gauge vacuum-assisted biopsy, and excision showed DCIS grade III.

Notes

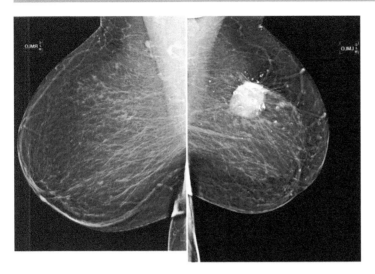

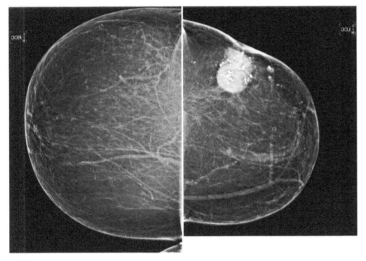

History: A 71-year-old woman returns for routine imaging 9 years after breast conservation therapy for infiltrating ductal carcinoma in the left breast.

1. What is the differential diagnosis for this mammogram? (Choose all that apply.)
   A. Calcified mass in the left breast, consistent with hematoma or seroma plus fat necrosis at the lumpectomy site
   B. Calcified mass in the left breast, highly suspicious for recurrent cancer at the lumpectomy site
   C. Calcified mass in the left breast; cannot exclude recurrent cancer at the lumpectomy site
   D. Calcified fibroadenoma

2. What is the next step in the management of this patient?
   A. Perform MRI to evaluate for neovascularity in the mass.
   B. Compare prior films.
   C. Perform ultrasound.

3. When prior mammograms are compared, the mass is stable, and the coarse calcifications have increased in and around the mass. What is the Breast Imaging Reporting and Data System (BI-RADS) category and next step?
   A. BI-RADS 4—recommend biopsy
   B. BI-RADS 2—1-year follow-up mammogram
   C. BI-RADS 0—need additional magnification views
   D. BI-RADS 3—short-interval follow-up

4. If the mass is palpable, does that change your management?
   A. Yes, a palpable mass at the lumpectomy site should be biopsied.
   B. Yes, any palpable mass in a cancer patient should be biopsied.
   C. No, this is a firm calcified hematoma at the lumpectomy site; it is superficial in the breast and would be expected to be palpable.
   D. No, but ultrasound should be performed to evaluate a palpable mass at the lumpectomy site.

Postoperative Hematoma

1. A and C
2. B
3. B
4. C

References
Bloomer WD, Berenberg AL, Weissman BN: Mammography of the definitively irradiated breast. *Radiology* 1976;118:425-428.

Brenner RJ, Pfaff JM: Mammographic features after conservation therapy for malignant breast disease: serial findings standardized by regression analysis. *AJR Am J Roentgenol* 1996;167:171-178.

Cross-Reference
Ikeda D: *Breast Imaging: THE REQUISITES*, 2nd ed, Philadelphia: Saunders, 2010, pp 307-318.

Comment

Breast conservation therapy is an alternative to mastectomy. Surgical excision of the tumor (lumpectomy) and radiation therapy to the whole breast, and sometimes to the chest wall and axilla, are performed. Some patients are treated with localized, rather than whole-breast, radiation. Expected changes that are seen in the treated breast include:

- Increased interstitial markings throughout the breast and skin thickening due to edema
- Architectural distortion at the lumpectomy site
- Hematoma or seroma at the lumpectomy site
- Calcifications within the surgical bed and radiation field due to fat necrosis

These findings may be seen in the first follow-up mammogram after radiation therapy is completed (usually 6 months after completion). All findings usually decrease in prominence over time during the next 5 years, except for calcifications of fat necrosis, which commonly persist.

In this patient (see the figures), the surgical seroma/hematoma did not resolve over time. Nine years after surgery and radiation, the hematoma is the same size. This is a relatively uncommon result after breast conservation therapy. The majority of hematomas resolve spontaneously. In this patient, calcifications consistent with fat necrosis developed at the hematoma site, which is commonly seen.

Hematomas that develop at the lumpectomy site need not be aspirated. They may be quite difficult to aspirate owing to organization of the clot with fibrin. If they are symptomatic, painful, or inflamed, surgical drainage may be indicated.

Ultrasound of the lumpectomy site can be performed if there is concern that the developing mass at the site may be tumor rather than fluid collection. However, the complex appearance of the hematoma and developing fat necrosis can be confused with malignancy. Extensive calcification in the wall of the hematoma/seroma, as in this case (see the figures), can cause dense shadowing on ultrasound, limiting interpretation. MRI can be used to evaluate fat necrosis, but this can be tricky because fat necrosis can enhance. The mammogram is the single best tool for evaluating and managing the patient with a postoperative hematoma and fat necrosis.

Notes

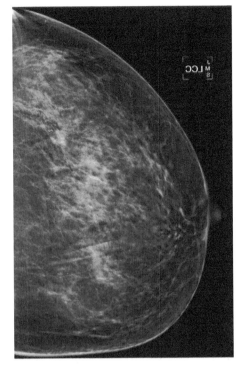 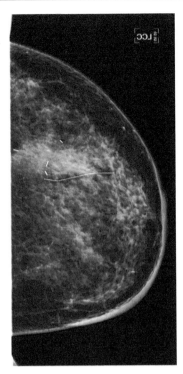 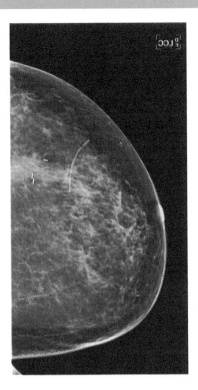

History: A 47-year-old woman developed a malignant mass in her left breast and was treated with breast conservation therapy (surgery and whole-breast irradiation). Images are shown on the day of needle biopsy, immediately after treatment, and 2 years after treatment.

1. What is the differential diagnosis for the appearance of the breast in the second figure?
   A. Inflammatory breast cancer
   B. Infection in the breast (mastitis)
   C. Expected changes after breast conservation therapy
   D. Recurrent cancer

2. What are the findings expected on mammography after breast conservation therapy?
   A. Infection
   B. Edema
   C. Calcifications indicating recurrent cancer
   D. Malignancy developing in the contralateral breast

3. What does the mammogram 2 years after completion of therapy demonstrate?
   A. Increase in skin edema
   B. Enlargement of the biopsy cavity
   C. Decreased edema
   D. Increase in fat necrosis calcifications

4. Why are magnification views performed after breast conservation therapy?
   A. To evaluate the seroma at the lumpectomy site
   B. To evaluate for residual and recurrent malignancy
   C. To evaluate punctate calcifications seen after radiation therapy
   D. To evaluate typical fat necrosis calcifications

Breast Conservation Therapy

1. B, C, and D
2. B
3. C
4. B

References

Brenner RJ, Pfaff JM: Mammographic features after conservation therapy for malignant breast disease: serial findings standardized by regression analysis. *AJR Am J Roentgenol* 1996;167:171-178.

Dershaw DD, Shank B, Reisinger S: Mammographic findings after breast cancer treatment with local excision and definitive irradiation. *Radiology* 1987;164:455-461.

Cross-Reference

Ikeda D: *Breast Imaging: THE REQUISITES*, 2nd ed, Philadelphia: Saunders, 2010, p 318.

Comment

To conserve the breast after breast cancer has been diagnosed, local therapy is performed. This includes surgical excision of the malignancy usually followed by radiation therapy. (In some cases of very early disease, radiation therapy might not be given.) Radiation can be given as whole-breast irradiation or as partial-breast irradiation to the tumor site.

This patient had an 8-mm infiltrating ductal carcinoma, initially seen on screening mammogram. Ultrasound exam detected the small mass in the upper outer quadrant of the left breast. Biopsy was performed with ultrasound guidance, with a clip placed on completion of the biopsy (see the figures). She then had surgical excision followed by whole-breast irradiation. The mammogram in the second figure is a view of her left breast after surgery and radiation (breast conservation therapy).

After therapy there are expected changes in the breast that are important to recognize. A mass is usually present at the lumpectomy site. This represents the biopsy cavity filled with serous fluid (seroma) and blood (hematoma). There may be surgical clips at the site, placed at the time of surgery. There are often architectural distortion at the surgical site and skin retraction from the scar. Clips and distortion might also be seen in the axilla if axillary node surgery was performed.

The breast will also show changes from irradiation, which initially is predominantly the result of edema. In the skin this appears as skin thickening, and in the interstitial tissues of the breast this is seen as thickening of the white trabecular markings in the breast. About 25% of patients develop calcifications at the lumpectomy site, which may be benign punctate types, rim-type calcifications indicating fat necrosis, or suture calcifications. Fat necrosis can develop, seen as lucent mass, spiculated density, and calcifications. In this patient, shown in the second figure immediately after treatment, skin and trabecular thickening is present, as well as a mass and distortion at the lumpectomy site.

With time, generally up to 3 years, in most patients the changes resolve, as is seen in the last figure. Calcifications of fat necrosis can increase as time progresses. Edema and cavity size should not increase over time, and they usually resolve, as in this patient. However, these findings can remain stable over time in a small proportion of patients.

Notes

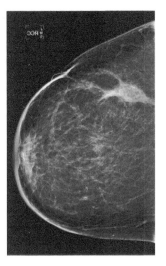
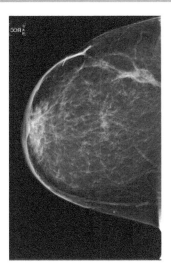
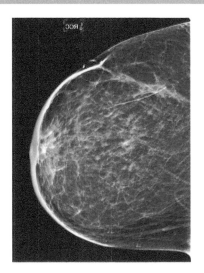

History: A 51-year-old woman was diagnosed with mucinous carcinoma in the outer right breast. She was treated with breast conservation therapy including lumpectomy and external-beam radiation therapy. Annual follow-up mammograms are shown, beginning with the third year after treatment.

1. What should be included in the differential diagnosis based on the images shown? (Choose all that apply.)
   A. Recurrent cancer in the right breast at the lumpectomy site
   B. Fat necrosis at the lumpectomy site
   C. Skin thickening suggestive of lymphovascular invasion
   D. Normal postlumpectomy and radiation changes

2. Which of the following is *not* an expected appearance of the breast 2 years after lumpectomy and radiation?
   A. Mass at the lumpectomy site
   B. Dystrophic calcifications
   C. Architectural distortion
   D. Increased density at the surgical site compared with previous mammogram

3. What is the benefit of radiation given to women being treated for breast cancer?
   A. Radiation reduces the recurrence rate at the surgical site.
   B. Radiation reduces recurrences away from the surgical site.
   C. The overall survival of women with lumpectomy and radiation is better than survival of women having mastectomy.
   D. The reduced recurrence rate is mitigated by the complications of slower healing and edema.

4. What is the MRI appearance of the lumpectomy site after conservation therapy?
   A. Seroma or hematoma that is hyperintense on T2, thin-rim enhancement after contrast
   B. Focal areas of irregular enhancement due to fat necrosis, increasing over time
   C. Increased enhancement throughout the breast caused by chemotherapy
   D. Enhancement of the skin caused by radiation therapy

C A S E 9 5

Postoperative Breast

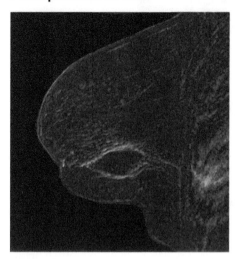

1. B and D
2. D
3. A
4. A

References

Brennan S, Liberman L, Dershaw DD, et al: Breast MRI screening of women with a personal history of breast cancer. *AJR Am J Roentgenol* 2010;195(2):510-516.

Carvelho BP, Frasson AL, Santo MM, et al: Mammography findings following electron intraoperative radiotherapy or external radiotherapy for breast cancer treatment. *Eur J Radiol* 2011;79(2):e7-e10.

Dershaw DD: Mammography in patients with breast cancer treated by breast conservation (lumpectomy with or without radiation). *AJR Am J Roentgenol* 1995;164(2):309-316.

Krishnamurthy R, Whitman GJ, Stelling CB, et al: Mammographic findings after breast conservation therapy. *Radiographics* 1999;19 (Spec No):S53-S62.

Mitnick J, Roses DF, Harris MN: Differentiation of postsurgical changes from carcinoma of the breast. *Surg Gynecol Obstet* 1988;166 (6):549-550.

Cross-Reference

Ikeda D: *Breast Imaging: THE REQUISITES*, 2nd ed, Philadelphia: Saunders, 2010, p 307.

Comment

Breast conservation therapy is commonly used as a treatment of breast cancer. The term *breast conservation therapy* includes lumpectomy and radiation therapy, often external-beam, whole-breast radiation therapy. Lumpectomy is wide excision of the tumor, with the excisional cavity left to fill in with fluid. Radiation therapy begins several weeks after surgery and continues for about 6 weeks.

This treatment causes changes in the breast, and it is important for the radiologist to understand the changes that are seen in routine healing and to differentiate those changes from the findings seen with recurrent cancer. Evidence of recurrence is rare before 18 months. Mammography has been the imaging method of choice for postoperative surveillance, but ultrasound and MRI are also useful to supplement the mammogram.

Mammogram findings after surgery and radiation therapy include masses, fluid collections, increased breast density, skin thickening, architectural distortion, and calcifications. Radiation therapy exacerbates these findings and delays their resolution. The masses seen may represent hematoma, seroma, abscess, fat necrosis, or fibrosis. These findings evolve over time, with decrease in the size of the mass until stable. Any changes after stabilization, in particular, increased masslike density and pleomorphic calcifications, should be viewed with suspicion.

This patient underwent breast conservation therapy 6 years ago for a 7-mm mucinous carcinoma. The first mammogram view shown is from her follow-up mammogram 3 years after treatment and shows a focal oval mass at the lumpectomy site, with increased interstitial markings and skin thickening (see the figures). On the next mammogram, 1 year later, the mass is smaller and less dense (see the figures). These changes are continual, as shown over 4 years (see the figures). There is no evidence of developing mass or microcalcifications. The patient has skin thickening, particularly apparent in the anterior breast; this is common after radiation therapy and may persist. Normal skin thickness is 2 mm; after radiation therapy, the skin thickness may measure 10 mm. This skin thickening is initially due to small vessel damage and later is due to fibrotic change.

This patient does not have calcifications, but they are commonly seen after therapy; 28% of patients develop calcifications at the surgical site within 12 months of treatment. These are benign dystrophic calcifications, or fat necrosis, and rarely suture calcifications. If the calcifications are few and punctate, they can usually be followed. If pleomorphic calcifications are seen, this may be due to fat necrosis, but biopsy may be needed to exclude recurrence. The ability of mammography to detect recurrence has been estimated at 25% to 45%. Ultrasound and MRI are also used to increase the detection rate. MRI is sensitive for the differentiation between scar and recurrence.

MRI can be used to evaluate for residual disease and to screen high-risk women. The American Cancer Society guidelines for screening breast MRI found no convincing evidence to support screening women with a personal history of breast cancer if they had no other risk factors. However, a recent study found detection of recurrent cancer in 12% of biopsy specimens of developing MRI abnormalities in patients with previous breast conservation therapy. The fourth figure is an MRI scan of a different patient who had breast conservation therapy. The seroma cavity is bordered by a rim of uniformly thin enhancement, consistent with healing. There is no evidence of recurrence. MRI evidence of residual or recurrent disease includes thick, irregular enhancement around the seroma, or an enhancing mass.

Notes

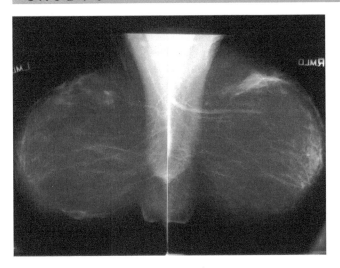

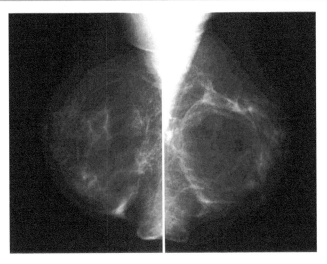

History: Asymptomatic 45-year-old woman, with two sets of screening mammograms 2 years apart.

1. What is the differential diagnosis for this set of mammograms? (Choose all that apply.)
   A. The patient had cancer and had bilateral lumpectomies.
   B. The patient has had bilateral reduction mammaplasty.
   C. The patient has lost weight.
   D. The patient has undergone pregnancy and lactational changes.

2. What are the expected changes on the mammogram for this circumstance?
   A. Architectural distortion
   B. Punctate calcifications
   C. Fat lucency
   D. All of the above

3. Is there an increased risk of malignancy with this surgery?
   A. Yes, any surgery increases the risk of cancer.
   B. Yes, the scar tissue can mask malignancy.
   C. No, there is no increased risk.
   D. Yes, women with larger breasts have inherently higher risk than women with smaller breasts.

4. What is a common problem after reduction mammaplasty?
   A. Palpable lump along the scars
   B. Increased cyclic pain before menses
   C. Nipple discharge
   D. Increased "heaviness" of the breasts

Reduction Mammaplasty

1. B and C
2. D
3. C
4. A

References

Douglas-Jones AG, Varma M: Screening at breast reduction: more than a little extra work. *BMJ* 2009;338:b2342.

Muir TM, Tresham J, Fritschi L, Wylie E: Screening for breast cancer post reduction mammoplasty. *Clin Radiol* 2010;65(3):198-205.

Tarone RE, Lipworth L, Young VL, McLaughlin JK: Breast reduction surgery and breast cancer risk: does reduction mammaplasty have a role in primary prevention strategies for women at high risk of breast cancer? *Plast Reconstr Surg* 2004;113(7):2104-2110.

Cross-Reference

Ikeda D: *Breast Imaging: THE REQUISITES*, 2nd ed, Philadelphia: Saunders, 2010, pp 360-346.

Comment

Reduction mammaplasty is a relatively common surgery performed on the breast for cosmetic reasons. Usually, this is done to reduce the size and weight of the breast, but it may also be performed to "lift" the breast. The surgeon makes incisions in the breast, removes breast tissue, and then may replace the nipple higher on the mound of the breast. The incisions most commonly used are a vertical scar from the nipple to the inframammary fold, a transverse incision along the inframammary fold, and a circumareolar incision if the nipple is moved up.

The incisions made in the breast will lead to scar formation and not uncommonly to fat necrosis. The scar tissue can develop calcifications. The most common mammography findings after reduction surgery are architectural distortion, punctate calcifications, focal fat lucency, and lines of density along the scars, as seen in this case (see the figures). Also, skin thickening may be seen in the lower breast, at the scar, and the ducts might appear to terminate lower than the nipple because the nipple has been moved up.

Technologists should always chronicle any breast surgery on the patient's history form before performing the mammogram.

Some patients present with a palpable lump after reduction mammoplasty, often along the scar tissue. Mammographic views of the palpable finding should be performed, and if fat necrosis is seen, no further workup is necessary. The patient might want to be seen by her plastic surgeon for reassurance. If the mammogram shows no signs of fat necrosis, ultrasound of the palpable finding should be performed. Fat necrosis on ultrasound may have the appearance of a hypoechoic round mass with a thick echogenic border, but ultrasound appearance can be variable. Fat lucency is required on the mammogram to dismiss the palpable finding as fat necrosis. If there is uncertainty about the etiology of the palpable mass, biopsy should be considered.

Notes

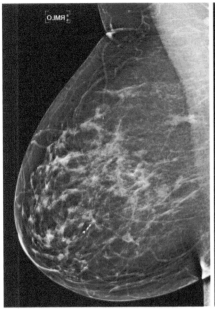
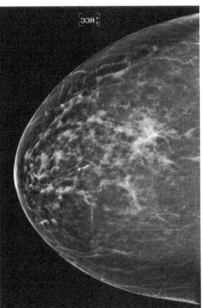
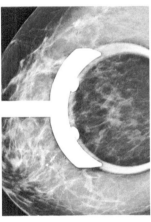
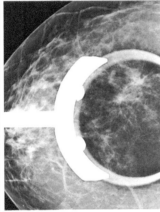

History: A 64-year-old asymptomatic woman underwent a routine screening mammogram. She has a family history of breast cancer in her daughter, diagnosed at age 37, and in her grandmother, age unknown. She is recalled for additional views.

1. What should be included in the differential diagnosis for the images shown? (Choose all that apply.)
   A. Radial scar
   B. Invasive ductal carcinoma (IDC)
   C. Invasive lobular carcinoma (ILC)
   D. Ductal carcinoma in situ (DCIS)

2. Why is the distortion better seen on one view?
   A. The craniocaudal (CC) view has more compression.
   B. The tumor grows in single-file lines of cells and does not induce a reaction in the surrounding stroma.
   C. The mediolateral oblique (MLO) view does not include the far medial and lateral breast.
   D. The MLO view is technically more difficult to perform and is more limited.

3. Which of the following is *not* the reason that ILC is detected at a larger size than IDC?
   A. ILC does not form a mass that is well seen on two views.
   B. ILC is often seen as an asymmetric density, on only one view.
   C. ILC is not typically palpable.
   D. ILC does not typically cause a desmoplastic reaction in the surrounding tissues.

4. Which of the following statements is true about ILC?
   A. ILC has a higher risk of bilaterality compared with IDC.
   B. ILC has a lower risk of bilaterality compared with IDC.
   C. The prognosis for ILC is worse than for IDC.
   D. Treatment of ILC is more likely to require chemotherapy.

CASE 97

Invasive Lobular Carcinoma

1. A, B, and C
2. B
3. D
4. A

References

Brem RF, Ioffe M, Rapelyea JA, et al: Invasive lobular carcinoma: detection with mammography, sonography, MRI, and breast-specific gamma imaging. *AJR Am J Roentgenol* 2009;192(2):379-383.

Lopez JK, Bassett LW: Invasive lobular carcinoma of the breast: spectrum of mammographic, US, and MR imaging findings. *Radiographics* 2009;29(1):165-176.

Michael M, Garzoli E, Reiner CS: Mammography, sonography and MRI for detection and characterization of invasive lobular carcinoma of the breast. *Breast Dis* 2009;30:21-30.

Cross-Reference

Ikeda D: *Breast Imaging: THE REQUISITES*, 2nd ed, Philadelphia: Saunders, 2010, p 101.

Comment

The mammogram shown demonstrates how ILC can be difficult to detect because it may be seen on only one view. When seen on one view, it is more commonly seen on the CC view, as in this patient (see the figures). The features most commonly seen on mammography are an equal-density developing asymmetry with distortion, or a spiculated mass. Calcifications are rare (seen in 1% to 11% of cases). Growth of the tumor is insidious, spreading in a single file of cells and not inciting a desmoplastic reaction. These features explain why the tumor is so difficult to detect on mammography. In one study, ILC was missed on the mammogram in 21% of patients. It is detected at a later stage owing to its difficulty in detection. In one study, 14% were larger than 5 cm at detection compared with 9% of IDC being larger than 5 cm at detection.

ILC represents approximately 10% of all breast cancers and is much less common than IDC. It is more commonly multifocal, multicentric, and bilateral. Bilateral rate is approximately 10% to 15%. For this reason, the ipsilateral and contralateral breasts must be evaluated for additional sites of disease; this evaluation is commonly done with MRI.

When ILC is suspected on mammography, spot compression views should be obtained (see the figures). On ultrasound, there is typically a hypoechoic shadowing mass that is similar to IDC. On MRI, ILC usually enhances, but it may not enhance more than the surrounding glandular tissue, leading to a false-negative study.

Notes

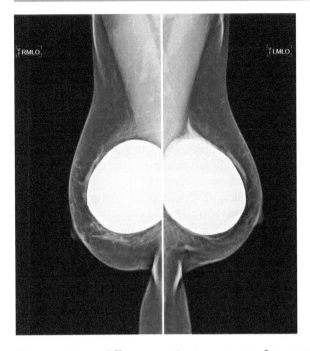

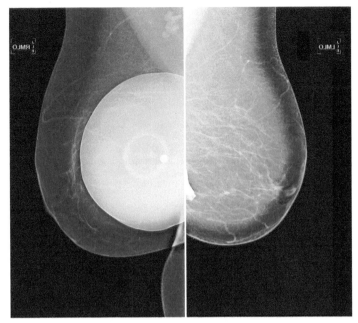

History: Two different patients present for routine screening.

1. What is the differential diagnosis for both patients? (Choose all that apply.)
   A. Both have saline implant leak.
   B. Both have silicone implant leak.
   C. Both patients have a rupture of the left implant.
   D. Patient A has an extracapsular rupture; patient B has a complete collapse of her implant.

2. Are the implants in these two patients subpectoral or subglandular?
   A. Both patients have subpectoral implants.
   B. Patient A has subglandular; patient B has subpectoral.
   C. Both patients have subglandular implants.
   D. Patient A has subpectoral implants; patient B has subglandular.

3. How does a silicone leak manifest itself?
   A. The implant shell collapses, and the silicone gel might stay contained within the fibrous capsule or might leak from the capsule.
   B. The implant shell does not collapse but rather holds the silicone gel in place.
   C. The implant shell collapses, and the silicone always leaks into the breast tissue.
   D. Silicone leaks are always seen on the mammogram.

4. How does a saline implant leak manifest itself?
   A. The saline stays in place, inside the fibrous capsule.
   B. The shell collapses, and the saline is quickly reabsorbed.
   C. The saline very slowly leaks from the implant over a period of years.
   D. The breast size remains the same after rupture.

Implant Leak

1. C and D
2. C
3. A
4. B

References

Berg WA, Caskey CI, Hamper UM, et al: Diagnosing breast implant rupture with MR imaging, US, and mammography. *Radiographics* 1993;13(6):1323-1336.
Caskey CI, Berg WA, Hamper UM, et al: Imaging spectrum of extracapsular silicone: correlation of US, MR imaging, mammographic, and histopathologic findings. *Radiographics* 1999;19:39-51.

Cross-Reference

Ikeda D: *Breast Imaging: THE REQUISITES*, 2nd ed, Philadelphia: Saunders, 2010, pp 341-346.

Comment

These two patients illustrate the appearance of implant rupture. Patient A has subglandular silicone implants (see the first figure). To judge the location of the implant, look for the implant's position relative to the pectoral muscle. If it is anterior to the muscle, as in the first set of figures, it is in the subglandular or prepectoral position. In the mammogram of patient A, there is a wispy area of silicone-density material adjacent to the superior aspect of the left silicone implant. This material is seen external to the contour of the implant; it is silicone that has escaped the confines of the silicone implant shell, as well as the confines of the fibrous capsule.

In the mammogram of patient B (see the second figure) an intact saline implant is seen in prepectoral position in the right breast. On the left side, there is a triangular density near the chest wall. This represents the collapsed saline implant.

Implants are essentially bags, usually made of silicone, with silicone gel, saline, or other material (peanut oil was used for a brief period) inside the shell. The bag is placed inside the body, either in front of the pectoralis muscle (see the figures) or posterior to the muscle. The anterior position is easier to place, but it more commonly leads to implant contracture. The contracture is due to constriction of the fibrous capsule, which is made by the host, as a foreign body reaction to the implanted silicone bag. This capsule is essentially fibrous tissue and has a tendency to constrict.

When discussing silicone implant rupture, it is important to classify the rupture as intracapsular or extracapsular. In the first instance, the bag ruptures, and the silicone gel is held in place by the host's fibrous capsule. This might not be recognized mammographically because the shape may be the same. It can be seen on MRI and can also be recognized on ultrasound. In the case of extracapsular rupture of a silicone implant, the silicone gel escapes from the fibrous capsule and extrudes into the breast tissue. It can then be picked up by the lymphatics and deposited into the lymph nodes (*not* seen in this patient). This can be recognized on mammography as in this case, on ultrasound ("snowstorm" appearance in the breast tissue), and on MRI.

In saline implant rupture, such distinction is not necessary. If the bag ruptures, the saline is reabsorbed by the body. The saline is not retained inside the capsule. The collapsed bag is seen. Patients who have saline implants do not need ultrasound or MRI for evaluation of the implant. The mammogram is diagnostic. Usually, the clinical exam is diagnostic, because the breast size decreases dramatically.

Notes

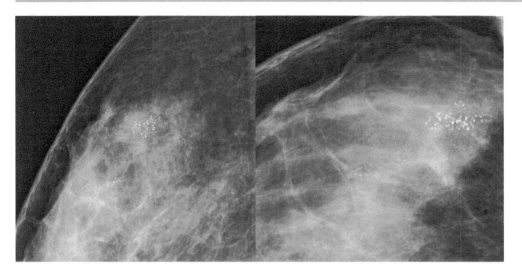

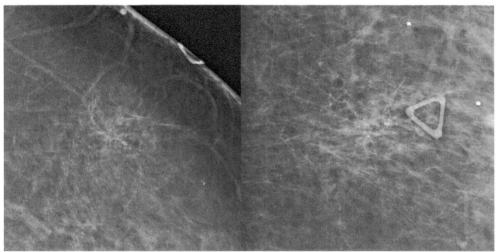

History: Two patients have mammograms. The first patient is 45 years old and asymptomatic; she had a screening mammogram and is recalled for additional views (see the first figure). The second patient is 60 years old and has not had a mammogram for 3 years; she feels a lump in her left breast and comes in for evaluation (see the second figure).

1. What should be included in the differential diagnosis for these two patients? (Choose all that apply.)
   A. Fibrocystic change with sclerosing adenosis
   B. Ductal carcinoma in situ (DCIS)
   C. Invasive ductal carcinoma
   D. Atypical ductal hyperplasia

2. What terminology would you use to describe the form and distribution of calcification in the first patient?
   A. Punctate and clustered
   B. Coarse and fine heterogeneous, in segmental distribution
   C. Fine linear branching, segmental
   D. Clusters of pleomorphic calcifications in a regional distribution

3. What terminology would you use to describe the form and distribution of calcification in the second patient?
   A. Clustered, round, and amorphous
   B. Linear calcifications in a regional distribution
   C. Fine linear branching calcifications in a focal cluster
   D. Amorphous calcifications in a cluster

4. Which of the following is *not* a reason to use the lexicon for describing calcifications?
   A. The form of the calcifications suggests the grade of DCIS.
   B. The lexicon describes the level of concern for the mammographic finding.
   C. The terminology describes the extent of the abnormality for the surgeon.
   D. It is a good academic exercise.

CASE 99

Ductal Carcinoma In Situ in Two Patients

1. B and C
2. B
3. C
4. D

References

Allred DC: Ductal carcinoma in situ: terminology, classification, and natural history. *J Natl Cancer Inst Monogr* 2010;2010 (41):134-138.

Kuerer HM, Albarracin CT, Yang WT, et al: Ductal carcinoma in situ: state of the science and roadmap to advance the field. *J Clin Oncol* 2009;27(2):279-288.

Menell JH, Morris EA, Dershaw DD, et al: Determination of the presence and extent of pure ductal carcinoma in situ by mammography and magnetic resonance imaging. *Breast J* 2005;11(6):382-390.

Schnitt SJ: Local outcomes in ductal carcinoma in situ based on patient and tumor characteristics. *J Natl Cancer Inst Monogr* 2010;2010 (41):158-161.

Yamada T, Mori N, Watanabe M, et al: Radiologic-pathologic correlation of ductal carcinoma in situ. *Radiographics* 2010;30 (5):1183-1198.

Cross-Reference

Ikeda D: *Breast Imaging: THE REQUISITES*, 2nd ed, Philadelphia: Saunders, 2010, pp 63-74.

Comment

The term *DCIS* encompasses a heterogeneous group of breast malignancies characterized by the clonal proliferation of epithelial cells originating in the terminal ductal lobular unit. It is a nonobligate precursor to invasive ductal carcinoma, which is lethal. The disease varies by the nuclear grade of the malignant epithelial cells and by the presence or absence of necrosis. When necrosis is present (also called *comedonecrosis*), the disease is more aggressive; the higher the nuclear grade (Van Nuys classification I, II, and III), the more aggressive. The local recurrence and chance of progression to invasive disease are related to the nuclear grade. Other histologic classifications used include cribriform, solid, papillary, and micropapillary forms. These types are typically less aggressive than the comedo type and usually well to moderately differentiated (grades I and II).

The distinctions are important in the management of the disease. There is a risk of local recurrence if the disease is incompletely resected at breast conservation therapy. The risk is increased in patients who have a high nuclear grade and comedonecrosis, patients who present with a lump or bloody nipple discharge, and young patients. The radiologist must recognize the characteristics of suspicious calcifications and the disease extent and obtain adequate biopsy samples of all of the lesions seen.

The first patient had coarse and fine heterogeneous calcifications in multiple groupings in the right upper outer breast (see the figures). These appeared within a segmental distribution. The histologic classification of coarse and fine heterogeneous calcifications is variable but tends to be low and intermediate nuclear grade. The patient may be able to be treated with breast conservation therapy, with relatively low risk of recurrence.

The first patient underwent ultrasound of the right breast, which showed several hypoechoic areas associated with calcifications, consistent with DCIS. Ultrasound can be used to evaluate for the presence of an associated mass and to target biopsy. In this patient, biopsy was performed with ultrasound guidance, and a diagnosis of DCIS, solid and cribriform types, nuclear grade II, was made, concordant with the imaging findings.

The second patient presented with a palpable mass. DCIS can be palpable if associated with stromal fibrosis around the intraductal malignancy, or if DCIS is present in an existing mass, such as fibroadenoma. The mammogram showed fine linear branching calcifications in a focal area and no mass (see the figures). This type of calcification has been shown to be associated with high–nuclear grade DCIS and necrosis, which has a higher incidence of local recurrence. Stereotactic biopsy results were concordant with the appearance of the calcifications: grade III DCIS with comedonecrosis.

Notes

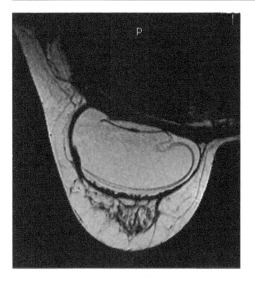

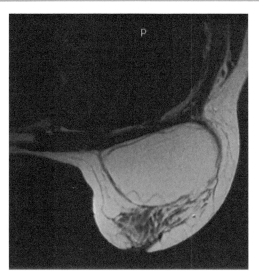

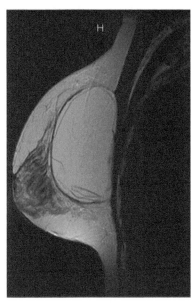

History: A 56-year-old woman presents with pain in both breasts. Silicone implants were placed 10 years ago.

1. What is the differential diagnosis based on the MR images?
   A. Bilateral intracapsular silicone implant rupture
   B. Bilateral extracapsular silicone implant rupture
   C. Bilateral intracapsular saline implant rupture
   D. Bilateral intact silicone implants

2. What imaging modality is the most sensitive for detecting intracapsular rupture?
   A. Mammography
   B. Ultrasound
   C. Breast-specific gamma imaging (BSGI)
   D. MRI

3. What term is *not* used to describe intracapsular rupture on MRI?
   A. Keyhole sign
   B. Noose sign
   C. Stepladder sign
   D. Linguine sign

4. What is the most important feature of intracapsular implant rupture diagnosis on MRI?
   A. Silicone on both sides of the implant capsule
   B. Folding of the implant capsule
   C. The position of the implant in front of the pectoralis muscle
   D. T2-bright fluid around the implant capsule

MRI of Intracapsular Rupture of Silicone Implant

1. A
2. D
3. C
4. A

References

Collis N, Litherland J, Enion D, Sharpe DT: Magnetic resonance imaging and explantation investigation of long-term silicone gel implant integrity. *Plast Reconstr Surg* 2007;120(5):1401-1406.

Di Benedetto G, Cecchini S, Grassetti L, et al: Comparative study of breast implant rupture using mammography, sonography, and magnetic resonance imaging: correlation with surgical findings. *Breast J* 2008;14(6):532-537.

Gabriel SE, Woods JE, O'Fallon WM, et al: Complications leading to surgery after breast implantation. *N Engl J Med* 1997;336:679-682.

Cross-Reference

Ikeda D: *Breast Imaging: THE REQUISITES*, 2nd ed, Philadelphia: Saunders, 2010, pp 351-354.

Comment

Implants are common. One estimate is that 2.5 million women in the United States have implants. Implants are placed for cosmetic augmentation (approximately 80%) and for reconstruction after mastectomy (approximately 20%). Implants consist of an envelope made of silicone elastomer membrane or shell, filled with saline or silicone gel. The patient's host response to the implant is to form a fibrous capsule around it.

Complications of silicone implants are common. Women can present with pain, capsular contracture, inflammation, and infection. Rupture of the implant is not unusual, and it can occur within the host's fibrous capsule (intracapsular), or it can break through the fibrous capsule (extracapsular). In intracapsular rupture, only the implant shell is ruptured. In extracapsular rupture, both the implant shell and the fibrous capsule rupture. In one retrospective study, 24% of women with implants (both silicone and saline) had a complication needing a surgical procedure during the first 5 years after receiving the implants. Women having implants for reconstruction were more likely to need reoperation, compared with women having cosmetic augmentation.

MRI is the most sensitive imaging study for evaluating implant rupture. Extracapsular rupture may be seen on the mammogram as dense material outside the confines of the implant capsule, and it can be recognized on ultrasound as the "snowstorm" appearance. However, intracapsular rupture is not well seen on the mammogram, and it can be difficult to recognize on ultrasound (the stepladder sign is not always obvious). When intracapsular rupture is pronounced, the silicone shell is collapsed, and it is seen floating free in the silicone gel. This is the stepladder sign in ultrasound and the linguine sign in MRI (see the figures). When the rupture is of a lesser degree, the implant shell is seen pulled slightly away from the fibrous capsule in loops or nooses, and silicone is seen on both sides of the silicone shell (see the figures).

Folds in the implant shell are common and must be differentiated from rupture of the shell. Look for the presence of silicone on both sides of the shell; this will not be present with folds. Also common is water-density fluid surrounding the capsule in intact implants. This will not be seen on a water-saturated, fat-saturated sequence, where only silicone is bright. It is not related to rupture.

In this patient, there is bilateral intracapsular silicone implant rupture (see the figures).

Notes

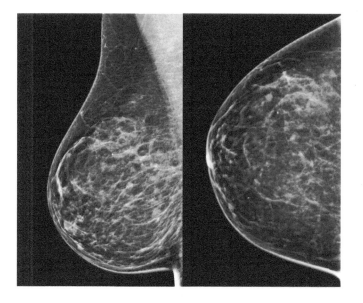

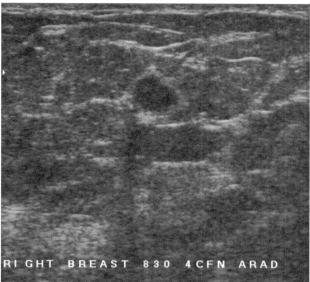

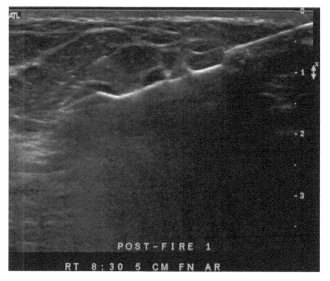

History: A 62-year-old woman presents for routine screening mammogram. The right breast only is shown; the finding is new since her last mammogram. She has a family history of breast cancer in her mother at age 62.

1. What should be included in the differential diagnosis of the right mammogram? (Choose all that apply.)
   A. Simple cyst
   B. Complex cystic mass
   C. Papilloma
   D. Fibroadenoma

2. What differentiates central and peripheral papillomas?
   A. They are the same lesion but in different locations.
   B. Peripheral papillomas are more likely to manifest with bloody nipple discharge.
   C. Peripheral papillomas arise from the terminal ductal lobular unit and are more likely to have associated malignancy.
   D. Both types are equally likely to be multiple.

3. What is unusual about the location of the mass on the mammogram and the location noted on ultrasound?
   A. The mass on the mammogram is in the upper outer quadrant, and it is located at the 8:30 position on ultrasound, which is below the nipple.
   B. The mass is lateral on the mammogram, and the 8:30 position is in the medial breast.
   C. Nothing—the locations of the mass on the mammogram and ultrasound are concordant.
   D. The mass on the mammogram and the mass on ultrasound are not one and the same, and a 90-degree lateral mammographic view is recommended to give the true orthogonal location.

4. What is the next step in management of a peripheral papilloma on core biopsy?
   A. Bilateral breast MRI
   B. Surgical excision
   C. Whole-breast ultrasound
   D. "Mirror-image" biopsy

Peripheral Papilloma with Ductal Carcinoma In Situ

1. A, B, and C
2. C
3. C
4. A

References

Al Sarakbi W, Worku D, Escobar PF, et al: Breast papillomas: current management with a focus on a new diagnostic and therapeutic modality. *Int Semin Surg Oncol* 2006;3:1.

Brookes MJ, Bourke AG: Radiological appearances of papillary breast lesions. *Clin Radiol* 2008;63(11):1265-1273.

Ibarra JA: Papillary lesions of the breast. *Breast J* 2006;12(3):237-251.

Leung JW: MR imaging in the evaluation of equivocal clinical and imaging findings of the breast. *Magn Reson Imaging Clin N Am* 2010;18(2):295-308.

Muttarak M, Lerttumnongtum P, Chaiwun B, et al: Spectrum of papillary lesions of the breast: clinical, imaging, and pathologic correlation. *AJR Am J Roentgenol* 2008;191(3):700-707.

Cross-Reference

Ikeda D: *Breast Imaging: THE REQUISITES*, 2nd ed, Philadelphia: Saunders, 2010, pp 120-383.

Comment

Papillary masses have various manifestations in the breast. The most commonly encountered is large duct papilloma, which is in the central, subareolar breast, is rarely palpable, and often manifests with nipple discharge. These are typically benign, and their surgical management is controversial.

Peripheral papilloma arises from the terminal ductal lobular unit, which is the location that gives rise to epithelial proliferation, including atypical ductal hyperplasia, ductal carcinoma in situ, and invasive ductal carcinoma. There is a higher association with malignancy in peripheral papilloma compared with large duct papilloma. In one large study, more than 37% of peripheral papillomas were associated with malignancy. They manifest less often with nipple discharge (about 20% of the time) and are more frequently palpable.

When a new mass is seen on routine mammography (see the figures), additional work-up is needed. The patient is recalled for additional spot compression views. Ultrasound is then performed to identify if there is a cystic or solid mass to correspond to the mammographic finding (see the figures). If the mass is cystic but has a thick wall, papillary projections, or thick internal septations, malignancy is suspected, and a biopsy is performed. If the mass is solid, biopsy is performed (see the figures). Biopsy can be averted only if the mass is typical of a simple cyst. Color flow Doppler should be used to ensure that the mass is not an anechoic solid tumor. Cyst aspiration can be performed if there is any doubt. The mass in the patient in the present case was a papilloma with associated ductal carcinoma in situ on 12-gauge vacuum core biopsy.

Papillomas on mammography manifest as round masses, with or without calcifications, as in the patient in this case, but also can manifest as foci of microcalcifications, clusters of nodules, and asymmetric density. Although additional abnormalities are not seen on this patient's mammogram, bilateral MRI may be performed to assess for additional disease. On MRI, papillomas are typically small round masses with brisk early enhancement and washout on kinetic curve.

Notes

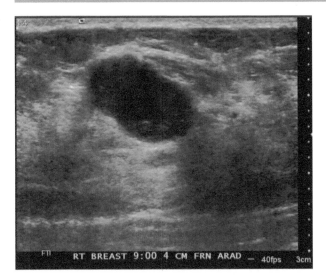
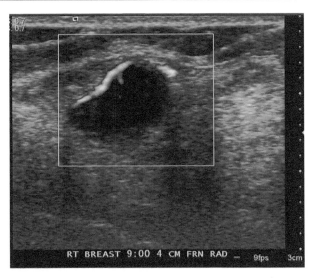

History: A 46-year-old woman has a family history of breast cancer in her sister at age 40. She has had multiple benign breast biopsies. She underwent breast MRI for high-risk screening, and multiple masses were seen, most consistent with fibroadenomas. One of the masses seen on MRI had brisk early enhancement and was considered indeterminate. She then had a targeted ultrasound with vacuum-assisted ultrasound-guided biopsy.

1. What should be included in the differential diagnosis for the mass in the right breast? (Choose all that apply.)
   A. Infiltrating ductal carcinoma
   B. Fibroadenoma
   C. Normal lymph node
   D. Ductal carcinoma in situ

2. What is the next step in management?
   A. Additional imaging with breast-specific gamma imaging
   B. Surgical referral
   C. Follow-up ultrasound examination in 6 months
   D. Needle biopsy using ultrasound guidance

3. Why is Doppler assessment useful before core biopsy?
   A. It adds no useful information if biopsy is to be performed anyway.
   B. If a mass is avascular on Doppler, no biopsy is indicated.
   C. It can help map the location of arteries and veins within the mass.
   D. A very vascular mass should not be biopsied with percutaneous technique.

4. Which of the following is *not* an advantage of vacuum-assisted, ultrasound-guided needle biopsy?
   A. The cores in a vacuum-assisted biopsy are larger.
   B. Ultrasound guidance is easier for the patient than stereotactic biopsy.
   C. There is no radiation exposure during an ultrasound-guided procedure.
   D. The ultrasound-guided procedure cannot cause a pneumothorax.

Vacuum-Assisted Biopsy

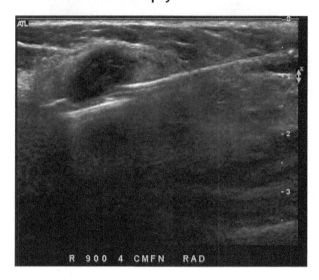 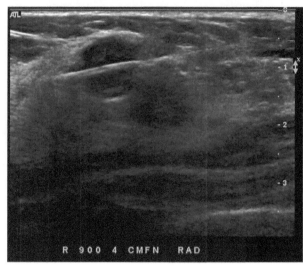

1. A and B
2. D
3. C
4. D

References

Chon N, Moon WK, Cha JH, et al: Sonographically guided core biopsy of the breast: comparison of 14-gauge automated gun and 11-gauge directional vacuum-assisted biopsy methods. *Korean J Radiol* 2005;6(2):102-109.

Parker SH, Klaus AJ, McWey PJ, et al: Sonographically guided directional vacuum-assisted breast biopsy using a handheld device. *AJR Am J Roentgenol* 2001;177(2):405-408.

Philpotts LE, Hooley RJ, Lee CH: Comparison of automated versus vacuum-assisted biopsy methods for sonographically guided core biopsy of the breast. *AJR Am J Roentgenol* 2003;180(2):347-351.

Cross-Reference

Ikeda D: *Breast Imaging: THE REQUISITES*, 2nd ed, Philadelphia: Saunders, 2010, p 215.

Comment

Ultrasound-guided core biopsy is a cost-effective, efficient method for determining the histology of an indeterminate lesion seen on ultrasound (see the figures). Compared with stereotactic guidance, it is more comfortable for the patient, uses no specialized equipment such as the stereotactic table, has no ionizing radiation, and is generally faster. The needle is seen in "real time" during the procedure. It is possible to evaluate for blood vessels using color Doppler (see the figures).

Some specific aspects of the ultrasound-guided procedure must be taken into consideration, making this procedure more difficult to learn than stereotactic biopsy. The location of the needle insertion site, relative to the mass, is important (see the figures). The needle must be seen at all times when in the breast and must be kept away from the chest wall to prevent pneumothorax. Ideally, the needle is inserted in such a way that it can be kept roughly parallel to the skin (see the figures).

The automated core biopsy device uses a spring to advance the needle into the lesion. The needle typically projects out 2.5 cm when the spring is activated. Multiple insertions are used to obtain the tissue needed compared with the single insertion of a vacuum device. The vacuum-assisted device is generally placed into or below the lesion (see the figures), and cores of tissue are taken after the vacuum device has "pulled" the tissue into the cutting slot of the needle (see the figures). Because there is no "throw" of the needle, there is a lower chance of the needle inadvertently penetrating the chest wall or lung. The vacuum device samples are larger for the same gauge needle compared with the automated device cores.

With image-guided biopsy, there is a possibility of false-negative diagnosis. The false-negative rate of ultrasound-guided biopsy is very low, 0.5% to 1%, whether using a 14-gauge automated core device or larger vacuum-assisted device. There is also the possibility of underestimation of disease, whether obtaining a core diagnosis of atypical ductal hyperplasia when ductal carcinoma in situ exists or obtaining a core diagnosis of ductal carcinoma in situ when invasive disease is present. The underestimation rate is lower (36% vs. 55% in one large series) for the vacuum-assisted device compared with the automated spring-activated device for calcified lesions. For this reason, the vacuum-assisted device is preferred when performing biopsy for calcifications, using either stereotactic or ultrasound guidance.

This patient's mass was a fibroadenoma.

Notes

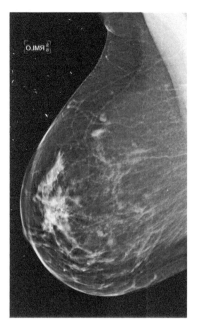

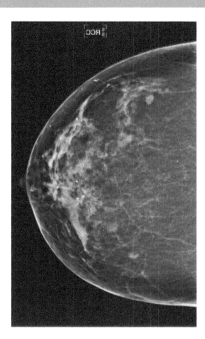

History: A 53-year-old woman with no history of prior breast surgery undergoes routine screening mammogram.

1. What should be included in the differential diagnosis for the distortion in the right upper breast? (Choose all that apply.)
   A. Infiltrating ductal carcinoma
   B. Radial scar
   C. Infiltrating lobular carcinoma
   D. Fibroadenoma

2. If this finding were stable over many years and at the site where a benign biopsy had been performed, what would be your BI-RADS (Breast Imaging Reporting and Data System) score of this mammogram?
   A. BI-RADS 1—normal
   B. BI-RADS 2—benign
   C. BI-RADS 4—suspicious
   D. BI-RADS 5—highly suspicious

3. What is the next step in management of this finding on screening mammogram?
   A. MRI to check for abnormal enhancement
   B. Spot compression views or spot magnification views
   C. Follow-up mammogram at 6 months
   D. Referral to a surgeon for excision

4. After additional views, the distortion is more obvious, and distortion is also seen on ultrasound. What is the next step?
   A. Referral to a surgeon for excision
   B. Needle core biopsy with vacuum-assisted technique
   C. Fine-needle aspiration biopsy using ultrasound
   D. Needle core biopsy using the smallest gauge needle available, owing to risk of bleeding

C A S E 1 0 3

Radial Scar

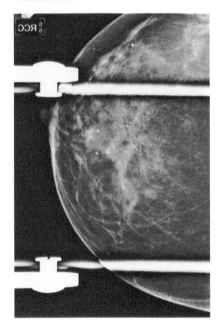
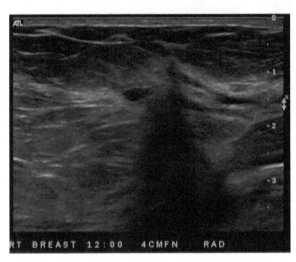

1. A, B, and C
2. B
3. B
4. B

References
Brenner RJ, Jackman RJ, Parker SH, et al: Percutaneous core needle biopsy of radial scars of the breast: when is excision necessary? *AJR Am J Roentgenol* 2002;179(5):1179-1184.
Linda A, Zuiani C, Furlan A, et al: Radial scars without atypia diagnosed at image-guided needle biopsy: how often is associated malignancy found at subsequent surgical excision, and do mammography and sonography predict which lesions are malignant? *AJR Am J Roentgenol* 2010;194(4):1146-1151.

Cross-Reference
Ikeda D: *Breast Imaging: THE REQUISITES*, 2nd ed, Philadelphia: Saunders, 2010, p 111.

Comment

Radial scar is a pathologic abnormality consisting of a central sclerotic core, with radiating bands of proliferating ducts and lobules, which may entrap surrounding fat. A radial scar is also called a *complex sclerosing lesion*. Atypical cells may be within the benign stromal cells. The radiating bands of stromal cells cause the spiculated appearance on mammography, an appearance that overlaps with invasive carcinoma (see the figures).

When a spiculated mass is seen and there is no history of benign surgery at the site, work-up should proceed with additional spot compression or magnification views (see the figures), and histology must be obtained. A radial scar is a benign lesion but is associated with atypia and malignancy: atypical ductal hyperplasia, ductal carcinoma in situ, atypical lobular hyperplasia, and lobular carcinoma in situ. In the past, surgical excision was recommended instead of needle core biopsy because of fear of sampling error, missing the associated atypia, or malignancy. In addition, the lesion can be misinterpreted as a tubular carcinoma by the pathologist because of similar features. It is also thought that the lesion may be a precursor to tubular carcinoma.

Because invasive carcinoma is a possibility with this appearance, performing needle biopsy before surgery is beneficial. Knowledge of the pathology before definitive surgery allows the surgeon to plan to perform the necessary excision and possible lymph node surgery in one step, rather than needing multiple surgical procedures. Core biopsy should be performed with vacuum assistance (9-gauge, 10-gauge, or 11-gauge needle) with multiple cores taken to increase the diagnostic yield of the biopsy. Ultrasound can be used to guide the biopsy if the lesion is seen. These lesions often appear subtle on mammography and may be better seen on ultrasound.

This patient underwent needle core biopsy with vacuum assistance, and histology showed a complex sclerosing lesion. The lesion was excised after a needle localization procedure. Final histology of the excised tissue included markedly atypical lobular hyperplasia, bordering lobular carcinoma in situ, and a complex sclerosing lesion (radial scar).

Notes

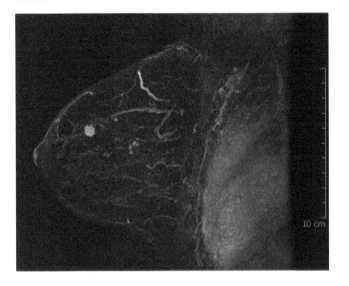

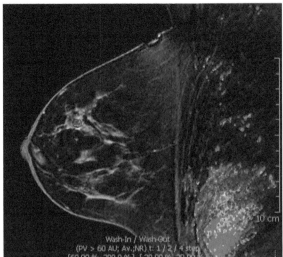

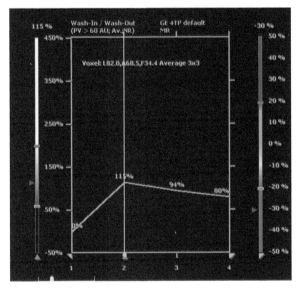

History: A 46-year-old woman underwent breast MRI for screening because of a strong family history of early-onset breast cancer.

1. What should be included in the differential diagnosis for the MRI views and time-intensity curve shown? (Choose all that apply.)
   A. Papilloma
   B. Breast cancer
   C. Fat necrosis
   D. Fibroadenoma

2. What do the colors on a computer-assisted detection (CAD) image of the breast denote?
   A. Margin analysis
   B. The presence of malignancy
   C. The wash-out pattern
   D. Suspicious shapes of masses

3. What is the effect of CAD on breast MRI interpretation?
   A. Increased sensitivity for suspicious lesions
   B. Increased time spent in reviewing hundreds of images for each MRI examination of the breast
   C. Decreased biopsy rate of benign breast lesions
   D. Increased specificity for breast cancer detection

4. What is the role of breast MRI in screening?
   A. All women should be screened with MRI because of low sensitivity of mammography.
   B. Women who have a 20% or greater lifetime risk of breast cancer are encouraged to undergo screening with breast MRI.
   C. Screening with MRI is reserved only for women who have had breast cancer previously.
   D. Screening MRI is best used in women with fatty breasts on mammography.

MRI of Breast Carcinoma

1. A, B, and C
2. C
3. A
4. B

References

Bassett LW, Dhaliwal SG, Eradat J, et al: National trends and practices in breast MRI. *AJR Am J Roentgenol* 2008;191(2):332-339.

Berg WA: Tailored supplemental screening for breast cancer: what now and what next? *AJR Am J Roentgenol* 2009;192(2):390-399.

Cross-Reference

Ikeda D: *Breast Imaging: THE REQUISITES*, 2nd ed, Philadelphia: Saunders, 2010, p 239.

Comment

Breast MRI has been shown to detect malignancies not detected on standard imaging with mammography and ultrasound. Because of its high cost, need for intravenous contrast agent and the inherent risk of the contrast agent, and other medical reasons for not tolerating MRI, use of MRI is best confined to patients at increased risk. The American Cancer Society has published guidelines for the groups of women who should be recommended for screening MRI. These include women with *BRCA1* or *BRCA2* mutation or first-degree relative with this mutation; 20% to 25% or greater lifetime risk for breast cancer; radiation to the chest between ages 10 and 30; history of Li-Fraumeni syndrome, Cowden disease, or Bannayan-Zonana syndrome; or first-degree relative with the aforementioned syndromes.

In this patient, a round mass with irregular margins was detected in the left breast on screening MRI (see the figures). The left breast 12 o'clock region was subsequently evaluated with ultrasound, and a suspicious lesion was found. Biopsy with needle core technique was performed. Histology showed well-differentiated invasive ductal carcinoma with tubular features. Mammography was negative, even after the location of the tumor was known.

MRI has been shown to increase the detection of breast cancer compared with mammography and ultrasound. Sensitivity of MRI is reported to be 94% to 100%, sensitivity of mammography alone is 25% to 59%, and sensitivity of mammography plus ultrasound is approximately 49% to 67%. The specificity of MRI is lower and may necessitate additional studies and biopsies. The use of CAD can increase the efficiency and sensitivity of the MRI reading because color coding is applied to breast lesions, allowing rapid assessment of the kinetics of the lesion. In the CAD system shown here, red color is applied to lesions with a rapid wash-in, wash-out curve; green color is assigned to lesions that have a plateau; and blue color is assigned to lesions that have persistent enhancement over time. This patient has a malignant mass with red on color assignment, indicating rapid wash-out.

Notes

Challenge

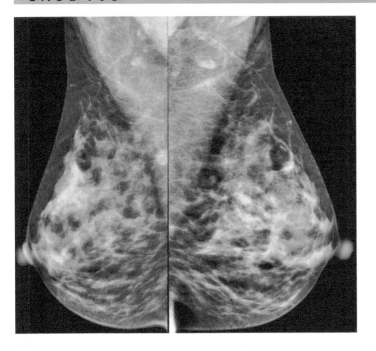

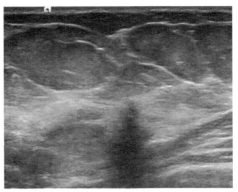

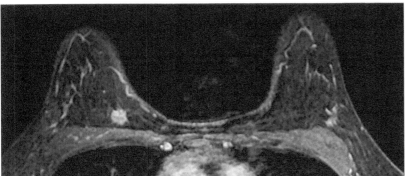

History: A 45-year-old African-American woman presents with a palpable area of concern in the upper inner right breast found on self-breast examination. She has no family history of breast cancer.

1. What should be included in the differential diagnosis? (Choose all that apply.)
   A. Invasive ductal carcinoma
   B. Ductal carcinoma in situ
   C. Fibroadenolipoma
   D. Granular cell tumor

2. Ultrasound-guided biopsy was performed and showed polygonal cells in bundles and cords, with abundant granular eosinophilic cytoplasm and stromal fibrosis. What is the next step in management?
   A. Repeat of ultrasound-guided biopsy
   B. Follow-up mammogram, ultrasound, and MRI in 6 months

C. Wide surgical excision
D. Lumpectomy and radiation therapy

3. Granular cell tumors may appear as any of the following except:
   A. Spiculated mass
   B. Partially circumscribed mass with calcifications
   C. Partially circumscribed mass without calcifications
   D. Partially ill-defined hypoechoic mass with posterior acoustic shadowing

4. Which of the following statements regarding granular cell tumors is true?
   A. They are typically found in the breast.
   B. They may mimic breast cancer both clinically and on imaging.
   C. They usually occur as an incidental finding on screening mammogram.
   D. They are a subtype of ductal breast carcinoma.

Granular Cell Tumor

1. A and D
2. C
3. B
4. B

References

Adeniran A, Al-Ahmadie H, Mahoney M, et al: Granular cell tumor of the breast: a series of 17 cases and review of the literature. *Breast J* 2004;10(6):528-531.

Porter GJ, Evans AJ, Lee AH, et al: Unusual benign breast lesions. *Clin Radiol* 2006;61(7):562-569.

Scaranelo AM, Bukhanov K, Crystal P, et al: Granular cell tumor of the breast: MRI findings and review of the literature. *Br J Radiol* 2007;80 (960):970-974.

Comment

Granular cell tumors are rare benign lesions, thought to derive from Schwann cells. They can be located in almost any tissue, but the most common site involved is the tongue. Approximately 5% to 8% of cases occur in the breast, and they are more common in premenopausal African-American women.

Granular cell tumors mimic breast cancer both clinically and on imaging. Clinically, they usually manifest as a firm, painless, palpable mass, usually fixed to the pectoral fascia, which may cause retraction of the skin. However, in contrast to breast carcinomas, which usually occur in the upper outer quadrant, granular cell tumors are predominantly found in the upper inner quadrant of the breast (area of cutaneous innervation by the supraclavicular nerve).

The appearance on mammography is more frequently a poorly defined or spiculated mass, without calcifications. On ultrasound, they may appear as an irregular or spiculated mass with posterior acoustic shadowing and less frequently as a circumscribed mass. Reported MRI findings of granular cell tumors in sites other than the breast show variable T2 signal intensity (from low or intermediate to high compared with the adjacent muscle) and low to intermediate signal on T1-weighted images; both homogeneous and peripheral enhancement have been described after contrast agent administration (see the figures).

Biopsy should be performed to obtain a definitive diagnosis. Although these are benign lesions, treatment is wide local excision, owing to their potential local recurrence. Rare malignant cases have been reported.

Notes

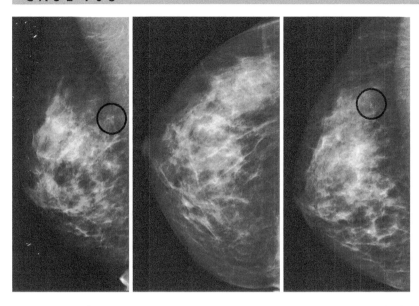 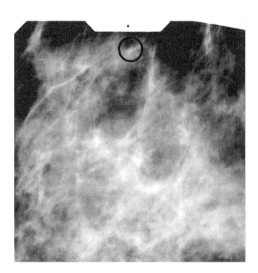

History: A 54-year-old woman presents for screening mammogram.

1. What should be included in the differential diagnosis for the calcifications in the far posterior upper outer right breast? (Choose all that apply.)
   A. Fibrocystic change
   B. Atypical ductal hyperplasia
   C. Ductal carcinoma in situ
   D. Invasive ductal carcinoma

2. Which of the following situations does *not* make stereotactic biopsy difficult (requiring special positioning of the patient) or technically impossible?
   A. Thin breast
   B. Central cluster of microcalcifications measuring 2 to 3 mm
   C. Microcalcifications located close to the chest wall
   D. Microcalcifications located in the axillary tail of the breast

3. Which of the following is *not* a special maneuver in patient and breast positioning during stereotactic biopsy to improve visualization of posterior or axillary tail microcalcifications?
   A. Pull the breast, gently but firmly, through the opening of the stereotactic table.
   B. Encourage the patient to relax the chest muscles as much as possible.
   C. Place the patient's arm through the breast opening of the table.
   D. Roll the patient into a supine position.

4. Which of the following is *not* a limitation of stereotactic biopsy compared with ultrasound-guided biopsy?
   A. Compression of the breast is a necessity.
   B. The patient must remain still during the biopsy procedure.
   C. The patient must lie on her stomach.
   D. The patient is typically lying supine.

Difficult Stereotactic Biopsy—Calcifications in the Axillary Tail of the Breast

1. A, B, and C
2. B
3. D
4. D

References

Jackman RJ, Marzoni FA Jr: Stereotactic histologic biopsy with patients prone: technical feasibility in 98% of mammographically detected lesions. *AJR Am J Roentgenol* 2003;180(3):785-794.

Verkooijen HM, Peeters PH: Borel Rinkes IH, et al; COBRA Study Group: Risk factors for cancellation of stereotactic large core needle biopsy on a prone biopsy table. *Br J Radiol* 2001;74 (887):1007-1012.

Cross-Reference

Ikeda D: *Breast Imaging: THE REQUISITES*, 2nd ed, Philadelphia: Saunders, 2010, p 215.

Comment

Stereotactic biopsy is the method used when indeterminate or suspicious calcifications are seen on a mammogram (see the figures). If there is no associated mass, these lesions may be seen only on the mammogram. To obtain a biopsy specimen of these lesions, stereotactic biopsy, a mammographically derived procedure, is performed. This procedure may be performed with a special add-on unit that is attached to the regular mammogram device, and the procedure is completed with the patient sitting in a chair. A specially designed table may also be used. On this table, the patient lies prone, and the breast is pulled through a round opening in the table. The biopsy is performed below the patient, by a radiologist sitting on a chair.

In 2003, nearly 2000 stereotactic biopsies and reasons for incomplete and canceled studies were reviewed.

When stereotactic biopsies were canceled for technical reasons, most were canceled because the lesion was too close to the chest wall. Lesions close to the chest wall and in the axillary tail of the breast are difficult to position in the stereotactic window for biopsy. However, maneuvers can be used to visualize posterior lesions better so that they can be sampled stereotactically.

The breast should be pulled, gently but firmly, as completely as possible down through the opening in the stereotactic table. The patient should be encouraged to relax the chest muscles as much as possible. If the lesion cannot be seen, the patient's arm can be placed through the breast opening of the table, which drops more of the axillary area into position for biopsy. The patient also can be rolled into a slightly decubitus position, with the side of interest down.

Biopsy specimens of calcifications in the axillary tail may be easier to obtain from the mediolateral oblique (MLO) or mediolateral approach rather than the craniocaudal (CC) approach. From the lateral approach, the calcifications are closer to the skin (see the figures). A biopsy clip should be placed at the site of biopsy after the procedure, so that if excision is needed, the area can be easily localized. Placement of a clip is especially important in difficult biopsies and if the cluster of microcalcifications is too small because it may be completely removed on the core biopsy. Specimen radiograph should be performed prior to clip placement, to ensure that the target has been sampled.

The mammogram obtained after biopsy in this case shows the clip at the site where the microcalcifications had been present. Histopathology of the calcifications on biopsy was atypical ductal hyperplasia, which should be surgically excised.

Notes

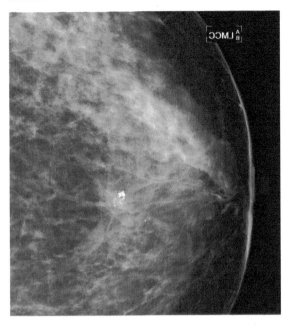
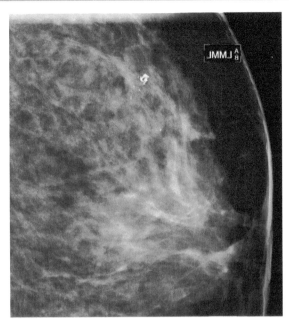
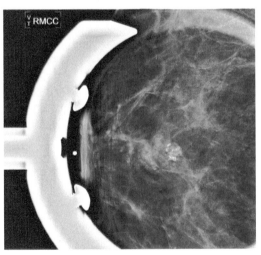
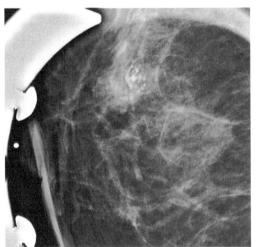

History: Two patients undergo routine screening mammograms. New calcifications are seen in the subareolar breast in each patient. Magnification views are shown.

1. What should be included in the differential diagnosis for both patients? (Choose all that apply.)
   A. PASH
   B. Ductal carcinoma in situ (DCIS)
   C. Intraductal papilloma
   D. Fibroadenoma

2. What is the next step in management?
   A. Follow-up diagnostic mammogram in 1 year with magnification views
   B. Short-interval follow-up magnification views in 6 months
   C. Surgical consultation
   D. Image-guided vacuum-assisted needle biopsy

3. The needle biopsy result for both patients showed intraductal papilloma. Which of the following is *not* recommended?
   A. Annual mammogram
   B. Short-interval follow-up magnification views in 6 months
   C. Surgical consultation
   D. Follow-up ultrasound examination in 6 months

4. What symptom is commonly associated with subareolar intraductal papilloma?
   A. Pain
   B. Palpable lump
   C. Nipple retraction
   D. Bloody nipple discharge

Calcified Subareolar Masses

1. B, C, and D
2. D
3. A
4. D

References

Al Sarakbi W, Worku D, Escobar PF, et al: Breast papillomas: current management with a focus on a new diagnostic and therapeutic modality. *Int Semin Surg Oncol* 2006;3:1.

Bernik SF, Troob S, Ying BL, et al: Papillary lesions of the breast diagnosed by core needle biopsy: 71 cases with surgical follow-up. *Am J Surg* 2009;197(4):473-478.

Liberman L, Tornos C, Huzjan R, et al: Is surgical excision warranted after benign, concordant diagnosis of papilloma at percutaneous breast biopsy? *AJR Am J Roentgenol* 2006;186(5):1328-1334.

Skandarajah AR, Field L, Yuen Larn Mou A, et al: Benign papilloma on core biopsy requires surgical excision. *Ann Surg Oncol* 2008;15(8): 2272-2277.

Cross-Reference

Ikeda D: *Breast Imaging: THE REQUISITES*, 2nd ed, Philadelphia: Saunders, 2010, p 120.

Comment

A papilloma is a tumor that arises from ductal epithelium. The term *papilloma* includes solitary papilloma (as in this case, see the figures), multiple papillomas, and juvenile papillomatosis. Intraductal papilloma is classified as a benign tumor of the breast, although the condition of multiple peripheral papillomas confers an increased risk of malignancy. Solitary papillomas, as in this case, are typically found in large ducts in the retroareolar breast and are less likely to be associated with DCIS. A solitary papilloma in a large duct is the most common presentation of all papillary lesions and affects an older age group compared with multiple peripheral papillomas.

Surgical consultation is recommended for women who have a biopsy result showing papilloma because there is an increased incidence of DCIS within the papilloma, which may not be found on a needle biopsy sample. This risk is reported to be 20%. There is some controversy surrounding this issue if a benign papilloma is found at core biopsy. However, if atypia or malignancy is present in the core specimen, surgical excision is universally recommended. There seems to be no statistical difference between 11-gauge and 14-gauge needle in the cancer yield in excisional biopsy in benign papillomas.

Papillomas may twist on the fibrovascular stalk and can cause bloody or clear spontaneous nipple discharge. Papilloma is the most common cause of pathologic nipple discharge (in 40% to 70% of women). However, most women with an intraductal papilloma are asymptomatic. Detection on mammogram is limited because these masses are contained within a duct that appears outwardly normal. When calcifications are present, mammographic detection increases (see the figures). A papilloma may also appear on mammogram as a well-defined mass.

Notes

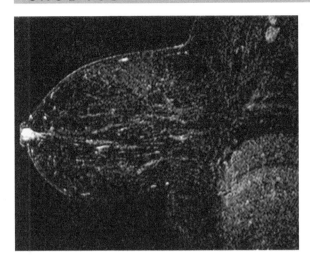
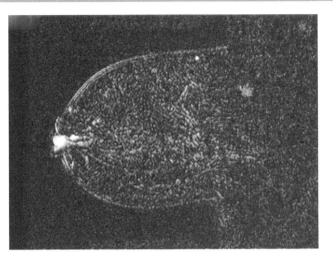
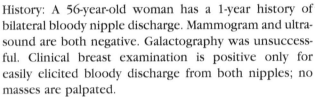

History: A 56-year-old woman has a 1-year history of bilateral bloody nipple discharge. Mammogram and ultrasound are both negative. Galactography was unsuccessful. Clinical breast examination is positive only for easily elicited bloody discharge from both nipples; no masses are palpated.

1. What should be included in the differential diagnosis of the bilateral, post–contrast subtraction MRI images shown? (Choose all that apply.)
   A. Bilateral intraductal carcinoma
   B. Bilateral papilloma
   C. Bilateral duct ectasia with debris
   D. Bilateral nipple adenoma

2. What is the management of this imaging finding?
   A. Targeted ultrasound with biopsy
   B. Surgical excision
   C. Follow-up in 6 months because these masses are likely benign
   D. MRI-guided biopsy

3. Is MRI useful in this clinical setting?
   A. No, because approximately 25% of papillomas do not enhance
   B. No, because galactography can provide the same information
   C. Yes, because MRI can provide the location and number of enhancing masses
   D. No, because the surgeon can perform central duct excision

4. Which of the following is *not* pathologic nipple discharge?
   A. Blackish and greenish discharge from multiple orifices
   B. Spontaneous watery discharge
   C. Serous and spontaneous
   D. Dark maroon and spontaneous

C A S E 1 0 8

MRI of Nipple Discharge

1. A, B, and D
2. B
3. C
4. A

References

An HY, Kim KS, Yu IK, et al: Image presentation. The nipple-areolar complex: a pictorial review of common and uncommon conditions. *J Ultrasound Med* 2010;29(6):949-962.

Ballesio L, Maggi C, Savelli S, et al: Role of breast magnetic resonance imaging (MRI) in patients with unilateral nipple discharge: preliminary study. *Radiol Med* 2008;113(2):249-264.

Daniel BL, Gardner RW, Birdwell RL, et al: Magnetic resonance imaging of intraductal papilloma of the breast. *Magn Reson Imaging* 2003;21(8):887-892.

Nicholson BT, Harvey JA, Cohen MA: Nipple-areolar complex: normal anatomy and benign and malignant processes. *Radiographics* 2009;29(2):509-523.

Yau EJ, Gutierrez RL, DeMartini WB, et al: The utility of breast MRI as a problem-solving tool. *Breast J* 2011;17(3):273-280.

Cross-Reference

Ikeda D: *Breast Imaging: THE REQUISITES*, 2nd ed, Philadelphia: Saunders, 2010, p 383.

Comment

Nipple discharge should be clinically evaluated because it may be a symptom of breast cancer. However, most causes of nipple discharge are benign. Pathologic nipple discharge includes spontaneous discharge that is unilateral, persists, and can range from clear (watery) to serous to bloody. Nonpathologic discharge is typically elicited only on squeezing the nipple; benign discharge can be milky, green, or gray to black. Nonpathologic discharge typically occurs in more than one orifice of the nipple and may be bilateral.

Masses that can cause nipple discharge include papillary masses arising in the lactiferous ducts, ranging from benign papilloma to papillary DCIS to invasive papillary cancer. Other masses include nipple adenoma, which is a proliferation of tubules in the duct, and DCIS and invasive ductal carcinoma.

MRI can be useful in the diagnosis of pathologic nipple discharge when standard diagnostic imaging fails. Intraductal masses may be the cause of discharge, and if the mass is not calcified, it is unlikely to be seen on mammography. Ultrasound is useful to evaluate the cause of discharge, but debris in the duct can look like a mass. With ultrasound, it is helpful to orient the transducer along the long axis of the duct. Galactography is the standard interventional method of evaluating discharge. It may be technically difficult to cannulate the duct, and distal nipple masses, such as in this patient (see the figures), can block the placement of the cannula.

Papillomas do not consistently enhance on MRI. Approximately 75% are seen after contrast injection, and kinetics range from slow, persistent enhancement to a malignant profile. Other findings on MRI include an enlarged duct, with fluid hyperintense on T2 images, with an intraductal hypointense mass.

Biopsy may be performed with imaging guidance if the lesion is seen on ultrasound or contains calcifications that can be targeted for stereotactic biopsy. Biopsy of masses in the nipple is technically difficult using any imaging modality, and these masses should be surgically excised.

Notes

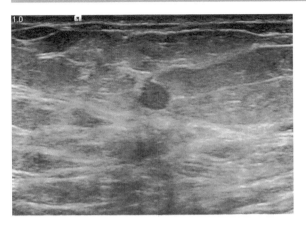
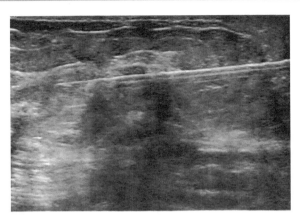
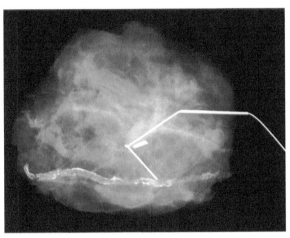

History: A 44-year-old woman is scheduled for surgery to remove a mass in the left breast after core biopsy.

1. What should be included in the differential diagnosis for the ultrasound image of the mass in the left breast? (Choose all that apply.)
   A. Invasive ductal carcinoma
   B. Fibroadenoma
   C. Granular cell tumor
   D. Papillary lesion

2. Which of the following statements regarding the best selection of imaging modality to guide needle localization is *false*?
   A. Masses are generally localized under ultrasound guidance.
   B. Calcifications are generally localized under mammographic guidance.
   C. Areas of non-masslike enhancement are generally localized under MRI guidance.
   D. Needle localization can be performed only under mammographic guidance.

3. Which of the following are the correct steps, *in order,* to perform ultrasound-guided needle localization?
   A. Selection of the skin entry site, ultrasound identification of the lesion, hook wire placement, needle placement and adjustment

B. Ultrasound identification of the lesion, selection of the skin entry site, needle placement and adjustment, hook wire placement
   C. Ultrasound identification of the lesion, needle placement and adjustment, hook wire placement, selection of the skin entry site
   D. Ultrasound identification of the lesion, selection of the skin entry site, hook wire placement, needle placement and adjustment

4. Which of the following statements regarding ultrasound-guided needle localization is true?
   A. It may not be necessary to send mammogram films to the operating room.
   B. Obtaining a radiograph of the specimen is unnecessary.
   C. The specimen radiograph is evaluated by the surgeon in the operating room.
   D. The surgeon does not need to be notified of the specimen radiograph findings.

Ultrasound-Guided Needle Localization

1. A, C, and D
2. D
3. B
4. A

References

DePalo AJ: Surgical considerations in needle localization procedures. *Semin Surg Oncol* 1991;7(5):253-256.

Homer MJ, Smith TJ, Safaii H: Prebiopsy needle localization: methods, problems, and expected results. *Radiol Clin North Am* 1992;30(1):139-153.

Klimberg VS: Advances in the diagnosis and excision of breast cancer. *Am Surg* 2003;69(1):11-14.

Kopans DB, Swann CA: Preoperative imaging-guided needle placement and localization of clinically occult breast lesions. *AJR Am J Roentgenol* 1989;152(1):1-9.

Cross-Reference

Ikeda D: *Breast Imaging: THE REQUISITES*, 2nd ed, Philadelphia: Saunders, 2010, p 200.

Comment

Needle localization procedures are less frequently performed at the present time because of the wide acceptance of percutaneous core biopsies. The most common indication for needle localization is excision of nonpalpable high-risk lesions or carcinoma diagnosed at core biopsy. Another indication is to aid in the excision of a nonpalpable lesion when biopsy with imaging guidance cannot be performed.

Needle localization may be performed under mammographic, ultrasound, or MRI guidance. The selection of the guiding modality should be based on the ease of seeing the lesion. Generally, calcifications are localized under mammographic guidance, masses are localized under ultrasound guidance, and areas of non-masslike enhancement are localized under MRI guidance.

For ultrasound-guided needle localization, the patient is positioned so that the skin entry site for placement of the localizing needle and hook wire is as close to the lesion as possible. The needle length is chosen by measuring the distance from the closest skin surface to the site of the lesion on the ultrasound screen. After the lesion is identified and the skin entry site has been selected, the skin is cleansed and anesthetized, and the needle is placed into the breast, parallel to the chest wall (see the figures). Needle placement into the lesion is confirmed by ultrasound in orthogonal planes (needle parallel and perpendicular to the transducer) in real time during the procedure. The needle is adjusted so that the tip is at or just beyond the lesion. The hook wire is placed through the needle and secured in the breast tissue. Some surgeons prefer to keep the needle in the breast to aid in localizing the lesion in the operating room, whereas other surgeons prefer to remove the needle and keep only the wire in the breast. Some surgeons prefer blue dye to be injected into the lesion to aid removal.

The ultrasound images are sent to the operating room, with the lesion circled. Some surgeons prefer that mammographic films also be sent to the operating room to serve as additional guidance. A specimen radiograph is obtained in every case (see the figures), but the lesion may not be evident radiographically, and ultrasound of the specimen may be necessary to confirm that the lesion has been removed. To aid the surgeon, a metal BB may be placed on the skin at the needle insertion site before the radiograph is taken. An "X" may be marked on the patient's skin overlying the mass because the needle is not placed through the skin directly over the mass.

The radiologist must review the specimen to ensure that the lesion has been removed (or sampled, depending on the case). The surgeon is notified of the findings, and if the lesion has not been removed or adequately sampled, the surgeon should be directed to obtain more tissue.

Notes

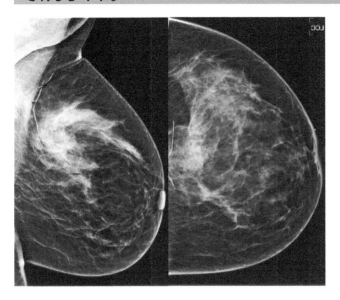
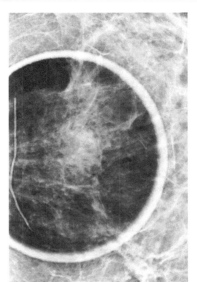
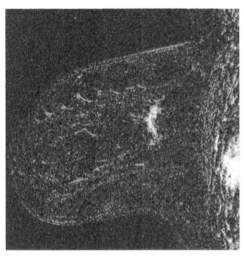

History: A 44-year-old woman had invasive lobular carcinoma (ILC) diagnosed 3 years previously, was treated with breast conservation therapy, and is asymptomatic. She now presents for her annual mammogram.

1. What should be included in the differential diagnosis for the images shown? (Choose all that apply.)
   A. Normal postoperative mammogram and MRI
   B. Recurrent carcinoma at the lumpectomy site
   C. Fat necrosis at the lumpectomy site
   D. Residual disease at the lumpectomy site

2. Is ILC more likely to have recurrence compared with invasive ductal carcinoma not otherwise specified (IDC NOS)?
   A. Yes, because this tumor is more likely multifocal and multicentric
   B. Yes, because ILC is typically larger at diagnosis compared with IDC
   C. No, the recurrence rates are similar
   D. Yes, because of the tumor biology of cells infiltrating in single file in ILC

3. What is the management of recurrent disease?
   A. Mastectomy
   B. Lumpectomy
   C. Bilateral mastectomy
   D. Surgery and additional radiation therapy

4. What is the most common presentation of recurrent disease after breast conservation?
   A. Mass and/or calcifications away from the lumpectomy site, within 3 years of treatment
   B. Mass and/or calcifications at the lumpectomy site, on the first mammogram after treatment
   C. Mass and/or calcifications in the opposite breast, 3 years or more after treatment
   D. Mass and/or calcifications at the lumpectomy site, 18 months or more after treatment

Invasive Lobular Carcinoma with Recurrence

1. B, C, and D
2. C
3. A
4. D

References

Arpino G, Bardou VJ, Clark GM, et al: Infiltrating lobular carcinoma of the breast: tumor characteristics and clinical outcome. *Breast Cancer Res* 2004;6(3):R149-R156.

McGahan LJ, Wasif N, Gray RJ, et al: Use of preoperative magnetic resonance imaging for invasive lobular cancer: good, better, but maybe not the best? *Ann Surg Oncol* 2010;17(Suppl 3):255-262.

Singletary SE, Patel-Parekh L, Bland KI: Treatment trends in early-stage invasive lobular carcinoma: a report from the National Cancer Data Base. *Ann Surg* 2005;242(2):281-289.

Cross-Reference

Ikeda D: *Breast Imaging: THE REQUISITES*, 2nd ed, Philadelphia: Saunders, 2010, pp 314, 324.

Comment

ILC is more difficult to detect on mammography, ultrasound, and MRI compared with IDC. It is more likely to spread through the breast in single files of cells, inciting little desmoplastic reaction by the host. For this reason, ILC is larger at diagnosis compared with IDC NOS, more likely to need reoperation because of positive margins at surgery, and more likely to necessitate mastectomy at the time of surgery for lumpectomy because of positive margins. It is also more commonly multifocal and multicentric and more likely to have contralateral breast involvement.

The above-mentioned characteristics do not affect the recurrence rate or the disease-free survival. In one large series reviewing more than 50,000 cases of early breast cancer, the recurrence rate of ILC was slightly lower than the recurrence rate of IDC NOS, although this was not clinically significant. The two breast cancer types should be considered to have essentially the same clinical outcome; the failure rate of breast cancer treatment for both types is approximately 1% per year.

The patient in this case was 41 years old at the time of diagnosis, making her younger than the average patient with ILC (average age is 65 years). She had a normal screening mammogram and felt a palpable mass in her left breast 2 months later (false-negative mammogram is common with ILC). At the time of the work-up for the palpable mass, the diagnostic mammogram was negative, and ultrasound showed an 8-mm mass. Ultrasound is more sensitive than mammography in ILC but tends to underestimate the size of the tumor, as in this patient. MRI was negative; no enhancement was seen at the tumor site. No enhancement is rare for infiltrating cancers but more common with ILC than with IDC. When MRI shows ILC as an enhancing mass, it more accurately shows tumor size than mammography and ultrasound. At surgery, this patient required two reexcisions to obtain clear margins, which is more common with ILC than with IDC.

At 3 years after surgery, mammogram showed increased density at the lumpectomy site (see the figures); follow-up imaging had been unremarkable at 1 year after lumpectomy. MRI (see the figures) showed a new area of non-masslike enhancement at the lumpectomy site. Ultrasound and ultrasound-guided core biopsy were performed and showed ILC at the lumpectomy site, consistent with recurrence. The patient underwent mastectomy.

Notes

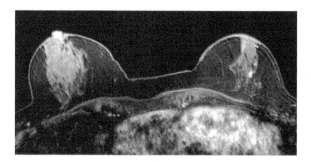

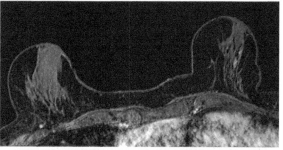

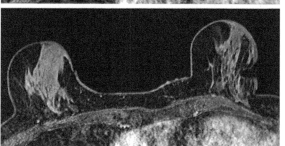

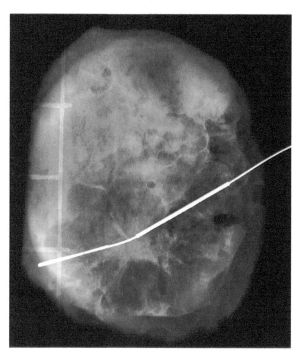

History: A 37-year-old woman who is *BRCA*-positive has a tiny irregular mass in the outer left breast found on screening MRI. The mass showed avid enhancement with gadolinium and was new compared with prior MRI studies. It was visible only on MRI.

1. What should be included in the differential diagnosis for the mass in the left breast? (Choose all that apply.)
   A. Invasive ductal carcinoma
   B. Hematoma
   C. Fibroadenoma
   D. Papillary lesion

2. Indications for MRI-guided needle localization include all of the following *except:*
   A. Areas of non-masslike enhancement
   B. Cluster of amorphous microcalcifications
   C. Lesions not visible on mammography or ultrasound
   D. Lesions visible on MRI, with equivocal results on mammogram and ultrasound

3. Which of the following statements regarding MRI-guided needle localization procedures is true?
   A. The patient is positioned supine within a dedicated breast coil.
   B. No special positioning of the breast is required.
   C. The needle should be placed at the site of the lesion.
   D. Adequate placement of the hook wire is confirmed after the patient is released from compression.

4. Which of the following statements is *false*?
   A. A two-view mammogram is performed after MRI-guided localization.
   B. Obtaining a radiograph of the specimen is unnecessary.
   C. The specimen radiograph is evaluated by the radiologist.
   D. The surgeon is notified of the specimen radiograph findings.

MRI-Guided Needle Localization

1. A, C, and D
2. B
3. C
4. B

References

Klimberg VS: Advances in the diagnosis and excision of breast cancer. *Am Surg* 2003;69(1):11-14.
Kuhl CK: Interventional breast MRI: needle localisation and core biopsies. *J Exp Clin Cancer Res* 2002 Sep;21(3 Suppl):65-68.
Van den Bosch MA, Daniel BL: MR-guided interventions of the breast. *Magn Reson Imaging Clin N Am* 2005;13(3):505-517.

Cross-Reference

Ikeda D: *Breast Imaging: THE REQUISITES*, 2nd ed, Philadelphia: Saunders, 2010, p 275.

Comment

Needle localization procedures generally are less frequently performed because of the wide acceptance of percutaneous core biopsies. MRI-guided needle biopsy and needle localization procedures are performed in lesions not clearly visible on either mammogram or ultrasound, such as areas of non-masslike enhancement. MRI-guided needle biopsy could be performed with a clip marker placed in the breast after biopsy. The clip can be localized mammographically if excision is needed.

In this case, the lesion was only seen on MRI, had irregular margins, showed avid enhancement with gadolinium with rapid washout, and was new compared with prior MRI examinations (see the figures). MRI-guided biopsy could have been performed, but the patient requested excision.

For MRI-guided needle localization, the patient is positioned prone within a dedicated breast coil, and the breast is gently compressed with a special compression paddle that includes a grid and a needle guide. Compression minimizes motion and allows consistent lesion location, but overly tight compression should be avoided because tight compression may hinder or delay enhancement of the lesion. After positioning, the patient is scanned, and when the lesion is identified, it is triangulated in a similar way as on mammographic guided localization (this can be done manually or with computer-assisted detection [CAD]). The needle is placed at the site of the lesion, and the hook wire is released (see the figures). Adequate placement of the hook wire is confirmed with MRI before the patient is released from compression.

The needle localization procedure can be done from a lateral or medial approach. Some breast coils allow medial access, whereas others offer only a lateral approach, which can be problematic when the lesion is located in the medial aspect of the breast because the distance from the skin would not be the shortest, and the available needle localization devices may not reach the lesion.

A two-view mammogram is performed to show the location of the wire in the breast, even if the lesion was not previously visible mammographically. Surgeons may need this mammogram in the operating room to help plan the surgical procedure. The mammogram may reveal an abnormality that was not seen before localization. Also, these images provide a baseline for mammograms after biopsy.

A specimen image cannot be obtained with MRI. However, a mammographic specimen radiograph is performed. The radiologist reviews the specimen and notifies the surgeon of the findings. In this case, a small spiculated mass was visualized within the specimen (see the figures). Histologically, this mass was a 5-mm invasive ductal carcinoma.

Notes

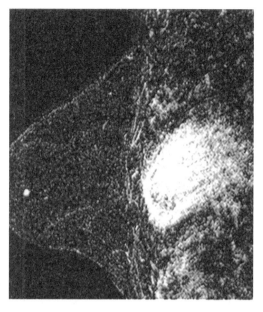
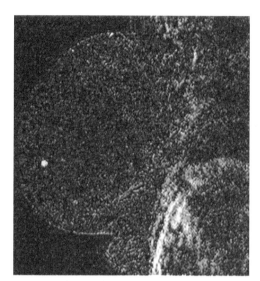
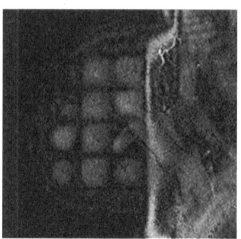
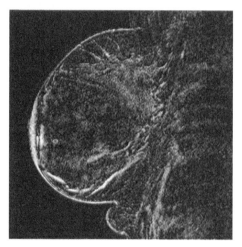

History: A 60-year-old woman has a history of right breast cancer, diagnosed as ductal carcinoma in situ (DCIS), 11 years before. She has extremely dense breasts on mammogram and is followed annually with mammogram and MRI. Previous MRI examinations have been negative.

1. What should be included in the differential diagnosis for the left breast MRI post–contrast subtraction images shown? (Choose all that apply.)
   A. Infiltrating ductal carcinoma
   B. Papilloma
   C. DCIS
   D. Complicated cyst

2. What is the next step in management for this developing lesion?
   A. Because the mass is tiny, repeat MRI in 6 months.
   B. Because the morphology of the mass is benign, return the patient to routine evaluation.

C. Perform targeted ultrasound to check for the presence of a mass; if none, perform follow-up MRI in 6 months.
D. Perform MRI-guided biopsy.

3. Which of the following statements about MRI-guided biopsy is *not* true?
   A. In contrast to stereotactic biopsy, the patient does not have to remain still during the procedure.
   B. The breast is in compression.
   C. A grid is used to help localize the mass.
   D. A vacuum-assisted biopsy apparatus is preferred for sampling.

4. Which of the following is *not* an appearance of DCIS on MRI?
   A. Clumped enhancement
   B. Focal mass
   C. Normal breast
   D. Large mass with spiculated margins

C A S E 1 1 2

MRI-Guided Biopsy

1. A, B, and C
2. D
3. A
4. D

References

Han BK, Schnall MD, Orel SG, et al: Outcome of MR-guided breast biopsy. *AJR Am J Roentgenol* 2008;191(6):1798-1804.

Lehman CD: Magnetic resonance imaging in the evaluation of ductal carcinoma in situ. *J Natl Cancer Inst Monogr* 2010;2010(41):150-151.

Orel SG, Rosen M, Mies C, et al: MR imaging-guided 9-gauge vacuum-assisted core-needle breast biopsy: initial experience. *Radiology* 2006;238(1):54-61.

Strigel RM, Eby PR, Demartini WB, et al: Frequency, upgrade rates, and characteristics of high-risk lesions initially identified with breast MRI. *AJR Am J Roentgenol* 2010;195(3):792-798.

Cross-Reference

Ikeda D: *Breast Imaging: THE REQUISITES*, 2nd ed, Philadelphia: Saunders, 2010, pp 265, 277.

Comment

MRI is a well-established modality for evaluation of the breast in selected patients. The postmenopausal patient in the present case has a personal history of right breast cancer and has dense breasts, which limit mammographic interpretation. She has been evaluated with mammogram and supplementary MRI for several years (see the figures). On the most recent MRI, a new 5-mm mass was noted in the subareolar left breast (see the figures).

Targeted ultrasound, or "second-look" ultrasound, is a useful examination after MRI shows a suspicious mass. If the lesion is found on ultrasound, ultrasound-guided biopsy is faster to perform and more easily tolerated by the patient. However, the use of targeted ultrasound should be tailored to the patient and to the MRI finding. Very small masses, non-masslike enhancement, and ductal enhancement can be difficult to identify on ultrasound. If a mass is not seen on targeted ultrasound, the finding cannot be presumed benign; in one large series, 14% of such lesions were malignant.

MRI-guided biopsy can be performed relatively easily and is similar to stereotactic biopsy with certain important differences. The contrast medium washes out of the breast lesion quickly, so once the location of the mass is noted, the patient may not move because the mass cannot be retargeted without administering more contrast medium. As in stereotactic biopsy, the patient is placed in prone position. With MRI-guided biopsy, the breast is only slightly compressed (see the figures). The compression cannot be too tight because the contrast medium may be inhibited from entering the breast blood vessels. The compression paddle has a grid to facilitate the localization of the biopsy site within the breast. A marker is placed on the skin, in one of the grid openings (see the figures), and the contrast-enhanced study is performed. The x, y, and z coordinates of the lesion are noted on the image, and then the location is compared with the location of the marker (called a *fiducial*). The appropriate x and y lesion location is noted on the skin, and the distance to the lesion from the skin (the z axis) is calculated. This localization of the mass can be accomplished by a computer-assisted detection (CAD) system or can be done by hand.

The skin is cleansed, local anesthesia is given, and the biopsy trocar is placed, similar to a stereotactic biopsy. When the desired location is reached, the metal trocar is replaced by an MRI-compatible stylet, and images are obtained to check the location of the stylet (see the figures). If the location is accurate, the stylet is removed; the biopsy device is placed through the sheath, and the samples are taken. With a vacuum-assisted device, multiple samples can be taken easily without removing the device from the breast. A clip is placed after the samples are taken, and additional images are obtained to assess the biopsy cavity and location of the clip, relative to the location of the mass as initially noted at the beginning of the examination. A mammogram is obtained after the biopsy to document the clip location.

The malignancy rate of MRI-detected areas of abnormal enhancement is approximately 20% to 60%. Lesions that are found to be benign by MRI-guided biopsy should be followed in 6 months with repeat MRI to ensure that the finding is smaller or resolved. If the lesion is unchanged or larger on follow-up, biopsy of the mass should be repeated.

In this patient, the small mass was DCIS. DCIS can have multiple features on MRI, ranging from a small mass to clumped enhancement in a ductal distribution to segmental, non-masslike enhancement. Kinetics is variable, with a slow or a rapid initial increase, with persistence or plateau. In the older literature, 25% to 40% of DCIS that was seen on mammography was not recognized on MRI. However, newer studies show DCIS detection on MRI to be greater than 90%.

Notes

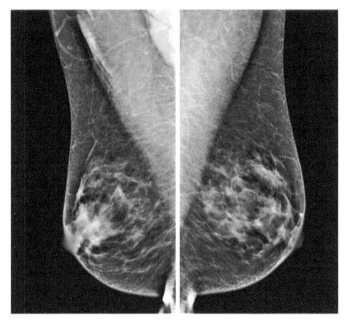

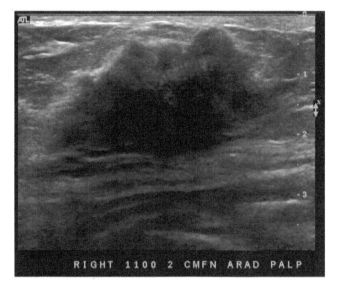

RIGHT 1100 2 CMFN ARAD PALP

History: A 43-year-old woman with juvenile-onset diabetes presents for a routine screening mammogram. A palpable mass is noted in the right subareolar breast by the technologist when positioning her for the mammogram.

1. What should be included in the differential diagnosis? (Choose all that apply.)
   A. Stromal fibrosis
   B. Diabetic mastopathy
   C. Ductal carcinoma in situ
   D. Invasive ductal carcinoma

2. Which of the following statements regarding diabetic mastopathy is true?
   A. It typically occurs in patients with type 2, non–insulin-dependent diabetes.
   B. Incidence is similar in women and men.
   C. Patients frequently have associated complications from diabetes, such as renal disease, retinopathy, and cardiac disease.
   D. The most common clinical presentation is an incidental mammographic finding.

3. Which of the following is *not* an imaging finding in diabetic mastopathy?
   A. Extensive microcalcifications on mammogram
   B. Poorly defined mass or dense focal asymmetry on mammogram
   C. Normal mammogram
   D. Poorly defined mass or areas of intense acoustic shadowing on ultrasound

4. Which of the following statements regarding diagnosis and management of diabetic mastopathy is *false*?
   A. Tissue diagnosis is necessary to exclude malignancy.
   B. Fine-needle aspiration is very accurate in providing a diagnosis of diabetic mastopathy.
   C. Core or excisional biopsies are often necessary for conclusive diagnosis of diabetic mastopathy.
   D. No specific treatment is necessary when diabetic mastopathy is diagnosed on biopsy.

Diabetic Mastopathy

1. A, B, and D
2. C
3. A
4. B

References

Camuto PM, Zetrenne E, Ponn T: Diabetic mastopathy: a report of 5 cases and a review of the literature. *Arch Surg* 2000;135(10):1190-1193.
Mackey SP, Sinha S, Pusey J, et al: Breast carcinoma in diabetic mastopathy. *Breast* 2005;14(5):392-398.
Neetu G, Pathmanathan R, Weng NK: Diabetic mastopathy: a case report and literature review. *Case Rep Oncol* 2010;3(2):245-251.
Thorncroft K, Forsyth L, Desmond S, et al: The diagnosis and management of diabetic mastopathy. *Breast J* 2007;13(6):607-613.

Cross-Reference

Ikeda D: *Breast Imaging: THE REQUISITES*, 2nd ed, Philadelphia: Saunders, 2010, p 400.

Comment

Diabetic mastopathy is an uncommon condition that occurs in patients with long-standing insulin-dependent diabetes. It is most often diagnosed in premenopausal women and has been reported only rarely in men. The most common presentation is a firm, palpable mass that may mimic carcinoma on breast examination, as in the patient in this case. Patients frequently have associated complications from diabetes, such as renal disease, retinopathy, and cardiac disease.

The mammographic findings in diabetic mastopathy are usually a poorly defined mass or a dense focal asymmetry (see the figures). Patients also may have mammographically detected vascular calcifications as a complication of long-standing diabetes. However, because many of these patients are young, the palpable mass may not be mammographically visible owing to surrounding dense breast tissue (see the figures). Ultrasound may show a poorly defined mass or areas of intense acoustic shadowing (see the figures).

The diagnosis of diabetic mastopathy may be suggested with the appropriate clinical history and ultrasound features, but tissue diagnosis is necessary to exclude malignancy. Fine-needle aspiration cytology has been reported to be nondiagnostic in half of lesions because diabetic fibrous tissue contains little cellular material. Core or excisional biopsies are often necessary for conclusive diagnosis of diabetic mastopathy. Core biopsy reveals thick bundles of collagen and periductal, lobular, and vascular inflammatory infiltrates.

An autoimmune etiology has been postulated for this condition. No association has been described between diabetic mastopathy and carcinoma. No specific treatment is necessary for this entity.

Notes

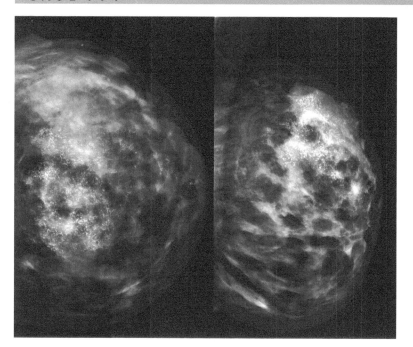 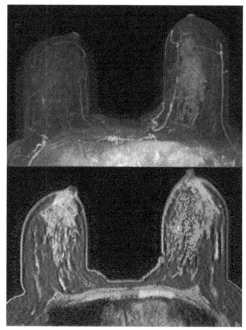

History: A 43-year-old woman presents with left bloody nipple discharge.

1. What should be included in the differential diagnosis? (Choose all that apply.)
   A. Papilloma
   B. Ductal carcinoma in situ (DCIS)
   C. Lobular carcinoma in situ
   D. Invasive ductal carcinoma

2. Which of the following statements regarding imaging of DCIS is *false*?
   A. The mammographic appearance consists of microcalcifications.
   B. The ultrasound appearance is characteristic and consists of an intraductal solid filling defect.
   C. The MRI appearance consists of non-masslike enhancement.
   D. DCIS can appear on mammography as a mass.

3. Signs of microinvasion or invasion in high-grade DCIS include all of the following *except:*
   A. Palpable mass on clinical examination
   B. Extensive linear, branching, pleomorphic, or casting calcifications

C. Irregular hypoechoic area or mass on ultrasound
D. Focal area of clumped non-masslike enhancement in a ductal distribution on MRI

4. Which of the following statements regarding management or prognosis of DCIS is true?
   A. When there are similar-appearing microcalcifications in different quadrants, biopsy of one cluster is enough to establish further management.
   B. The best imaging modality to guide percutaneous biopsy is ultrasound.
   C. When DCIS is diagnosed by needle core biopsy, the next step in management is the same as for invasive carcinoma.
   D. After adequate treatment, the recurrence rate of high-grade DCIS (comedocarcinoma) is low.

High-Grade Ductal Carcinoma In Situ

1. B and D
2. B
3. D
4. C

References

Estevez L, Alvarez I, Segui MA, et al: Current perspectives of treatment of ductal carcinoma in situ. *Cancer Treat Rev* 2010;36(7):507-517.

Mossa-Basha M, Fundaro GM, Shah BA, et al: Ductal carcinoma in situ of the breast: MR imaging findings with histopathologic correlation. *Radiographics* 2010;30(6):1673-1687.

Yamada T, Mori N, Watanabe M, et al: Radiologic-pathologic correlation of ductal carcinoma in situ. *Radiographics* 2010;30(5): 1183-1198.

Cross-Reference

Ikeda D: *Breast Imaging: THE REQUISITES*, 2nd ed, Philadelphia: Saunders, 2010, pp 65, 170.

Comment

DCIS is a type of noninvasive cancer in which the cancer cells have not extended beyond the basal membrane of a duct. DCIS accounts for approximately 20% to 30% of the cancers detected on screening mammogram.

DCIS is classified according to its nuclear grade as low, intermediate, and high grade and morphologically as cribriform, micropapillary, solid, and comedo subtypes. The presence or absence of necrosis is also important in classification of DCIS. High-grade DCIS (comedocarcinoma) is a poorly differentiated form of DCIS that tends to have continuous growth along the ductal system (other subtypes of DCIS have a higher incidence of discontinuous or skip-type growth patterns).

High-grade DCIS appears on mammography as linear, branching, pleomorphic, or casting microcalcifications (see the figures). Because of its tendency to have a continuous growth pattern, the linear branching calcifications seen on mammography may provide an accurate estimate of extent of disease.

DCIS is usually not seen on ultrasound. Occasionally—especially with newer equipment—microcalcifications can be visualized on ultrasound as hyperechoic dots, but the main contribution of ultrasound is to assess for possible additional invasive components (hypoechoic areas or mass or both).

On MRI, DCIS appears as non-masslike enhancement (usually clumped) in a linear, ductal, segmental, or regional distribution. MRI is useful to evaluate extent of disease, multifocality or multicentricity, and presence of contralateral disease. It may detect masses not seen on mammography, and it may show areas of noncalcified DCIS (see the figures).

To establish a diagnosis, stereotactic biopsy of microcalcifications is the best initial approach. When there are multifocal or multicentric areas of microcalcifications, biopsy specimens of any suspicious areas may be obtained to document extent of disease or at least the two most distant sites of microcalcifications. Ultrasound and MRI can be used to guide biopsy of a possible invasive component not detected with mammography.

As the volume of DCIS increases, the chance of microinvasion increases as well. When the extent of disease seen on mammography is 5 cm or greater, the likelihood of microinvasion is high enough that many surgeons perform a sentinel lymph node biopsy even though no invasion may have been documented histologically. Other symptoms and signs of microinvasion or invasion include palpable abnormality on self-examination or clinical examination, hypoechoic areas or mass on ultrasound, and enhancing mass on MRI.

Management of DCIS is the same as management of invasive carcinoma. Treatment includes surgery (lumpectomy or mastectomy), radiation therapy, and chemotherapy or hormonal therapy. Comedocarcinoma is associated with a higher rate of recurrence than other subtypes of DCIS because of the high nuclear grade and the radioresistance of the tumor.

Notes

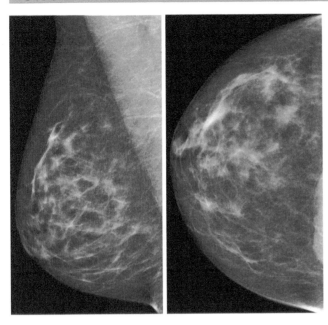

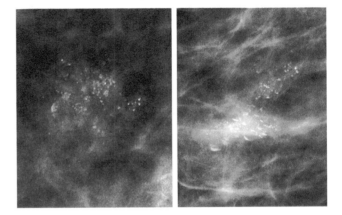

History: A 48-year-old woman presents for screening mammogram.

1. What should be included in the differential diagnosis for the calcifications in the lower outer right breast? (Choose all that apply.)
   A. Fibrocystic changes
   B. Atypical ductal hyperplasia (ADH)
   C. Ductal carcinoma in situ (DCIS)
   D. Lobular carcinoma in situ (LCIS)

2. Stereotactic biopsy revealed ADH, fibrocystic change, and columnar cell change. ADH is usually found associated with which type of calcifications?
   A. Popcorn calcification
   B. Pleomorphic microcalcifications
   C. Regional amorphous microcalcifications
   D. Fine, linear, branching microcalcifications

3. Which of the following statements regarding management of ADH is true?
   A. ADH does not require further management.
   B. When ADH is found at core needle biopsy, the next step in management is to repeat the needle biopsy to obtain more samples.
   C. When ADH is found at core needle biopsy, the next step in management is excisional biopsy at the site of ADH.
   D. When ADH is found at core needle biopsy, the next step in management is lumpectomy, radiation, and chemotherapy.

4. What is the role of biopsy clip placement after stereotactic biopsy?
   A. Biopsy clip placement after stereotactic biopsy of calcifications is unnecessary.
   B. A biopsy clip should be placed at the site of biopsy so that if excision is needed, the area can be easily localized.
   C. Patients with a clip placed after stereotactic biopsy with benign results do not need to continue having screening mammograms.
   D. A biopsy clip placed after stereotactic biopsy is used as a guide for radiotherapy.

CASE 115

Atypical Ductal Hyperplasia

1. A, B, and C
2. C
3. C
4. B

References

Jackman RJ, Birdwell RL, Ikeda DM: Atypical ductal hyperplasia: can some lesions be defined as probably benign after stereotactic 11-gauge vacuum-assisted biopsy, eliminating the recommendation for surgical excision? *Radiology* 2002;224(2):548-554.

Kohr JR, Eby PR, Allison KH, et al: Risk of upgrade of atypical ductal hyperplasia after stereotactic breast biopsy: effects of number of foci and complete removal of calcifications. *Radiology* 2010;255(3): 723-730.

Lomoschitz FM, Helbich TH, Rudas M, et al: Stereotactic 11-gauge vacuum-assisted breast biopsy: influence of number of specimens on diagnostic accuracy. *Radiology* 2004;232(3):897-903.

Villa A, Tagliafico A, Chiesa F, et al: Atypical ductal hyperplasia diagnosed at 11-gauge vacuum-assisted breast biopsy performed on suspicious clustered microcalcifications: could patients without residual microcalcifications be managed conservatively? *AJR Am J Roentgenol* 2011;197(4):1012-1018.

Cross-Reference

Ikeda D: *Breast Imaging: THE REQUISITES*, 2nd ed, Philadelphia: Saunders, 2010, p 230.

Comment

ADH is in the spectrum of hyperplastic changes of the breast that range from usual ductal hyperplasia to DCIS. ADH refers to the proliferation of monomorphic epithelial cells within the duct. ADH is found in approximately 5% of all biopsy specimens obtained for any type of calcifications but is frequently found associated with regional amorphous calcifications (approximately 20%). In this case, the patient had a focal area of clustered heterogeneous microcalcifications (see the figures) and was recalled for additional magnification views. On the additional views, some of the calcifications layer (suggestive of milk of calcium), but other calcifications are more irregular and raise concern for atypia or DCIS (see the figures). When a cluster of microcalcifications exhibits both benign and suspicious features, management should be based on the most suspicious features.

A patient with ADH diagnosed by core biopsy should always undergo excisional biopsy because of the high incidence of histologic underestimation of DCIS. When an 11-gauge vacuum-assisted core needle is used, there is an underestimation of malignancy of approximately 25% when ADH is the core needle diagnosis. Lesions on which core biopsies are performed and that are interpreted as ADH show various histology on excision, including fibrocystic change, ADH, DCIS, and invasive ductal carcinoma.

A biopsy clip should be placed at the site of biopsy so that the area can be easily localized if excision is needed. A clip is especially important if the cluster of microcalcifications is small because the microcalcifications may be completely removed on the core biopsy. Complete removal of all mammographic evidence of the microcalcifications at core biopsy does not obviate the need for excision. The goal of stereotactic biopsy is not complete removal, but rather adequate sampling of the lesion. In this patient, after excisional biopsy with complete removal of the lesion, the histopathology was low-grade DCIS. The vacuum-assisted core biopsy result was an underestimation of the disease present. Approximately 75% of underestimation of ADH is DCIS. The patient went on to definitive management of stage 0 breast cancer.

Notes

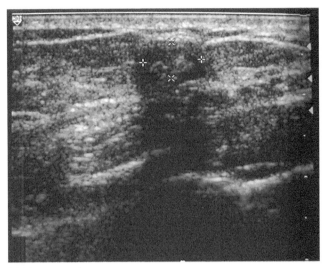

Initial presentation.

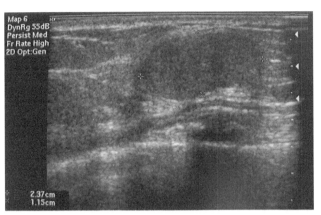

Six months later.

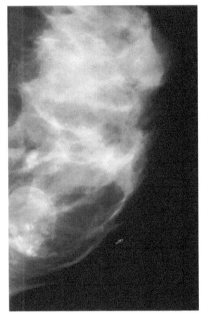

Six months later.

History: A 38-year-old woman in her third trimester of pregnancy presents with a palpable mass. Her family history is significant for breast cancer in her mother.

1. What should be included in the differential diagnosis for the initial presentation? (Choose all that apply.)
   A. Invasive ductal carcinoma
   B. Ductal carcinoma in situ
   C. Fibroadenoma
   D. Lactating adenoma

2. Why did the patient undergo ultrasound evaluation only at initial presentation?
   A. Because ultrasound is always the first step in evaluating a palpable mass
   B. Because of the patient's age
   C. Because the patient is pregnant
   D. Because of her family history

3. Which of the following is *not* a reasonable option for further evaluation?
   A. Fine-needle aspiration
   B. Core biopsy
   C. Surgical excision
   D. Short-term follow-up

4. The patient underwent needle core biopsy. She complained of a persistent lump at the biopsy site 6 months later, larger than the original mass (mammogram and ultrasound are shown). The differential diagnosis includes all of the following *except:*
   A. Lactating adenoma
   B. Milk fistula
   C. Galactocele
   D. Invasive ductal carcinoma

CASE 116

Milk Fistula and Galactocele: Complication of Core Biopsy during Lactation

1. C and D
2. C
3. C
4. D

References

Kim MJ, Kim EK, Park SY, et al: Galactoceles mimicking suspicious solid masses on sonography. *J Ultrasound Med* 2006;25(2):145-151.

Parker SH, Stavros AT, Dennis MA: Needle biopsy techniques. *Radiol Clin North Am* 1995;33(6):1171-1186.

Sawhney S, Petkovska L, Ramadan S, et al: Sonographic appearances of galactoceles. *J Clin Ultrasound* 2002;30(1):18-22.

Schackmuth EM, Harlow CL, Norton LW: Milk fistula: a complication after core breast biopsy. *AJR Am J Roentgenol* 1993;161(5):961-962.

Scott-Conner CEH: Diagnosing and managing breast disease during pregnancy and lactation. *Medscape Womens Health* 1997;2(5):1.

Cross-Reference

Ikeda D: *Breast Imaging: THE REQUISITES*, 2nd ed, Philadelphia: Saunders, 2010, pp 379-380.

Comment

This patient presented with a palpable mass in the left breast. Ultrasound was performed as the initial examination because she was in the third trimester of pregnancy at the time of detection of the mass (see the figures). A needle core biopsy of the 0.7-cm palpable mass in the left upper inner breast was performed, and histology of the mass showed a lactating adenoma. No immediate complications were seen. Several weeks after biopsy, the patient returned with a palpable mass, larger than the original palpable finding. Ultrasound of the new finding showed a well-circumscribed, oval mass consistent with a complex cyst, likely a galactocele resulting from milk fistula, 2.4 cm in diameter (see the figures).

The patient was reassured that this should resolve spontaneously, and she was followed by ultrasound. The mass decreased in size and resolved completely after several months.

The most common palpable masses in pregnant and lactating women are lactating adenomas and fibroadenomas; lactating adenomas account for 70% of masses undergoing biopsy in this population. A lactating adenoma is most often seen in ultrasound as a well-circumscribed, oval, hypoechoic mass, parallel to the chest wall (see the figures). However, a lactating adenoma can have a more suspicious appearance, with shadowing and irregular margins, making malignancy more difficult to exclude.

Although the mass had benign features on ultrasound examination, this patient was concerned about the possibility of malignancy and requested a biopsy. This is an acceptable approach in a probably benign lesion, BI-RADS (Breast Imaging Reporting and Data System) 3. Any intervention in the breast carries a possibility of complications, although complications of needle core biopsy are unusual (approximately 1% to 2% in many published series). The most common complications are hematoma and infection. An additional complication that can occur in the third trimester of pregnancy or during lactation is milk fistula (see the figures). Damage to the ducts by the needle causes leaking of duct contents (milk) into the biopsy cavity, which may result in the formation of a galactocele, which appears as a mixed-density, partially lucent mass on mammogram (see the figures). The ultrasound appearance is commonly a mass with thin echogenic walls and homogeneous hypoechoic internal echoes (see the figures).

Notes

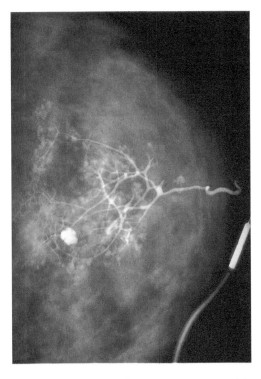

History: A 51-year-old woman presents with spontaneous clear yellow discharge from one opening of the left nipple. Her galactogram is shown.

1. What is the differential diagnosis from this single image of a galactogram? (Choose all that apply.)
   A. Malignant mass communicating with duct
   B. Multiple small intraductal papillomas
   C. Normal galactogram
   D. Normal ducts, forceful injection during galactogram

2. Why is contrast seen in the faint rounded areas adjacent to the ducts?
   A. Contrast has entered lobules.
   B. Contrast has extravasated from the ducts into the adjacent stroma.
   C. There is malignancy in the lobules (ILC).
   D. There is an abnormal mass in the terminal duct lobular unit (TDLU), allowing contrast into the lobules.

3. Does this exam answer the question of the etiology of the discharge?
   A. Yes, the duct is normal, so the discharge must be normal.
   B. No, because the duct is normal, it is probably not the discharging duct.
   C. Yes, a normal galactogram allows you to follow the discharge expectantly.
   D. Yes, because there is one duct in the nipple, this normal galactogram indicates a nonsuspicious discharge.

4. What is the best next step in managing this discharge?
   A. Repeat the galactogram.
   B. Perform MRI without IV contrast.
   C. Perform a mammogram to evaluate for intraductal mass.
   D. Recommend that the patient return in 6 months for re-evaluation.

Normal Galactogram

1. C and D
2. A
3. B
4. A

References

Cardenosa G, Doudna C, Eklund GW: Ductography of the breast: technique and findings. *Am J Roentgenol* 1994;162:1081-1087.

Slawson SH, Johnson BA: Ductography: how to and what if? *Radiographics* 2001;21(1):133-150.

Cross-Reference

Ikeda D: *Breast Imaging: THE REQUISITES*, 2nd ed, Philadelphia: Saunders, 2010, pp 383-389.

Comment

This is an example of a galactogram of a normal duct. There are no suspicious features. In this normal exam, shown in the figure, the ducts are thin, with smooth walls, regular branching, and no filling defects. Abnormal ducts are enlarged and can have irregular duct walls, abrupt termination of ducts, and filling defects.

This example (see the figure) shows the effect of maximal pressure exerted during the galactogram. The contrast has entered the lobules. The rounded areas of contrast outside the ducts in this patient represent contrast that has entered the lobules, called *lobular blush*. This is not extravasation, which occurs when the cannula perforates the side wall of the duct and a pool of contrast occurs outside the duct lumen and which is to be avoided. The rounded area of contrast is likely a cyst in communication with the duct.

Galactography is performed when there is a clinically suspicious discharge, which is a unilateral, spontaneous, clear, yellow, pink, or bloody discharge. Patients with this type of discharge often have an underlying cancer (up to 33%). Benign causes of discharge, such as papilloma, are more common than malignancy. It is not necessary to perform galactography for nipple discharge that is bilateral, nonspontaneous, and occurring in multiple duct orifices and that is green, gray, amber, or milky.

Notes

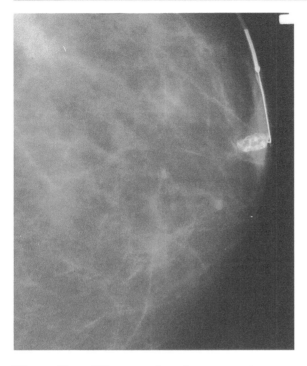
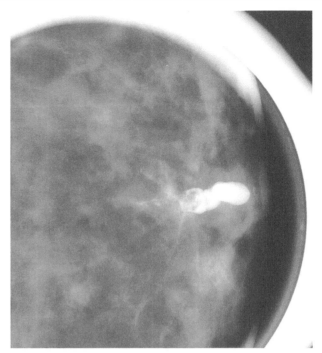

History: Two different patients have a spontaneous, non-bloody unilateral nipple discharge emanating from one nipple orifice.

1. What is the differential diagnosis for these two different patients? (Choose all that apply.)
   A. Malignant intraductal mass
   B. Apocrine metaplasia within ducts
   C. Intraductal papilloma
   D. Air bubbles in the contrast column

2. What is the purpose of the galactogram?
   A. To identify whether intraductal masses are malignant
   B. To treat nipple discharge
   C. To identify the presence of abnormal cells in duct fluid
   D. To depict the extent of intraductal masses

3. What other modalities can be used to evaluate nipple discharge?
   A. Contrast CT
   B. Ultrasound
   C. MRI without contrast
   D. Mammography alone is the best imaging modality for breast ducts

4. What type of discharge is evaluated with galactography?
   A. Nonspontaneous clear yellow discharge from multiple openings of one nipple
   B. Milky spontaneous discharge from both breasts
   C. Bloody discharge from multiple openings in both breasts in a woman who has just delivered a baby
   D. Spontaneous discharge that is not milky from one opening of one nipple

Intraductal Mass

1. A and C
2. D
3. B
4. D

References

Cardenosa G, Doudna C, Eklund GW: Ductography of the breast: technique and findings. *AJR Am J Roentgenol* 1994;162: 1081-1087.

Orel SG, Dougherty CS, Reynolds C, et al: MR imaging in patients with nipple discharge: initial experience. *Radiology* 2000;216:248-254.

Slawson SH, Johnson BA: Ductography: how to and what if? *Radiographics* 2001;21:133.

Cross-Reference

Ikeda D: *Breast Imaging: THE REQUISITES*, 2nd ed, Philadelphia: Saunders, 2010, p 383.

Comment

The steps in evaluating patients with spontaneous nipple discharge are controversial. First, the type of discharge and its true spontaneous nature must be determined. Many women can express discharge from their nipples on manipulation, but true spontaneous discharge is uncommon and requires a work-up regardless of the nature of the discharge. If the discharge is bilateral and milky, prolactin levels are usually checked. However, if the discharge is bloody, clear, or serous and is from a single duct and truly spontaneous, further evaluation is necessary. This may be carried out with surgical exploration of the duct or radiologically, with ultrasound, MRI, and/or galactography.

The purpose of a galactogram is to locate any intraductal lesions and map out the extent of the disease in the discharging duct. The procedure is generally simple. The discharging duct must be localized. Often, this requires a hot compress or heating pad to be placed on the nipple to relax the musculature of the nipple. Adequate lighting and magnification are commonly necessary to identify the opening of the duct. Often, the patient is able to demonstrate a trigger point in the breast that initiates the discharge. Once the discharging duct is localized, a 30-gauge blunt-tip sialogram cannula is gently placed into the duct orifice. The cannula is attached to tubing and a Luer lock syringe is filled with water-soluble contrast. The tubing must be checked carefully so that no air bubbles are present because bubbles injected into the ductal system can mimic intraductal lesions. The Luer lock apparatus will help prevent additional air from entering the tubing system once it has been filled and the initial bubbles have cleared. The contrast is instilled into the duct until the patient feels fullness in the breast or the contrast is seen spilling retrograde from the duct orifice. The procedure should not be painful. If the patient experiences any pain or burning when the contrast is injected, the injection should be stopped because the contrast might have extravasated outside of the ductal system into the surrounding parenchyma. Once a lesion or lesions have been mapped, the areas may be localized for surgical excision.

There is a wide spectrum of findings on galactography, but most significant are intraductal filling defects (see the figures), obstruction with blunt termination of the contrast (see the figures), or wall irregularity or distortion (see the figures). There is a significant overlap in the galactogram findings seen with papillomas and carcinomas. However, the greater the irregularity of the ductal architecture, the higher the likelihood that there is a malignancy. Any of these findings are suspicious and a biopsy is recommended. The first figure shows a lobulated distal intraductal mass that was shown to be a papilloma at excision. The second figure was a small intraductal carcinoma.

This case is courtesy of Emily F. Conant, M.D., Professor and Chief, Division of Breast Imaging, Hospital of the University of Pennsylvania, Philadelphia, Pennsylvania.

Notes

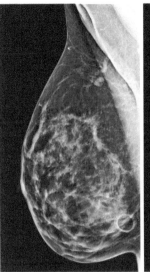
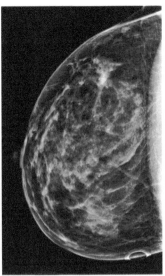

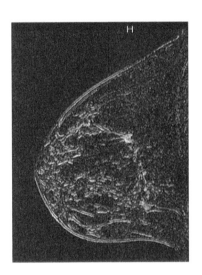
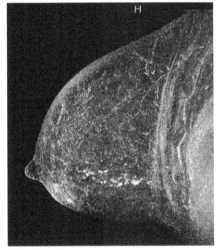

Contralateral breast.

History: A 40-year-old woman had an area of distortion seen in the right upper outer breast on routine baseline screening mammogram. Biopsy was performed, and bilateral MRI was performed.

1. What should be included in the differential diagnosis of the right breast abnormality? (Choose all that apply.)
   A. Infiltrating ductal carcinoma
   B. Radial sclerosing lesion
   C. Focal fibrosis
   D. Infiltrating lobular carcinoma

2. Which indication for MRI after a needle biopsy of carcinoma is *incorrect*?
   A. MRI may reveal multifocal disease not seen on mammogram.
   B. MRI may reveal multicentric disease not seen on mammogram.
   C. MRI is used to image the axilla, which is poorly seen on mammogram.
   D. MRI may reveal contralateral malignancy not seen on mammogram.

3. What is the most likely histology causing the enhancement in the contralateral left breast?
   A. Ductal carcinoma in situ
   B. Fibrocystic change
   C. Invasive lobular carcinoma (ILC)
   D. Fat necrosis

4. What is the next step in management after MRI in this patient?
   A. Follow-up MRI of the left breast in 6 months
   B. Ultrasound of the left breast to look for any evidence of a mass to correspond to the MRI enhancement
   C. MRI-guided biopsy of the left breast
   D. Positron emission mammography

Invasive Lobular Carcinoma, Contralateral Disease

1. A, B, and D
2. C
3. A
4. C

References

Dixon JM, Anderson TJ, Page DL, et al: Infiltrating lobular carcinoma of the breast: an evaluation of the incidence and consequence of bilateral disease. *Br J Surg* 1983;70(9):513-516.

Fortunato L, Mascaro A, Poccia I, et al: Lobular breast cancer: same survival and local control compared with ductal cancer, but should both be treated the same way? Analysis of an institutional database over a 10-year period. *Ann Surg Oncol* 2012;19(4):1107-1114.

Lopez JK, Bassett LW: Invasive lobular carcinoma of the breast: spectrum of mammographic, US, and MR imaging findings. *Radiographics* 2009;29(1):165-176.

Mann RM, Hoogeveen YL, Blickman JG, et al: MRI compared to conventional diagnostic work-up in the detection and evaluation of invasive lobular carcinoma of the breast: a review of existing literature. *Breast Cancer Res Treat* 2008;107(1):1-14.

Quan ML, Sclafani L, Heerdt AS, et al: Magnetic resonance imaging detects unsuspected disease in patients with invasive lobular cancer. *Ann Surg Oncol* 2003;10(9):1048-1053.

Cross-Reference

Ikeda D: *Breast Imaging: THE REQUISITES*, 2nd ed, Philadelphia: Saunders, 2010, pp 265, 305.

Comment

ILC accounts for 8% to 14% of breast cancers. However, it is more difficult to detect—and is more frequently multicentric, multifocal, and bilateral—compared with the more common infiltrating ductal carcinoma.

When ILC is found on a mammogram (see the figures), the next step in management after needle biopsy is MRI. This study helps diagnose the extent of disease. Extent of disease includes assessment of the size of the known tumor, which may be larger than expected based on the mammogram. It has been shown that positive margins after surgery are much more common in ILC compared with infiltrating ductal carcinoma, exceeding 50%, likely owing to the pattern of spread of this insidious tumor. If tumor size is measured on MRI before surgery, this can aid the surgeon in surgical planning.

Extent of disease also includes whether there is additional tumor in that quadrant or elsewhere in the same breast (multifocal or multicentric disease). In a meta-analysis, MRI showed additional ipsilateral disease in 32% of patients. MRI of the opposite breast should also be performed. The same meta-analysis showed contralateral disease seen only on MRI in 7%. MRI may show a different enhancement pattern for ILC than for infiltrating ductal carcinoma because ILC may be slower to enhance and fail to have wash-out kinetics. This enhancement pattern is similar to background fibroglandular tissue and may be difficult to detect. The most common enhancement pattern seen in ILC is the irregular or spiculated mass, seen in approximately 30% to 40% (see the figures). It may also manifest as a mass surrounded by multiple smaller masses or foci or multiple enhancing foci with enhancing interconnecting strands.

In the patient in this case, the ipsilateral disease is unifocal (see the figures). The enhancement pattern in the ipsilateral breast seen in the second figure mimics the mammographic appearance. There is enhancement in the contralateral breast, which is of some concern for malignancy. The enhancement pattern in the contralateral breast is different, consisting of a stippled area of non-masslike enhancement that extends from anterior to posterior in a linear distribution (see the figures). This pattern suggests a ductal process, possibly ductal carcinoma in situ. The next step in management of the contralateral breast is MRI-guided needle biopsy.

Notes

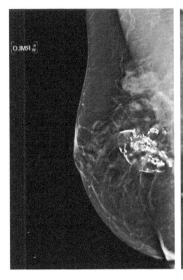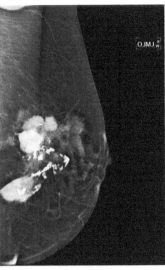

History: A 71-year-old patient presents for routine mammography. She gives a history of having silicone implants and experiencing rupture of the left implant. Her implants were removed 8 years ago. This is her first mammogram after the surgery.

1. What is the differential diagnosis for this mammogram? (Choose all that apply.)
   A. High-density irregular masses in the left breast, possible malignancy
   B. Pleomorphic calcifications in both breasts, suspicious for ductal carcinoma in situ (DCIS)
   C. Dense masses in the left breast, possible metastatic disease
   D. Dense material in the left breast, consistent with silicone granulomas

2. What additional work-up is needed?
   A. Magnification views of the calcifications bilaterally
   B. Ultrasound of the left breast dense masses
   C. MRI of the breasts
   D. B and C

3. What is the etiology of silicone granulomas?
   A. Silicone gel that has leaked from the implant is walled off by inflammation
   B. Occurs in patients with intact silicone implants and TB or sarcoid
   C. Caused by fat necrosis, related to silicone implant surgery
   D. Seen in women with intact silicone implants and multiple fibroadenomas

4. Would MRI help in this case?
   A. No, because the masses will enhance whether they are silicone granuloma or malignant masses.
   B. Yes, because the masses will not enhance if they are silicone granulomas.
   C. Yes, but contrast enhancement is not needed for silicone evaluation in this patient.
   D. Yes, but mammography and ultrasound are diagnostic, so MRI is not needed.

Explanted Ruptured Silicone Implants

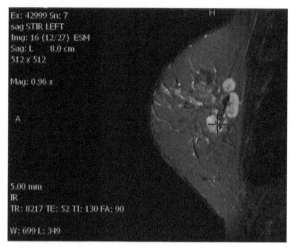

Left breast STIR image.

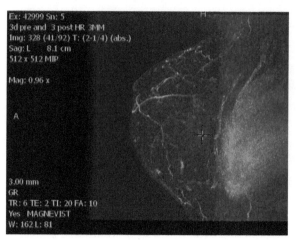

Left breast post–contrast MIP image.

1. A, C, and D
2. D
3. A
4. B

References

Berg WA, Nguyen TK, Middleton MS, et al: MR imaging of extracapsular silicone from breast implants: diagnostic pitfalls. *AJR Am J Roentgenol* 2002;178:465-472.

Robinson OG Jr, Bradley EL, Wilson DS: Analysis of explanted silicone implants: a report of 300 patients. *Ann Plast Surg* 1995;34:1-7.

Wang J, Shih TT, Li YW, et al: Magnetic resonance imaging of paraffinomas and siliconomas after mammoplasty. *J Formos Med Assoc* 2002;101(2):117-123.

Cross-Reference

Ikeda D: *Breast Imaging: THE REQUISITES*, 2nd ed, Philadelphia: Saunders, 2010, p 346.

Comment

Silicone implants consist of a silicone gel within a shell made of a polymer that might also contain silicone. The implants may be placed in front of (subglandular) or behind (subpectoral) the pectoralis muscle.

The body makes a fibrous capsule that surrounds the silicone implant. Silicone implants can rupture, and two broad types of rupture are recognized: intracapsular and extracapsular. These two designations describe whether the silicone that has escaped from the polymer shell is contained by the patient's fibrous capsule (intracapsular rupture) or escapes beyond the fibrous capsule and into the breast (extracapsular rupture). It can be difficult to recognize rupture on mammographic images, particularly intracapsular rupture. Ultrasound is more sensitive than mammography for the presence of rupture, and MRI is the most sensitive for the diagnosis of rupture, intracapsular or extracapsular.

Once a silicone implant has undergone extracapsular rupture, there is free silicone in the breast, which may be taken up by the lymphatics and deposited in the axillary lymph nodes. This can be seen as dense particles in the nodes, similar to calcium. The free silicone in the breast is walled off as granulomas, which can calcify, and in this patient, the granulomas are seen as dense masses in the left breast (see the figures). The silicone granuloma is also termed siliconoma. The implant capsule can also calcify, likely a reaction to gel bleed, and can be seen in mammograms with and without implant rupture.

When implants are removed, free silicone that is formed into granulomas might not be excised, as in this patient (see the figures). The capsule might or might not be removed. In this patient, the capsules, which have calcified, were not removed. The calcifications in the capsule are typically coarse and benign, as in this patient (see the figures), but the calcifications can be difficult to interpret if they are faint.

In this patient, the diagnosis of the left breast masses was not certain, and MRI was recommended. MRI demonstrates nonenhancing masses in the left breast (see the figures) that have increased signal on T1- and water-suppressed inversion recovery (STIR) T2-weighted images (see the figures), consistent with silicone granulomas. Biopsy is not indicated. This patient can be followed with annual mammography.

Notes

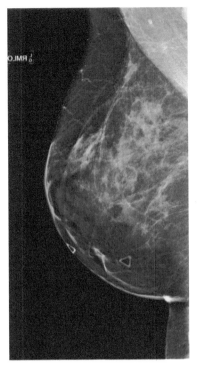

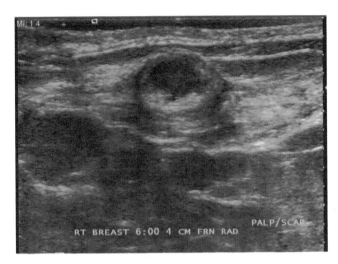

History: A 46-year-old woman had bilateral reduction surgery 2 years ago and now feels a palpable lump in her right lower breast at the 6 o'clock position.

1. What is the differential diagnosis for the mammographic and ultrasound images? (Choose all that apply.)
   A. Fibroadenoma
   B. Malignancy
   C. Fat necrosis
   D. Hematoma or seroma

2. Is this location typical for fat necrosis after breast reduction surgery?
   A. No, the location is usually in the upper outer quadrant.
   B. Yes, this is a typical location.
   C. No, this can occur anywhere in the breast; there is no typical location.
   D. No, the location is usually along the inframammary fold.

3. Why does fat necrosis occur after breast reduction surgery?
   A. Ischemia due to surgical disruption of blood supply
   B. Poor postoperative wound care
   C. Infection after surgery
   D. The breast has been made too small

4. What ultrasound appearance is seen in fat necrosis?
   A. The appearance is typically a complex cyst.
   B. There is always shadowing seen in oil cysts.
   C. Complex cystic mass with mural nodules is one appearance.
   D. The border of fat necrosis is typically smooth.

CASE 121

Palpable Mass after Reduction Surgery

1. B, C, and D
2. B
3. A
4. C

References

Miller CL, Feig SA, Fox JW: Mammographic changes after reduction mammoplasty. *AJR Am J Roentgenol* 1987;149:35-38.

Muir TM, Tresham J, Fritschi L, Wylie E: Screening for breast cancer post reduction mammoplasty. *Clin Radiol* 2010;65(3):198-205.

Cross-Reference

Ikeda D: *Breast Imaging: THE REQUISITES*, 2nd ed, Philadelphia: Saunders, 2010, p 360.

Comment

Breast reduction surgery is cosmetic surgery performed to reduce the size of the breasts. Commonly, patients who have this surgery have large, fatty, and pendulous breasts. The surgical incisions include a transverse incision along the inferior aspect of the breast, near the inframammary fold, and a vertical incision at the 6 o'clock position. The inferior breast tissue is removed, decreasing the volume of the breast. A keyhole incision around the edge of the areola may also be made to move the nipple superiorly on the breast mound.

Fat necrosis is often seen at the scar lines, particularly along the 6 o'clock vertical scar and the circumareolar scar. The patient might feel a palpable mass. Fat necrosis is caused by the trauma to the breast by the surgery: ischemia of the relatively poorly vascularized fatty tissue, interruption of blood vessels, and bleeding into the site. The mammographic features are more typical than the ultrasound features because of the appearance of fat lucency. Rim calcifications and thick, noncalcified fibrous walls can be seen surrounding the fat (see the figures). The encapsulated fat may be present as a palpable mass. The ultrasound features are more variable, and the fat necrosis can appear echogenic, can shadow, and can be a suspicious-appearing complex cyst with mural nodules (see the figures).

In this patient, the location and mammographic appearance are typical of fat necrosis, and the size of the ultrasound complex cyst matches the size of the lucent mass on mammogram. No further work-up is required. The findings can be given a Breast Imaging Reporting and Data System (BI-RADS) score of 2.

Notes

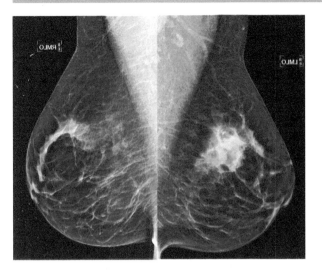

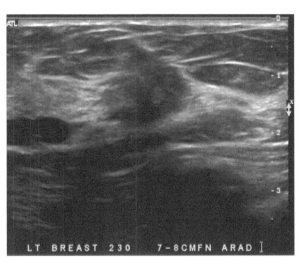

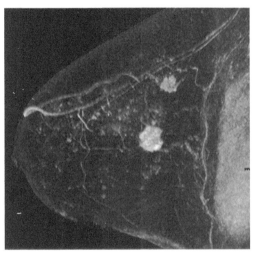

History: A 51-year-old woman is recalled for additional views and ultrasound after a routine screening mammogram shows a subtle change in the left breast asymmetry compared with previous mammogram.

1. What should be included in the differential diagnosis of the screening mammogram? (Choose all that apply.)
   A. Asymmetric gland tissue in the left upper outer breast
   B. Cyst in the left outer breast
   C. Malignant mass in the left outer breast
   D. Fat necrosis

2. What is the next step in management after mammogram and ultrasound?
   A. MRI
   B. Short-term follow-up for probably benign findings
   C. Fine-needle aspiration biopsy
   D. Needle core biopsy

3. Which of the following is *not* a reason to perform MRI?
   A. MRI should be performed before needle biopsy to ensure there is an enhancing mass.
   B. MRI can give information about the contralateral breast.
   C. MRI can establish the presence of multicentric disease.
   D. MRI can establish the presence of multifocal disease.

4. How is *multifocal disease* defined?
   A. Multifocal disease is additional cancer in the opposite breast.
   B. Multifocal disease is additional cancer in the same quadrant.
   C. Multifocal disease is additional disease in a separate quadrant.
   D. Multifocal disease refers to cancer that has spread to the ipsilateral lymph nodes.

Multifocal Disease Seen on MRI

1. A, B, and C
2. D
3. A
4. B

References

Houssami N, Ciatto S, Macaskill P, et al: Accuracy and surgical impact of magnetic resonance imaging in breast cancer staging: systematic review and meta-analysis in detection of multifocal and multicentric cancer. *J Clin Oncol* 2008;26(19):3248-3258.

Houssami N, Hayes DF: Review of preoperative magnetic resonance imaging (MRI) in breast cancer: should MRI be performed on all women with newly diagnosed, early stage breast cancer? *CA Cancer J Clin* 2009;59(5):290-302.

Lehman CD, Gatsonis C, Kuhl CK, et al; ACRIN Trial 6667 Investigators Group: MRI evaluation of the contralateral breast in women with recently diagnosed breast cancer. *N Engl J Med* 2007;356 (13):1295-1303.

Schell AM, Rosenkranz K, Lewis PJ: Role of breast MRI in the preoperative evaluation of patients with newly diagnosed breast cancer. *AJR Am J Roentgenol* 2009;192(5):1438-1444.

Schnall M: MR imaging evaluation of cancer extent: is there clinical relevance? *Magn Reson Imaging Clin N Am* 2006;14 (3):379-381.

Cross-Reference

Ikeda D: *Breast Imaging: THE REQUISITES*, 2nd ed, Philadelphia: Saunders, 2010, pp 300, 305.

Comment

MRI is performed for evaluation of both breasts before surgery in patients with a diagnosis of breast cancer; this is also termed *preoperative MRI*. In a meta-analysis, proponents of preoperative MRI showed that an additional lesion is seen in 16% of patients. The most common secondary lesion found is in the ipsilateral breast and may be in the same quadrant, a multifocal lesion, as in the patient in this case (see the figures). Additional lesions may also be seen in a different quadrant; this is termed *multicentric disease*. Less commonly (approximately 2% to 3%), additional lesions are found in the contralateral breast.

The location of the additional disease relative to the primary tumor is very important for surgical planning. Disease in the same quadrant may still be considered for breast conservation therapy, whereas disease in different quadrants may be treated with mastectomy. Patients who are being considered for partial breast irradiation may undergo MRI before treatment to determine if they qualify for this procedure. Partial breast irradiation is performed only in select patients.

Biopsy is indicated for additional lesions that are identified on MRI, just as biopsy was performed on the initial lesion before excision. Although MRI is very sensitive, its specificity is lower, and many lesions seen on MRI are benign and need no excision.

The need for additional time before surgery causing delay in treatment, additional biopsy procedures, and cost are several of the reasons cited against the use of preoperative MRI. Opponents also state that the detection of additional disease and the subsequent change in surgical management do not alter outcome; trials have not substantiated that patients who undergo preoperative MRI have a decrease in local recurrence. Preoperative MRI is still widely performed in patients with new diagnoses, in particular, patients with invasive lobular carcinoma, patients with dense breasts, patients with implants limiting the mammogram, and patients with a posterior lesion that may involve the chest wall.

Notes

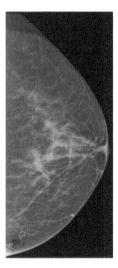
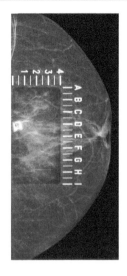
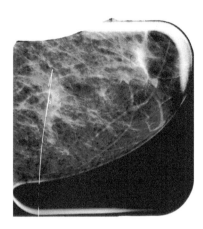
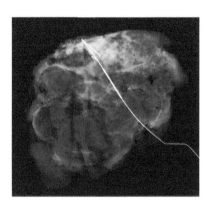

History: A 63-year-old woman is scheduled for surgery for removal of microcalcifications in the left lower breast after stereotactic guided biopsy.

1. What should be included in the differential diagnosis for the calcifications in the lower left breast? (Choose all that apply.)
   A. Fibrocystic change
   B. Atypical ductal hyperplasia
   C. Lobular carcinoma in situ
   D. Ductal carcinoma in situ

2. Which of the following statements regarding the best selection of imaging modality to guide needle localization is *false*?
   A. Needle localization can be performed only under mammographic guidance.
   B. Calcifications are generally localized under mammographic guidance.
   C. Masses are generally localized under ultrasound guidance.
   D. Areas of non-masslike enhancement are generally localized under MRI guidance.

3. What are the correct steps, in order, to perform mammography-guided needle localization?
   A. Needle placement, needle adjustment in the orthogonal plane, selection of the coordinates within the alphanumeric grid, hook wire placement

   B. Hook wire placement, needle adjustment in the orthogonal plane, needle placement, selection of the coordinates within the alphanumeric grid
   C. Selection of the coordinates within the alphanumeric grid, needle placement, needle adjustment in the orthogonal plane, hook wire placement
   D. Hook wire placement, selection of the coordinates within the alphanumeric grid, needle placement, needle adjustment in the orthogonal plane

4. Which of the following statements regarding mammography-guided needle localization is true?
   A. It is unnecessary to send mammogram films to the operating room.
   B. A radiograph of the specimen should always be obtained.
   C. The specimen radiograph is evaluated by the surgeon in the operating room.
   D. The surgeon does not need to be notified of the specimen radiograph findings.

Mammography-Guided Needle Localization

1. B, C, and D
2. A
3. C
4. B

References

DePalo AJ: Surgical considerations in needle localization procedures. *Semin Surg Oncol* 1991;7(5):253-256.

Homer MJ, Smith TJ, Safaii H: Prebiopsy needle localization: methods, problems, and expected results. *Radiol Clin North Am* 1992 Jan;30(1): 139-153.

Klimberg VS: Advances in the diagnosis and excision of breast cancer. *Am Surg* 2003;69(1):11-14.

Kopans DB, Swann CA: Preoperative imaging-guided needle placement and localization of clinically occult breast lesions. *AJR Am J Roentgenol* 1989;152(1):1-9.

Cross-Reference

Ikeda D: *Breast Imaging: THE REQUISITES*, 2nd ed, Philadelphia: Saunders, 2010, p 195.

Comment

Needle localization under mammographic guidance can be guided by mediolateral and craniocaudal (CC) images from the standard imaging equipment (see the figures) or can be guided stereotactically. This case illustrates the standard-imaging approach. Needle localizations are necessary to guide the surgeon accurately to a lesion that is nonpalpable and requires excision.

To expedite the localization procedure on the day of the surgery, a complete work-up of the lesions should have been performed in advance (e.g., magnification views, if needed, to establish the extent of microcalcifications) and triangulated on orthogonal imaging. The closest skin surface to the lesion is determined. Needle localization may be performed under mammographic, ultrasound, or MRI guidance. The selection of the guiding modality should be based on the ease of seeing the lesion. Generally, calcifications are localized under mammographic guidance, masses are localized under ultrasound guidance, and areas of non-masslike enhancement are localized under MRI guidance.

For mammography-guided needle localization, the most important step is positioning the patient so that the skin entry site for placement of the localizing needle and hook wire is from the closest skin surface.

The needle length is chosen by measuring the distance from the closest skin surface to the site of the lesion. The patient is placed in compression with the alphanumeric grid open over the appropriate skin surface. The patient is imaged, and the coordinates at the center of the lesion are chosen (in this case, ½ and D½; see the figures). The skin is cleansed and anesthetized, and the needle is placed into the breast. To ensure that the needle is placed into the lesion, an image of the needle hub superimposed over the shaft of the needle is obtained (see the figures).

The patient is removed from compression, and an orthogonal view is obtained showing the position of the tip of the needle relative to the lesion (see the figures). The needle depth is adjusted so that the tip of the needle is at or just beyond the lesion (in this case, the needle was placed slightly deep to the lesion and had to be withdrawn slightly). The hook wire is placed through the needle and secured in the breast tissue. Some surgeons prefer to keep the needle in the breast to aid in localizing the lesion in the operating room, whereas other surgeons prefer to remove the needle and keep only the wire in the breast. Two orthogonal films (usually a CC view and mediolateral or lateromedial view) showing the wire and its relationship to the lesion, with the lesion circled, are sent to the operating room to serve as a "map" for the surgeon.

The specimen radiograph is an essential component of mammography-guided needle localization (see the figures). The radiologist must review the specimen to ensure that the lesion has been removed (or sampled, depending on the case). The surgeon is notified of the specimen radiograph findings, and if the lesion has not been removed or adequately sampled, the surgeon should be directed to obtain more tissue. In this case, the surgeon had intended to remove the entire area of microcalcifications and biopsy clip and obtain clear margins for a lumpectomy. The specimen radiograph revealed that the microcalcifications are at the edge of the tissue, and the surgeon was directed to obtain more tissue. Communication from the radiologist assists the surgeon in obtaining clean margins and reducing the likelihood of reexcision.

Notes

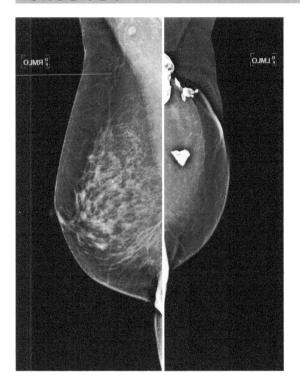

History: A 71-year-old woman who had a mastectomy for cancer with TRAM reconstruction 10 years previously now feels a mass in her reconstructed left breast.

1. What is the differential diagnosis for a palpable mass in a reconstructed breast? (Choose all that apply.)
   A. Recurrent breast cancer
   B. Calcified fat necrosis, Breast Imaging Reporting and Data System (BI-RADS) 2
   C. Fibroadenoma
   D. Simple breast cyst

2. What is the first imaging study in a patient who has a personal history of breast cancer and has a new lump?
   A. MRI
   B. Ultrasound
   C. Positron emission tomography (PET)
   D. Mammogram

3. Is the mammogram alone sufficient for diagnosis in a patient with palpable mass in a reconstructed breast?
   A. Yes, mammogram is sufficient if the palpable finding is an oil cyst.
   B. Yes, mammogram is sufficient if the mammogram is completely normal.
   C. No, ultrasound is always needed for a palpable finding.
   D. No, MRI is necessary to further evaluate the palpable mass.

4. Which description best fits fat necrosis calcifications?
   A. Fine, linear, branching
   B. Layering on 90-degree true lateral view
   C. Large, coarse, and irregular
   D. Large, cigar shaped

C A S E 1 2 4

Palpable Mass in Transverse Rectus Abdominis Myocutaneous (TRAM) Flap

1. C and D
2. C
3. C
4. D

References
Helvie MA, Bailey JE, Roubidoux MA, et al: Mammographic screening of TRAM flap breast reconstructions for detection of nonpalpable recurrent cancer. *Radiology* 1002;224:211.

Taboada JL, Stephens TW, Krishnamurthy S, et al: The many faces of fat necrosis in the breast. *AJR Am J Roentgenol* 2009;192:815-825.

Cross-Reference
Ikeda D: *Breast Imaging: THE REQUISITES*, 2nd ed, Philadelphia: Saunders, 2010, pp 75, 355.

Comment
One common method of breast reconstruction after mastectomy is the transverse rectus abdominis myocutaneous (TRAM) flap. Skin, fat, and rectus muscle are brought up from the abdomen to construct a breast mound. This procedure uses living tissue from the mastectomy patient (autogenous transplant).

Fat necrosis after a surgical procedure is not uncommon because areas of fat can lose their blood supply during the procedure. The area of fatty tissue death can calcify, and the calcifications can initially appear as rim types or as pleomorphic shapes that, in time, become coarse, often with associated fat lucency. On mammogram, fat necrosis is most commonly seen as oil cyst associated with coarse calcification (see the figures) but may also present with a focal asymmetry, spiculated density, or pleomorphic microcalcifications. The many appearances result from the cytologic makeup of the process: Fat cells degenerate and hemorrhage, which results in an oil cyst. Fibrosis can surround the oil cyst. It is the varying degree of fibrosis that causes the different appearances on the mammogram. In the cases with the least amount of fibrosis, the palpable mass is lucent (oil cyst), with developing peripheral calcifications forming early and coarse central calcifications forming later. With this appearance of a calcified oil cyst, the appearance is pathognomonic of fat necrosis, and no additional imaging or biopsy is needed. Fibrosis may be the only finding, with an irregular or spiculated density, and the calcifications can be pleomorphic. In these cases, the mammographic appearance overlaps with malignancy, and biopsy may be needed.

The mechanism of malignancy developing in the TRAM reconstruction includes residual cancer tissue, tumor seeding at the time of mastectomy, and tumor sequestered in lymphatics. It can also develop in remnants of native breast tissue not removed entirely at mastectomy. The patient who has undergone a mastectomy for malignant disease is at increased risk for developing a new breast cancer or a recurrence of the known cancer.

The patient in this example presented with a palpable finding, and a diagnostic mammogram of the TRAM flap was performed. Although it is controversial, it may be useful to perform routine screening mammography of the TRAM reconstruction at the time of the mammogram of the remaining breast. Helvie and colleagues noted that malignancy was found as nonpalpable lesions in the TRAM flap in 2% of cases, approximately the same rate of malignancy found after breast conservation therapy.

Notes

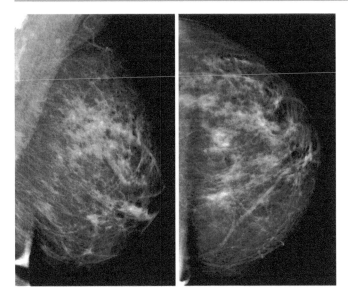

History: A 53-year-old asymptomatic woman presents for screening mammogram.

1. What should be included in the differential diagnosis for the calcifications in the upper inner left breast? (Choose all that apply.)
   A. Fibrocystic changes
   B. Atypical lobular hyperplasia
   C. Lobular carcinoma in situ (LCIS)
   D. Invasive lobular carcinoma

2. Stereotactic biopsy revealed benign calcifications associated with fibrocystic change and multiple adjacent foci of LCIS. Which of the following statements regarding LCIS and microcalcifications is true?
   A. Microcalcifications are a predisposing factor for the development of LCIS.
   B. Microcalcifications exclude the diagnosis of LCIS.
   C. Microcalcifications are pathognomonic of LCIS.
   D. Microcalcifications may or may not be associated with LCIS.

3. All of the following statements regarding LCIS and cancer are true *except:*
   A. LCIS is an important risk factor for future development of breast cancer.
   B. The risk for developing breast cancer in patients with LCIS is approximately 8 to 12 times the normal rate.
   C. Patients with LCIS are at increased risk for developing invasive lobular carcinoma only.
   D. Future cancer can develop in either breast.

4. Which of the following statements regarding management of LCIS is true?
   A. LCIS does not require further management.
   B. When LCIS is found at needle core biopsy, the next step in management is to repeat the needle biopsy to obtain more samples.
   C. When LCIS is found at needle core biopsy, the next step in management is excisional biopsy at the site of LCIS.
   D. When LCIS is found at needle core biopsy, the next step in management is lumpectomy, radiation, and chemotherapy.

CASE 125

Management of Lobular Carcinoma In Situ

1. A, B, and C
2. D
3. C
4. C

References

Anderson BO, Calhoun KE, Rosen EL: Evolving concepts in the management of lobular neoplasia. *J Natl Compr Canc Netw* 2006;4(5):511-522.

Berg WA, Mrose HE, Ioffe OB: Atypical lobular hyperplasia or lobular carcinoma in situ at core-needle breast biopsy. *Radiology* 2001; 218(2):503-509.

Hanby AM, Hughes TA: In situ and invasive lobular neoplasia of the breast. *Histopathology* 2008;52(1):58-66.

Simpson PT, Gale T, Fulford LG, et al: The diagnosis and management of pre-invasive breast disease: pathology of atypical lobular hyperplasia and lobular carcinoma in situ. *Breast Cancer Res* 2003;5(5):258-262.

Cross-Reference

Ikeda D: *Breast Imaging: THE REQUISITES*, 2nd ed, Philadelphia: Saunders, 2010, p 26.

Comment

LCIS is a high-risk lesion and an important risk factor for future development of breast cancer. The increased risk is for both breasts, not specifically at the site where the LCIS was found. In the patient in this case, biopsy specimens of the microcalcifications present in the left breast were obtained and shown to be fibrocystic change and multiple foci of LCIS (see the figures). The LCIS was not associated with the calcifications and was an incidental finding, as is often the case. A new spiculated mass was seen 3 years later in the contralateral breast (see the figures). Needle core biopsy showed invasive ductal carcinoma.

Patients with LCIS have an approximately 8 to 12 times increased risk of developing breast cancer. LCIS is detected on imaging-guided biopsy and at excisional biopsy for calcifications and masses, and it is usually an incidental finding. It has no imaging features of its own. The risk of subsequent cancer increases when multiple lobules of LCIS are seen on histopathology. LCIS is multicentric in 85% of cases and bilateral in 30% to 67% of cases. The pathology of the future cancer can be either ductal or lobular.

In the past in women diagnosed with LCIS, recommendations for surveillance included bilateral prophylactic mastectomy. That is no longer recommended, and annual screening mammogram is now recommended. Some recommendations include ultrasound as a screening tool, in addition to mammogram, particularly in women with dense breasts, but this is not universally accepted. MRI can be used as an adjunct to mammography but is not recommended, either for or against, in the 2007 American Cancer Society guidelines for screening MRI. Some patients with LCIS are given selective estrogen receptor modulator therapy, such as tamoxifen. Tamoxifen has been shown to reduce the risk of developing breast cancer by 50%.

Excisional biopsy is recommended in patients who have LCIS found at needle core biopsy because there is a 10% to 20% chance that DCIS or invasive cancer is near the site of LCIS, and the core biopsy did not represent the entire lesion. The same is true for core biopsy specimens showing atypical lobular hyperplasia and atypical ductal hyperplasia.

Notes

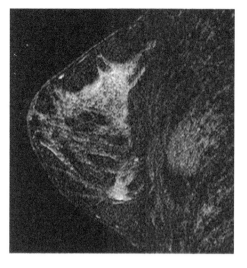
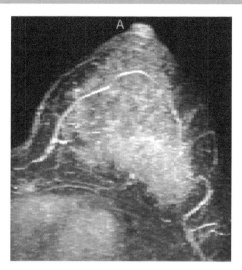
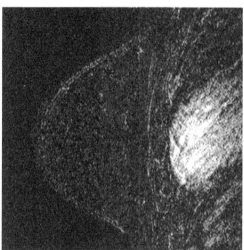
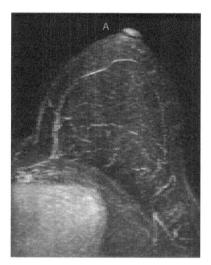

History: A 46-year-old woman with a greater than 20% lifetime risk of breast cancer based on personal history and family history of the disease undergoes screening MRI and follow-up MRI 6 months later.

1. What should be included in the differential diagnosis for the images shown? (Choose all that apply.)
   A. A woman scanned before and after tamoxifen therapy
   B. A woman scanned at two different times of the normal menstrual cycle
   C. Two different patients have been scanned
   D. Two scans from a postmenopausal patient

2. Which of the following is *not* an indication for screening MRI?
   A. A patient who is worried about breast cancer because her sister-in-law just received a diagnosis of breast cancer
   B. A woman with a 30% lifetime risk of breast cancer
   C. A woman whose sister carries the *BRCA1* gene mutation
   D. A woman with Cowden syndrome

3. Why is the timing of the MRI examination during the menses important?
   A. It is not important.
   B. The patient is more comfortable if scanned during the latter half of the cycle.
   C. Estrogen and progesterone levels are lower during the luteal phase, and this affects gland enhancement.
   D. The sensitivity of detecting small masses is greater during the follicular phase.

4. What is the next step in imaging management for this patient?
   A. Because MRI is normal, no further MRI should be performed.
   B. Annual screening with MRI should be performed; no mammogram is necessary.
   C. Annual MRI and mammography screening are needed.
   D. The patient needs no further screening.

CASE 126

MRI in Follicular and Luteal Menstrual Phase

1. A, B, and C
2. A
3. D
4. C

References

Chan S, Su MY, Lei FJ, et al: Menstrual cycle-related fluctuations in breast density measured by using three-dimensional MR imaging. *Radiology* 2011;261(3):744-751.

Delille JP, Slanetz PJ, Yeh ED, et al: Physiologic changes in breast magnetic resonance imaging during the menstrual cycle: perfusion imaging, signal enhancement, and influence of the T1 relaxation time of breast tissue. *Breast J* 2005;11(4):236-241.

Saslow D, Boetes C, Burke W, et al; American Cancer Society Breast Cancer Advisory Group: American Cancer Society guidelines for breast screening with MRI as an adjunct to mammography. *CA Cancer J Clin* 2007;57:75-89.

Cross-Reference

Ikeda D: *Breast Imaging: THE REQUISITES*, 2nd ed, Philadelphia: Saunders, 2010, p 268.

Comment

Screening MRI is recommended as an adjunct to screening mammogram for women who have *BRCA* gene mutation, who have a lifetime breast cancer risk based on risk assessment models of 20% or greater, or who have certain high-risk syndromes, such as Cowden syndrome and Li-Fraumeni syndrome. The patient in this case was diagnosed at age 40 with right breast cancer. Her grandmother and two maternal aunts were diagnosed with breast cancer in their thirties and forties. The patient has heterogeneously dense breasts on mammogram. Her lifetime risk is greater than 20%.

Our practice is to ask women younger than 55 about their last menstrual period before scheduling a breast MRI. This patient had not had a menses in several months and so was scheduled at the next available opening. MRI showed bilateral areas of non-masslike enhancement (see the figures). The enhancement has benign characteristics on time-intensity curve, with persistence over time, coded in blue on computer-assisted detection (CAD). This enhancement was believed to be due to the increased estrogen and progesterone levels of the luteal phase of the menstrual cycle, and follow-up was recommended.

The patient returned after her next menses; breast MRI was scheduled during days 7 to 14 of the menstrual cycle. The change in the appearance of the enhancement pattern is remarkable; there is no glandular enhancement (see the figures). This case illustrates the benefit of performing breast MRI during the follicular phase of the cycle if possible. It is much easier to detect a small enhancing mass against the background of nonenhancing glandular tissue compared with during the luteal phase against the background of areas of non-masslike enhancement.

Notes

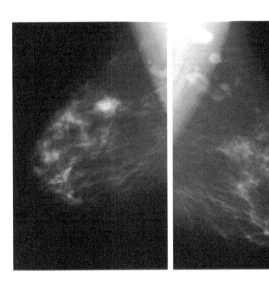

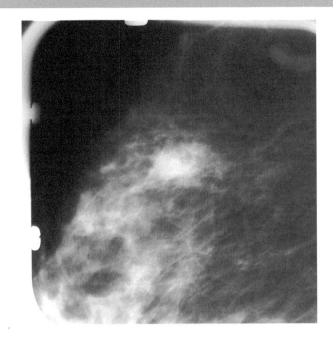

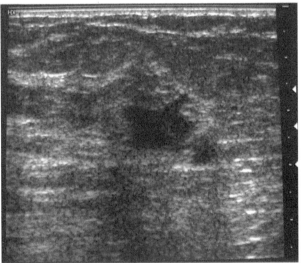

History: A 63-year-old woman presents for a screening mammogram.

1. What should be included in the differential diagnosis for the initial presentation? (Choose all that apply.)
   A. Invasive ductal carcinoma
   B. Ductal carcinoma in situ
   C. Adenoid cystic carcinoma
   D. Fibroadenoma

2. Which of the following is *not a rare* type of invasive breast cancer?
   A. Secretory carcinoma
   B. Adenoid cystic carcinoma
   C. Squamous cell carcinoma
   D. Ductal carcinoma not otherwise specified

3. Why is it useful to know the pathologic subtype of a breast cancer?
   A. It makes surgery easier.
   B. The pathologic subtype often predicts the prognosis of the cancer.
   C. Treatment may be unnecessary.
   D. Knowing the subtype of the breast cancer is of no use.

4. Which of the following is *not* characteristic of adenoid cystic carcinoma?
   A. It cannot be distinguished from other subtypes of breast cancer by imaging only.
   B. Metastases are infrequent.
   C. The prognosis is excellent.
   D. It affects younger women.

CASE 127

Adenoid Cystic Carcinoma

1. A and C
2. D
3. B
4. D

References

Glazebrook KN, Reynolds C, Smith RL, et al: Adenoid cystic carcinoma of the breast. *AJR Am J Roentgenol* 2010;194(5):1391-1396.

Khanfir K, Kallel A, Villette S, et al: Management of adenoid cystic carcinoma of the breast: a Rare Cancer Network Study. *Int J Radiat Oncol Biol Phys* 2012;82(5):2118-2124.

Santamaria G, Velasco M, Zanon G, et al: Adenoid cystic carcinoma of the breast: mammographic appearance and pathologic correlation. *AJR Am J Roentgenol* 1998;171(6):1679-1683.

Sperber F, Blank A, Metser U: Adenoid cystic carcinoma of the breast: mammographic, sonographic, and pathological correlation. *Breast J* 2002;8(1):53-54.

Thompson K, Grabowski J, Saltzstein SL, et al: Adenoid cystic breast carcinoma: is axillary staging necessary in all cases? Results from the California Cancer Registry. *Breast J* 2011;17(5):485-489.

Yerushalmi R, Hayes MM, Gelmon KA: Breast carcinoma—rare types: review of the literature. *Ann Oncol* 2009;20(11):1763-1770.

Cross-Reference

Ikeda D: *Breast Imaging: THE REQUISITES*, 2nd ed, Philadelphia: Saunders, 2010, p 131.

Comment

Adenoid cystic carcinoma is an unusual subtype of breast cancer, which accounts for less than 1% of all breast cancers. This subtype rarely spreads beyond the breast to the lymph nodes or to distant sites. The appearance on mammography and ultrasound is similar to other breast cancers, most often a lobulated mass (see the figures). It is important to know the cell type of breast cancers because the cell type often determines the clinical outcome. Adenoid cystic carcinoma has a better prognosis than other types. In a study of 28 patients with adenoid cystic carcinoma, the 5-year disease-free survival was 100%. This excellent prognosis affects treatment options. Axillary dissection and chemotherapy are unnecessary. However, the mass must be completely excised, or recurrence may occur in the breast. The average age of diagnosis is postmenopausal, age 65 years.

In the patient in this case, a developing irregular, high-density mass with microlobulated margins was seen in the upper outer quadrant of the right breast on routine screening mammogram (see the figures). The patient was 63 years old when the diagnosis was made; on pathology, this was a 2-cm mass that was predominantly in situ adenoid cystic cancer, with rare areas of invasion.

Notes

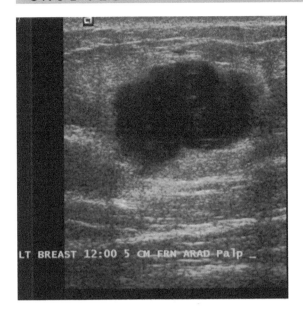

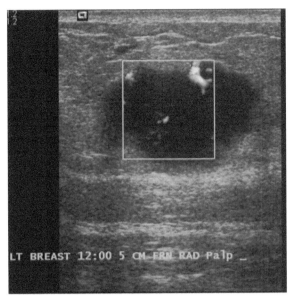

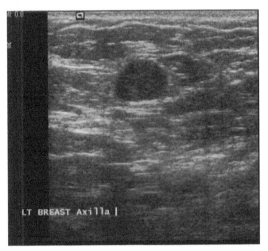

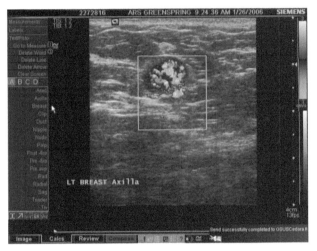

History: A 53-year-old woman presents for her baseline mammogram with a palpable left breast mass. After review of the mammogram, ultrasound was performed.

1. What should be included in the differential diagnosis for the lesion seen on ultrasound? (Choose all that apply.)
   A. Simple cyst
   B. Phyllodes tumor
   C. Mucinous carcinoma
   D. Medullary carcinoma

2. What is the next step in management of this palpable mass?
   A. MRI to differentiate benign from malignant
   B. Needle core biopsy
   C. Short-interval follow-up with ultrasound in 6 months
   D. PET/CT to evaluate for additional lesions

3. What are the special subtypes of infiltrating ductal carcinoma (IDC)?
   A. Medullary, mucinous, tubular, and papillary cancer
   B. Invasive ductal carcinoma not otherwise specified (IDC NOS)
   C. Ductal carcinoma in situ
   D. Lobular carcinoma in situ, atypical lobular hyperplasia, atypical ductal hyperplasia

4. Which of the following statements is true about medullary cancer?
   A. It is very rare—about 1% of all breast cancers.
   B. It has a worse prognosis than IDC NOS.
   C. It may manifest as a benign, soft mass.
   D. It is commonly found in men and women.

Medullary Cancer

1. B, C, and D
2. B
3. A
4. C

References

Meyer JE, Amin E, Lindfors KK, et al: Medullary carcinoma of the breast: mammographic and US appearance. *Radiology* 1989;170(1 Pt 1): 79-82.

Schrading S, Kuhl CK: Mammographic, US, and MR imaging phenotypes of familial breast cancer. *Radiology* 2008;246(1):58-70.

Cross-Reference

Ikeda D: *Breast Imaging: THE REQUISITES*, 2nd ed, Philadelphia: Saunders, 2010, p 114.

Comment

Medullary cancer is a subtype of IDC of the breast. It is uncommon, accounting for about 5% to 7% of IDCs. It is seen in slightly younger women compared with generic invasive ductal carcinoma, or NOS. It is well circumscribed, may be soft and mobile on examination, and may have features that suggest a benign etiology on mammography and ultrasound. On mammography, it may be round, oval, or lobulated. Calcifications are rare. On ultrasound, it is round, oval, or lobulated; is hypoechoic; has sharply circumscribed margins; and often has increased through-transmission of sound (see the figures).

On histology, medullary cancer comprises poorly differentiated cells, with a high nuclear grade. A lymphoplasmacytic reaction is seen in the tumor. It has a "pushing" margin, rather than an infiltrative margin, leading to its circumscribed edges, and no spiculation on mammography and ultrasound. It is common to find axillary node enlargement, but the nodes may be reactive rather than metastatic (see the figures). There is an overlap with the appearance of mucinous carcinoma, which is another tumor subgroup of IDC. The differential diagnosis also includes fibroadenoma, phyllodes tumor, and lymphoma.

In this case, the ultrasound features are inconsistent with a fibroadenoma because of the irregular, microlobulated margins. One suspicious ultrasound feature, such as the margins in this mass, means that the mass is a BI-RADS (Breast Imaging Reporting and Data System) 4, and biopsy is indicated. Color Doppler can help evaluate the vascularity of the mass (see the figures) and help differentiate a solid mass from a complex cyst. In this patient, axillary nodes were abnormal: round and hypoechoic, and intensely hypervascular (see the figures). However, the core biopsy of the axillary node revealed reactive cells and no metastases. This is not unusual in medullary carcinoma.

Notes

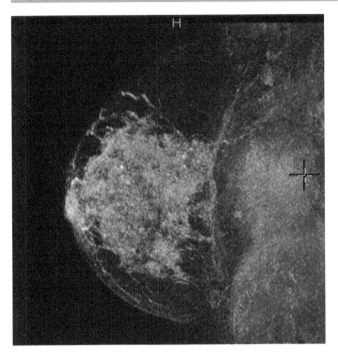

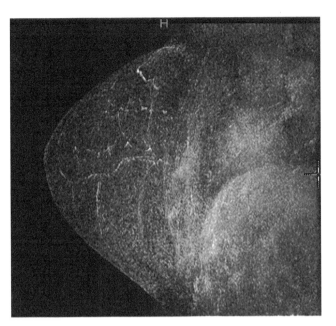

History: A 57-year-old woman underwent image-guided core biopsy, and stage IIIC invasive mammary carcinoma was diagnosed. MRI was performed for extent of disease. She underwent neoadjuvant chemotherapy, and follow-up MRI after chemotherapy.

1. What should be included in the differential diagnosis for the images shown? (Choose all that apply.)
   A. Complete clinical response to chemotherapy
   B. Decrease in size of enhancement after chemotherapy
   C. Improved pathologic response to chemotherapy
   D. Absence of residual disease

2. Which of the following statements about MRI after chemotherapy is *not* true?
   A. Chemotherapy has an antineovascularity effect.
   B. Chemotherapy can break up a larger tumor into smaller clumps of tumor.
   C. Tumor is completely eradicated if MRI is negative.
   D. Absence of residual tumor on MRI predicts improved survival.

3. Why is neoadjuvant chemotherapy used?
   A. To decrease the size of tumors before surgical treatment
   B. To negate the need for surgery
   C. To reduce the need for radiation therapy
   D. Because overall survival is higher in women who have neoadjuvant therapy compared with chemotherapy after surgery

4. Is this patient's first MRI consistent with inflammatory carcinoma?
   A. No, because there is no evidence of skin enhancement
   B. No, because the area of enhancement is too large
   C. Yes, because of the diffuse enhancement of the entire breast
   D. No, because there is no axillary adenopathy

CASE 129

Response to Neoadjuvant Chemotherapy

1. B and C
2. C
3. A
4. A

References

Chen JH, Feig B, Agrawal G, et al: MRI evaluation of pathologically complete response and residual tumors in breast cancer after neoadjuvant
chemotherapy. *Cancer* 2008;112(1):17-26.

Yuan Y, Chen X, Liu S, et al: Accuracy of MRI in prediction of pathologic complete remission in breast cancer after preoperative therapy:
a meta-analysis. *AJR Am J Roentgenol* 2010;195(1):260-268.

Cross-Reference

Ikeda D: *Breast Imaging: THE REQUISITES*, 2nd ed, Philadelphia:
Saunders, 2010, pp 273, 297.

Comment

Neoadjuvant chemotherapy is systemic treatment for
breast cancer that is given before definitive surgery.
The goal is to allow the patient to have breast conservation therapy, rather than mastectomy. Neoadjuvant chemotherapy is typically discussed when a patient presents
with locally advanced breast cancer, such as in the present case (see the figures).

Neoadjuvant chemotherapy is an alternative to adju-
vant chemotherapy, which is given after the cancer has
been resected. Both regimens have been shown to be
equivalent in overall survival and in the rate of development of distant metastases. Using chemotherapy before
surgery allows the clinician to gauge the response of
the patient to the therapy; this serves as an in vivo evaluation of the patient's response to the chemotherapeutic
regimen.

Pathologic response is measured at surgery. Complete
pathologic remission is the complete disappearance of
cancer in the primary tumor area. MRI predicts complete
pathologic response in approximately 70% of cases.
The patient in this case had absence of enhancement
on follow-up MRI but did not have a complete pathologic
response (see the figures).

Because chemotherapy targets tumor angiogenesis,
the MRI contrast agent may not reach the tumor, and
the enhancement may not accurately reflect the residual
tumor present. The radiologist should be cautious about
reporting a "complete response" and may want to report
only "response to treatment." MRI is about 90% specific
and about 60% sensitive for the presence of residual disease after chemotherapy but performs better than clinical
examination, mammography, and ultrasound.

Notes

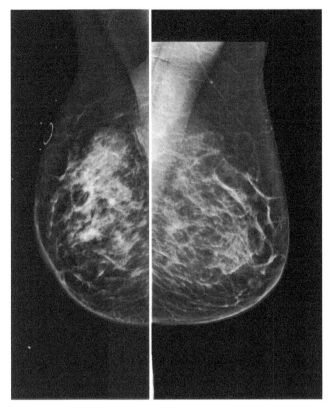
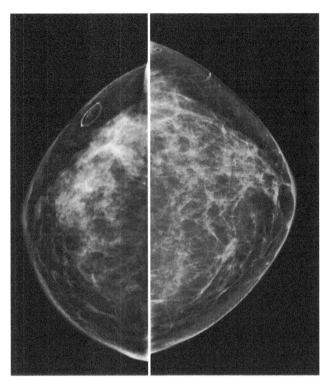

History: A 57-year-old woman presents for her baseline mammogram because of palpable mass in her right breast.

1. What is the differential diagnosis of the four-view mammogram? (Choose all that apply.)
   A. Normal mammogram
   B. Right breast diabetic mastopathy
   C. Right breast inflammatory cancer
   D. Right breast infiltrating lobular carcinoma

2. What is the next step?
   A. Ultrasound of the palpable concern
   B. Surgical consultation for biopsy of the palpable mass
   C. MRI
   D. Short-interval follow-up

3. What histologic type of breast cancer can manifest with increased density and a decrease in the size of the breast on the mammogram?
   A. Colloid-type cancer
   B. Medullary-type cancer
   C. Invasive lobular carcinoma
   D. Ductal carcinoma in situ (DCIS)

4. Diagnosis of a large malignancy in the right breast was made. Is breast MRI indicated? Why or why not?
   A. No, once the diagnosis is made, the patient should be referred for surgery as soon as possible.
   B. No, the patient will not be a candidate for breast conservation therapy owing to the large size of the malignancy, so MRI is not needed.
   C. Yes, MRI is useful to evaluate for extent of disease in the ipsilateral and contralateral breast.
   D. No, MRI is not needed because the patient should be advised to have bilateral mastectomy.

Invasive Lobular Cancer: The Shrinking Breast

1. B, C, and D
2. A
3. C
4. C

References

Harvey JA: Unusual breast cancers; useful clues to expanding the differential diagnosis. *Radiology* 2007;242:683-694.

Harvey JA, Fechner RE, Moore MM: Apparent ipsilateral decrease in breast size at mammography: a sign of infiltrating lobular carcinoma. *Radiology* 2000;214(3):883-889.

Jafri NF, Slanetz PJ: The shrinking breast: an unusual mammographic finding of invasive lobular carcinoma. *Radiology Case Reports* 2007;2:94.

Cross-Reference

Ikeda D: *Breast Imaging: THE REQUISITES*, 2nd ed, Philadelphia: Saunders, 2010, p 101.

Comment

This patient noted a palpable mass, but on review of the mammogram, no discrete mass was seen. The right breast appeared smaller than the left but was not smaller on clinical exam (compare the first and second figures). The right breast was also noted to have ill-defined areas of increased density throughout the central portion (see the figures).

Ultrasound was performed, and there was a large, ill-defined hypoechoic area measuring approximately 10 cm in diameter in the central breast. Ultrasound-guided needle biopsy was performed and showed infiltrating, poorly differentiated mammary carcinoma, with predominantly lobular features. Core biopsy of an axillary node showed metastatic disease.

Invasive lobular carcinoma (ILC) is less common than invasive ductal carcinoma (IDC), comprising less than 10% of all breast cancer. The cells of this cancer spread through the breast in single file or sheets, thus not forming a discrete mass, making it more difficult to detect on the mammogram. Because of this, ILC is more commonly missed on routine screening mammogram and manifests at a later stage than invasive ductal carcinoma. It also manifests more often as muticentric and bilateral disease than does IDC.

When ILC is large, the breast may appear to be shrinking on the mammogram. This is a mammographic finding, not a clinical finding, and may be due to the sheets of tumor cells causing decreased compressibility of the breast. The mammogram can show an irregular mass or asymmetry with ill-defined margins, as in this case.

Notes

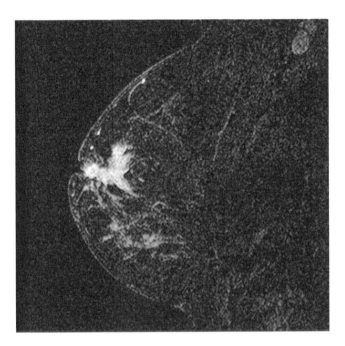

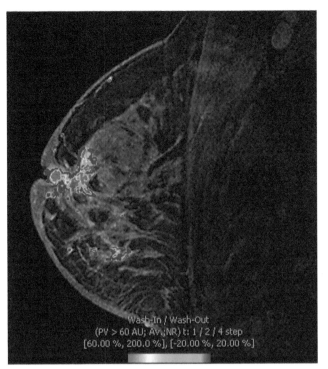

Wash-In / Wash-Out
(PV > 60 AU; Av.;NR) t: 1 / 2 / 4 step
[60.00 %, 200.0 %], [-20.00 %, 20.00 %]

History: A 51-year-old woman presents with nipple re-traction in the right breast. Mammogram shows a retracted nipple and skin thickening (not shown). Needle biopsy and bilateral MRI are performed.

1. What should be included in the differential diagnosis for the images shown? (Choose all that apply.)
   A. Papilloma
   B. Invasive ductal carcinoma
   C. Metaplastic carcinoma
   D. Invasive lobular carcinoma

2. What is metaplastic cancer?
   A. Synonymous with metastatic cancer, it means cancer that has spread outside the breast
   B. Cancer derived from two cell lines, also termed *carcinosarcoma*
   C. Relatively benign-acting tumor that is rare
   D. A rare cancer that has only mesenchymal cells and no epithelial cells

3. What is the next management step?
   A. Positron emission tomography (PET) scan to check for metastases
   B. Positron emission mammography to check for additional sites of cancer in both breasts
   C. Referral to surgical and medical oncology
   D. Strong recommendation that the patient return in 3 months for follow-up

4. Which of the following statements about breast sarcomas is *not* true?
   A. Sarcomas are unusual in the breast.
   B. Sarcomas spread hematogenously.
   C. Osteosarcomas can occur in the breast.
   D. Sarcomas in the breast generally have a good outcome.

Metaplastic Cancer

1. B and C
2. B
3. C
4. D

References

Feder JM, de Paredes ES, Hogge JP, et al: Unusual breast lesions: radiologic-pathologic correlation. *Radiographics* 1999;19(Spec No): S11-S26.

Hennessy BT, Giordano S, Broglio K, et al: Biphasic metaplastic sarcomatoid carcinoma of the breast. *Ann Oncol* 2006;17(4):605-613.

Wargotz ES, Norris HJ: Metaplastic carcinomas of the breast. III. Carcinosarcoma. *Cancer* 1989;64(7):1490-1499.

Cross-Reference

Ikeda D: *Breast Imaging: THE REQUISITES*, 2nd ed, Philadelphia: Saunders, 2010, p 398.

Comment

Metaplastic carcinoma is a rare form of breast cancer that accounts for less than 0.1% of all breast cancers. Also termed *carcinosarcoma,* it has carcinomatous (epithelial) and sarcomatous (mesenchymal) features. It is an aggressive form of cancer, behaving similarly to high-grade, receptor-negative adenocarcinomas.

Metaplastic cancer manifests clinically similar to invasive ductal carcinoma as a rapidly growing mass that may be centered on the nipple, as in the patient in this case (see the figures). Rapid wash-in and wash-out kinetics and nipple retraction are noted. The tumor may be locally aggressive, so breast conservation therapy may fail, and mastectomy may be the best surgical option. Chemotherapeutic agents given as neoadjuvant therapy are not as effective in metaplastic carcinoma compared with invasive ductal carcinoma. Recurrence can be rapid, and metastases to the lung are more common than to other organs, making the prognosis poor after metastatic spread occurs.

Notes

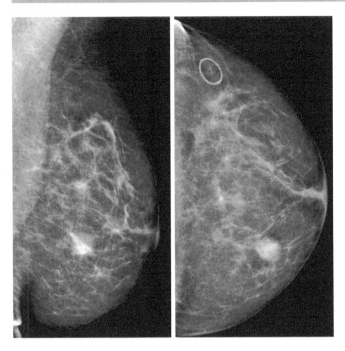

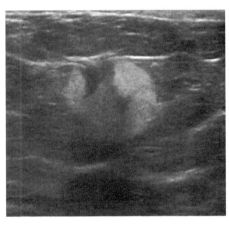

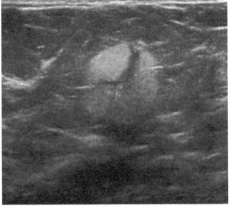

History: A 31-year-old woman presents with a new left palpable lump. Her past medical history is significant for acute myeloid leukemia that was diagnosed 5 years ago, relapsed 1 year ago, and now is in remission.

1. What should be included in the differential diagnosis? (Choose all that apply.)
   A. Lipoma
   B. Lymphoma
   C. Leukemia
   D. Pseudoangiomatous stromal hyperplasia

2. Which of the following statements regarding metastases to the breast is true?
   A. Metastases to the breast are common lesions.
   B. Metastases manifest only as bilateral lesions.
   C. The most common primaries include melanoma, lymphoma, lung, and ovarian.
   D. Breast involvement in leukemia is common.

3. Which of the following is *not* another name for leukemic infiltrates of the breast?
   A. Granulocytic sarcoma
   B. Extramedullary plasmacytoma
   C. Chloroma
   D. Extramedullary myeloblastoma

4. Which of the following is an imaging characteristic of leukemic infiltrates in the breast?
   A. They always occur as a single mass.
   B. They usually appear as a spiculated mass with microcalcifications on mammogram.
   C. They usually appear as a predominantly well-defined hypoechoic mass on ultrasound.
   D. On MRI, they are easily distinguishable from primary breast cancer.

Leukemic Infiltrate of the Breast

1. B, C, and D
2. C
3. B
4. C

References

Bayrak IK, Yalin T, Ozmen Z, et al: Acute lymphoblastic leukemia presented as multiple breast masses. *Korean J Radiol* 2009;10(5): 508-510.

Ginat DT, Puri S: FDG PET/CT manifestations of hematopoietic malignancies of the breast. *Acad Radiol* 2010;17(8):1026-1030.

Irshad A, Ackerman SJ, Pope TL, et al: Rare breast lesions: correlation of imaging and histologic features with WHO classification. *Radiographics* 2008;28(5):1399-1414.

Nishida H, Kinoshita T, Yashiro N, et al: MR findings of granulocytic sarcoma of the breasts. *Br J Radiol* 2006;79(945):e112-e115.

Noguera JJ, Martinez-Miravete P, Idoate F, et al: Metastases to the breast: a review of 33 cases. *Australas Radiol* 2007;51(2):133-138.

Cross-Reference

Ikeda D: *Breast Imaging: THE REQUISITES*, 2nd ed, Philadelphia: Saunders, 2010, p 117.

Comment

Metastases to the breast are uncommon lesions, accounting for 0.5% to 6.6% of all breast malignancies. They can manifest as unilateral or bilateral, single or multiple lesions. Although any malignancy has the potential to metastasize to the breast cancer, melanoma, lymphoma, oat cell carcinoma of the lung, and ovarian cancers are the most common primaries. Other primaries include rhabdomyosarcoma and leukemia. Breast involvement in leukemia is uncommon, with an estimated incidence of less than 1%. It usually occurs by hematologic spread and usually manifests in a setting of diffuse systemic disease. It typically involves younger patients than those with breast involvement in other lymphoproliferative neoplasms and can even affect children.

Leukemic infiltrates, also known as chloromas, extramedullary myeloblastomas, or granulocytic sarcomas, are essentially extramedullary solid tumors composed of granulocytic precursor cells. They are mainly associated with myelogenous leukemia, can occur during either leukemia relapse or remission, and may be the only presentation of the disease. In addition, radiotherapy to the breast can cause acute leukemia in the breast tissue.

Clinically, leukemic infiltrates can mimic primary breast tumors and can be misdiagnosed. Patients may present with single or multiple, unilateral or bilateral breast masses or enlargement, with or without axillary lymphadenopathy. Masses may be hard on palpation. The lesions usually regress after systemic therapy.

Leukemia can manifest on mammogram as a well-defined or ill-defined noncalcified mass or masses (see the figures), ovoid or irregular, or as diffusely increased breast density. The mammogram can also be unremarkable.

The ultrasound appearance is variable. The most frequent presentation is a predominantly well-defined hypoechoic mass, but tumors may also manifest as areas of mixed echogenicity with central anechoic and peripheral hyperechoic areas (see the figures), a large mass with spiculations or angular margins or both, or areas of marked low attenuation with or without acoustic shadowing. Some leukemic breast masses have shown increased vascularity with color Doppler.

MRI findings can be indistinguishable from findings of multicentric carcinoma or malignant lymphoma. The most common presentation is multiple enhancing masses with smooth edges and wash-out kinetics. MRI constitutes an accurate study for monitoring after treatment.

These tumors may manifest as single or multiple, unilateral or bilateral hypermetabolic breast masses on PET/CT (see the figures). They can be widespread and multifocal.

Notes

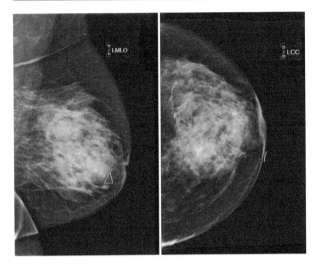

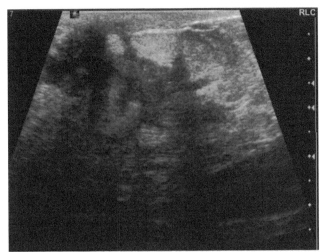

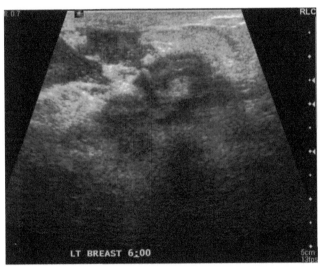

History: A 45-year-old woman presents with a palpable mass and warm, erythematous, tender skin in the central left breast.

1. What should be included in the differential diagnosis of the findings in the left breast on mammography and ultrasound? (Choose all that apply.)
   A. Abscess in the left breast
   B. Fibroadenoma
   C. Inflammatory breast cancer
   D. Hematoma

2. What is the next step in management?
   A. Biopsy to rule out inflammatory cancer
   B. MRI to evaluate for abnormal enhancement pattern of malignancy
   C. A trial of antibiotics
   D. Short-interval follow-up ultrasound in 1 to 2 weeks

3. What is the etiology of breast abscess?
   A. A source of infection is always found.
   B. It occurs exclusively in nursing mothers.
   C. Infection not related to breastfeeding is more commonly seen in smokers.
   D. There is typically a skin wound that undergoes secondary infection.

4. Why does inflammatory breast cancer mimic infection?
   A. Inflammatory breast cancer has tumor emboli in the dermal lymphatics.
   B. The cancer has become infected.
   C. The cancer spreads into the skin.
   D. Infection and inflammatory breast cancer manifest very differently.

Abscess

1. A, C, and D
2. C
3. C
4. A

References

Christensen AF, Al-Suliman N, Nielsen KR, et al: Ultrasound-guided drainage of breast abscesses: results in 151 patients. *Br J Radiol* 2005;78(927):186-188.

Hook GW, Ikeda DM: Treatment of breast abscesses with US-guided percutaneous needle drainage without indwelling catheter placement. *Radiology* 1999;213(2):579-582.

Cross-Reference

Ikeda D: *Breast Imaging: THE REQUISITES*, 2nd ed, Philadelphia: Saunders, 2010, p 140.

Comment

The appearance of breast abscess may be nonspecific. It manifests with findings similar to breast malignancy, and malignancy must always be excluded when a patient presents with a mass. The location of the mass near the nipple is characteristic of breast abscess. The margins of the abscess on mammography may be poorly delineated, as in this patient (see the figures). The mass in this patient merges with the background breast tissue, and the reason is clear on the ultrasound images. On ultrasound, the margins are infiltrative and irregular (see the figures) as the infection tracks along tissue planes. This ultrasound appearance is not unique to infection because malignancy can also manifest as an infiltrative process, rather than a well-defined mass (particularly infiltrating lobular carcinoma). On ultrasound, you may also find low-level, horizontal echoes in the fluid, which may indicate air (see the figures). Color Doppler may show hyperemia in the surrounding tissue.

The abscess may be drained percutaneously using ultrasound guidance. An 18-gauge needle may be needed if the infected fluid is thick, and repeated efforts may be needed. Antibiotics are also necessary, and a trial of antibiotics may serve to differentiate inflammatory breast cancer. If the patient improves after 10 days, biopsy of the mass to exclude cancer may be unnecessary. It is important to observe the patient closely until the mass is completely gone. If there is no improvement on antibiotics, inflammatory cancer must be considered possible, and biopsy must be performed.

In the case of abscess, particularly abscesses greater than 3 cm, percutaneous aspiration may not resolve the infection completely, and surgical incision and drainage may be needed. Rarely, a drain may be placed percutaneously by the radiologist.

Notes

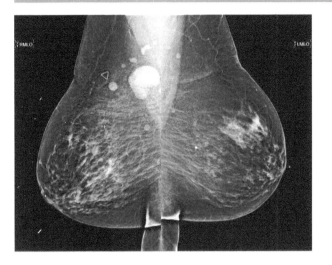

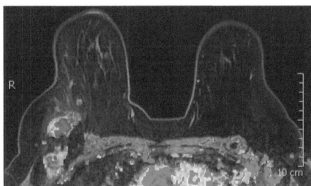

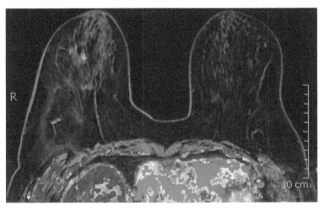

History: A 74-year-old woman with a palpable mass in the right axilla presents for a diagnostic mammogram.

1. What should be included in the differential diagnosis of the mammographic images shown? (Choose all that apply.)
   A. Enlarged right axillary nodes owing to metastatic breast cancer
   B. Enlarged axillary nodes owing to lymphoma
   C. Enlarged reactive axillary lymph nodes
   D. Normal mammogram

2. What is the next step in management?
   A. Right breast ultrasound
   B. Spot compression views of right breast
   C. Biopsy of axillary node
   D. MRI of the right breast

3. How common is axillary metastatic disease as the only manifestation of breast cancer?
   A. Very common—more than 50% of breast cancers manifest first with a metastatic node.

B. Common—it is the presentation in about 25% of breast cancer cases.
C. Less common—about 10% of breast cancers manifest first with a metastatic node.
D. Rare—about 1% of all breast cancers have this presentation.

4. If biopsy of the axillary node shows adenocarcinoma, what is the next step in management?
   A. PET/CT should be performed to evaluate for other sites of adenocarcinoma.
   B. The breast should be evaluated first when adenocarcinoma is found in an axillary node.
   C. Work-up of the colon should be done because colonic adenocarcinoma is the most common primary for axillary node metastases.
   D. Chest x-ray and, if needed, chest CT for lung evaluation should be obtained.

Axillary Node Presentation of Occult Breast Cancer

1. A, B, and C
2. C
3. D
4. B

References

Argus A, Mahoney MC: Indications for breast MRI: case-based review. *AJR Am J Roentgenol* 2011;196(3 Suppl):WS1-WS14.

Baron PL, Moore MP, Kinne DW, et al: Occult breast cancer presenting with axillary metastases. *Arch Surg* 1990;125(2):210-214.

Orel SG, Weinstein SP, Schnall MD, et al: Breast MR imaging in patients with axillary node metastases and unknown primary malignancy. *Radiology* 1999;212(2):543-549.

Cross-Reference

Ikeda D: *Breast Imaging: THE REQUISITES*, 2nd ed, Philadelphia: Saunders, 2010, p 396.

Comment

It is uncommon for breast cancer to manifest as a palpable axillary node as the only finding. More typically, when breast cancer has invaded the axillary nodes, its presence is not occult. A mass is palpable, or mammographic abnormalities are present by the time the tumor has spread. This presentation occurs in about 1% of all breast cancers (see the figures). In this case, a previous routine mammogram obtained 10 months before the current examination was normal with normal axillary nodes.

Biopsy of the node should be performed first because other etiologies exist for an enlarged palpable axillary node, including granulomatous disease, reactive node, and lymphoma. If adenocarcinoma is found on biopsy, the chances are quite small that the etiology is anything but breast cancer, and work-up of other adenocarcinomas is not needed. The mammogram should be carefully scrutinized for any evidence of abnormality, and additional views should be taken as needed. If no abnormality is seen, MRI is the best next step (see the figures).

According to two published reports, the likelihood of MRI detecting the primary cancer is 75% to 86%. If the cancer is found, patient management is altered. The patient would have likely gone on to mastectomy because the primary was not found. One third of the time, the primary tumor is not found in the mastectomy specimen, likely because it is difficult for the pathologist to examine every square centimeter of the entire breast specimen. Finding the primary tumor allows the patient to have possible breast conservation therapy. The patient in this case had multiple enlarged axillary nodes on MRI and a 1-cm invasive ductal carcinoma grade III on biopsy of the mass, seen in the 6:30 o'clock location on MRI.

Notes

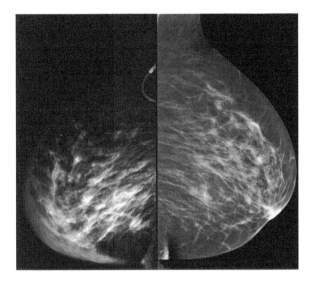

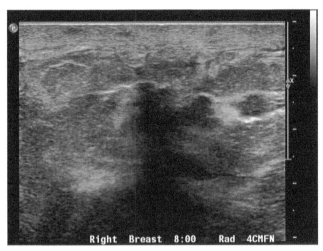

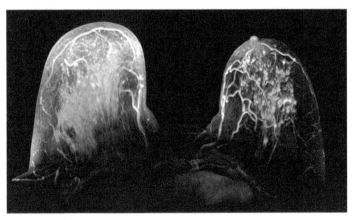

History: A 43-year-old woman with a history of colon cancer and chemotherapy presents with rapid onset of right breast enlargement, associated with peau d'orange and redness, with no discrete palpable mass.

1. What should be included in the differential diagnosis considering the clinical history and mammographic findings? (Choose all that apply.)
   A. Mastitis
   B. Ductal carcinoma in situ
   C. Congestive heart failure
   D. Inflammatory breast cancer

2. What is the best next diagnostic step?
   A. Follow-up mammogram, ultrasound, and MRI in 6 months
   B. PET/CT
   C. Percutaneous biopsy
   D. Surgical biopsy

3. Which of the following statements regarding inflammatory breast cancer is true?
   A. Invasive ductal carcinoma is the only cause of inflammatory breast cancer.
   B. Inflammatory breast cancer is very prevalent.
   C. It may be difficult to differentiate from infectious mastitis.
   D. The classic clinical presentation includes a discrete palpable mass.

4. What is the best treatment for inflammatory breast cancer?
   A. Mastectomy
   B. Lumpectomy and radiation therapy
   C. Chemotherapy
   D. Chemotherapy followed by mastectomy and radiation therapy

CASE 135

Inflammatory Breast Cancer

1. A, C, and D
2. C
3. C
4. D

References

Gunhan-Bilgen I, Ustun EE, Memis A: Inflammatory breast carcinoma: mammographic, ultrasonographic, clinical, and pathologic findings in 142 cases. *Radiology* 2002;223(3):829-838.

Robertson FM, Bondy M, Yang W, et al: Inflammatory breast cancer: the disease, the biology, the treatment. *CA Cancer J Clin* 2010;60 (6):351-375.

Yang WT: Advances in imaging of inflammatory breast cancer. *Cancer* 2010;116(11 Suppl):2755-2757.

Cross-Reference

Ikeda D: *Breast Imaging: THE REQUISITES*, 2nd ed, Philadelphia: Saunders, 2010, pp 175, 393.

Comment

Inflammatory breast cancer is an aggressive form of invasive carcinoma. It is a rare entity, accounting for 1% to 4% of all breast cancers. Clinically, inflammatory breast cancer is characterized by rapid onset of unilateral breast thickening, edema (which gives a *peau d'orange* ["orange peel"] appearance to the skin), and erythema but little or no pain and may be associated with a sensation of heat in the affected breast. It frequently manifests in younger patients, with early local and distant metastasis (55% to 58% have axillary adenopathy at presentation), and overall survival is lower compared with other forms of breast cancer. Bilateral involvement has been reported in 1% to 55% of cases.

Any tissue type of cancer may cause inflammatory carcinoma, but invasive ductal carcinoma is the most common. Histology shows tumor infiltration and emboli into the dermal lymphatics, often with nonlymphocytic reaction surrounding the large dilated vessels of the dermis.

The main differential diagnostic consideration is diffuse infectious mastitis, which has a similar clinical presentation except for the presence of fever, localized pain, and leukocytosis, which are not seen in inflammatory cancer. Skin changes in the breast can also be seen after breast surgery and radiation therapy, superior vena cava thrombosis, congestive heart failure, and lymphoma. Clinical history is important to eliminate these causes of breast erythema and edema.

Skin thickening, increased breast density, and trabecular thickening may be seen on mammogram, although the findings may be subtle (see the figures). Masses and calcifications may be present. Ultrasound is a useful imaging tool after mammography to evaluate skin changes and localize a specific parenchymal mass to guide biopsy. The most frequent ultrasound findings include heterogeneous infiltration of the breast tissue or a conglomerate of intraparenchymal masses with overlying skin and subcutaneous edema (see the figures). Lymph nodes can also be easily assessed with ultrasound. MRI can be performed if mammography and ultrasound are inconclusive. Findings on MRI include breast enlargement, diffuse skin thickening, edema, masses, and abnormal parenchymal enhancement (see the figures). MRI is also useful to evaluate tumor response to chemotherapy.

The definitive diagnosis of inflammatory carcinoma requires biopsy. The procedure should include a biopsy specimen of the skin and a specimen of any identifiable discrete mass. Biopsy can be performed with ultrasound guidance. MRI can be also used to guide biopsies of focal areas of suspicious enhancement.

The current standard management of inflammatory breast cancer consists of systemic chemotherapy followed by surgery and radiation therapy. Mastectomy with axillary lymph node dissection is the optimal surgical procedure because the presence of positive margins leads to a poorer prognosis.

Notes

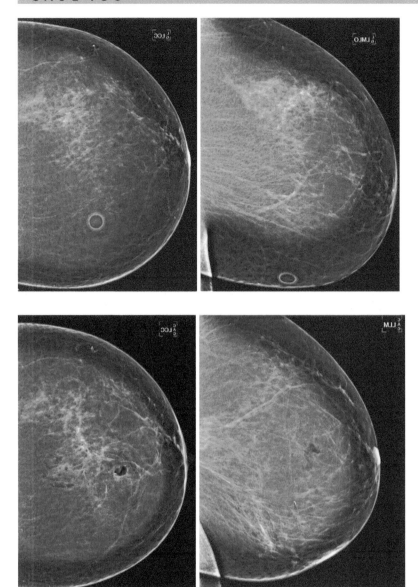

History: A 70-year-old woman developed microcalcifications in the left breast. She underwent stereotactic biopsy, with successful retrieval of all the calcifications.

1. What should be included in the differential diagnosis of the mammograms shown? (Choose all that apply.)
   A. Ductal carcinoma in situ
   B. Lobular carcinoma in situ
   C. Apocrine metaplasia
   D. Fibroadenoma

2. What is the next step in management of developing calcifications?
   A. Short-interval follow-up with magnification views
   B. Stereotactic biopsy
   C. Referral to a surgeon
   D. Consultation with a breast surgical specialist regarding advisability of biopsy

3. What would be a case in which a clip would *not* be needed after biopsy?
   A. The lesion is absolutely benign, and no surgery would be needed.
   B. The lesion is large.
   C. The microcalcifications are only moderately suspicious.
   D. The calcifications have been completely removed with the biopsy.

4. All of the following are reasons that clips become displaced after biopsy *except:*
   A. Compression of the breast during the biopsy
   B. Hematoma formation at the time of biopsy
   C. Clip migration secondary to very dense breast tissue
   D. Displacement within the biopsy track

Clip Displacement

1. A, C, and D
2. B
3. B
4. C

References

Esserman LE, Cura MA, DaCosta D: Recognizing pitfalls in early and late migration of clip markers after imaging-guided directional vacuum-assisted biopsy. *Radiographics* 2004;24(1):147-156.

Parikh JR: Delayed migration of Gel Mark Ultra clip within 15 days of 11-gauge vacuum-assisted stereotactic breast biopsy. *AJR Am J Roentgenol* 2005;185(1):203-206.

Cross-Reference

Ikeda D: *Breast Imaging: THE REQUISITES*, 2nd ed, Philadelphia: Saunders, 2010, p 223.

Comment

Needle biopsy is the appropriate management step for indeterminate or suspicious masses or calcifications in the breast (see the figures). When the lesions are small, it is possible that all radiographic evidence of the lesion is removed by the image-guided biopsy, particularly if vacuum-assisted technique is used. For this reason, the site of biopsy is marked after the procedure is completed. The most common way of marking the site is a metal clip or marker. These clips are made of stainless steel or titanium and may have adjacent echogenic absorbable gelatin sponge material (Gelfoam) to allow visualization under ultrasound and to facilitate hemostasis after biopsy. Earlier clips were made to clip the tissue; later devices are termed markers because they are designed to fall into the biopsy cavity.

The clip may be displaced after the biopsy in 20% of patients, according to one series. Clip displacement is most common with stereotactic biopsy, as the breast is compressed during the biopsy procedure and then the compression is released after the sampling. The "accordion effect" allows the clip to travel back along the biopsy track, in the direction of the skin insertion (along the z-axis). Hematoma formation at the time of biopsy can also cause the clip to become displaced.

It is important to obtain standard mammographic views of craniocaudal and lateral projections after the biopsy to assess the location of the clip (see the figures). In the patient in this case, the clip was displaced several centimeters inferiorly, along the z-axis, immediately after the biopsy. Clips can also become displaced several months after the biopsy. Clip displacement is more common in the loose stroma of a fatty breast than in a dense breast. The location of the clip related to the biopsy site should be mentioned in the biopsy report. If subsequent needle localization is needed, the biopsy site, not the clip location, needs to be localized and excised.

Notes

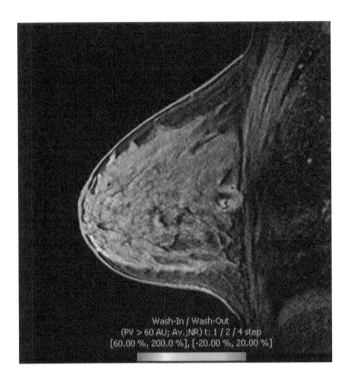

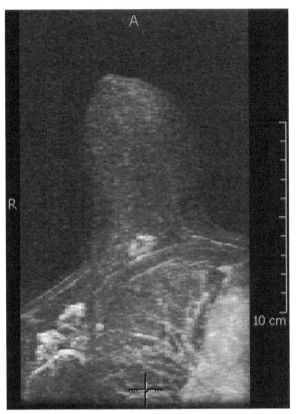

Wash-In / Wash-Out
(PV > 60 AU; Av.;NR) t: 1 / 2 / 4 step
[60.00 %, 200.0 %], [-20.00 %, 20.00 %]

History: In a 58-year-old woman, a posterior right breast mass has been diagnosed and evaluated with needle core biopsy and clip placement.

1. What should be included in the differential diagnosis based on MRI? (Choose all that apply.)
   A. Invasive ductal cancer in the posterior breast
   B. Enlarged lymph node
   C. Fibroadenoma in the posterior breast
   D. Complicated cyst

2. What is the relationship of the mass to the chest wall?
   A. The mass infiltrates the pectoralis muscle.
   B. The mass infiltrates the intercostal muscles.
   C. The mass abuts the pectoralis but does not invade it.
   D. The mass is posterior but is several centimeters away from the pectoralis.

3. What is the best imaging tool for evaluating the relationship of the posterior mass and the chest wall?
   A. Ultrasound
   B. MRI
   C. Mammography
   D. Positron emission mammography (PEM)

4. How does chest wall involvement affect staging of breast cancer?
   A. There is no effect on staging.
   B. Enhancement of the pectoralis muscle indicates stage IV disease.
   C. Enhancement of the intercostal muscles indicates at least stage IIIB disease.
   D. Tumor enhancement of both the pectoralis and the intercostal muscles increases stage.

C A S E 1 3 7

Posterior Mass on MRI

1. A, B, and C
2. C
3. B
4. C

References

Mahoney MC, Argus A: Indications for breast MRI: case-based review. *AJR Am J Roentgenol* 2011;196(3 Suppl):WS1-WS14.

Morris EA, Schwartz LH, Drotman MB, et al: Evaluation of pectoralis major muscle in patients with posterior breast tumors on breast MR images: early experience. *Radiology* 2000;214(1):67-72.

Orel SG, Schnall MD: MR imaging of the breast for the detection, diagnosis, and staging of breast cancer. *Radiology* 2001;220(1):13-30.

Cross-Reference

Ikeda D: *Breast Imaging: THE REQUISITES*, 2nd ed, Philadelphia: Saunders, 2010, p 271.

Comment

MRI is the best imaging tool for evaluating the extent of disease beyond the breast by direct extension into the pectoralis muscle and into serratus muscle and intercostal muscles. The distinction between extension into the pectoralis major muscle and into the underlying chest wall is important: Pectoralis extension alone does not affect staging, but chest wall involvement is designated as at least stage IIIB.

To diagnose muscle involvement, one should look for enhancement of the muscle—more than the physiologic enhancement normally seen in nearby areas of muscle. The enhancement may be a diffuse involvement or may show enlargement of the muscle. Obliteration of the fat plane between the malignant mass and the pectoralis major muscle is not a definite indication of involvement with tumor, and it may be seen in tumors that abut the pectoralis but do not involve it (see the figures).

Notes

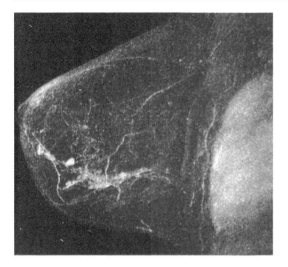
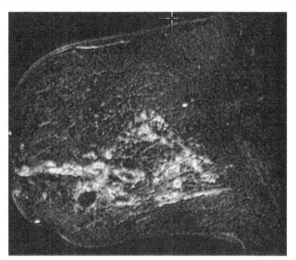
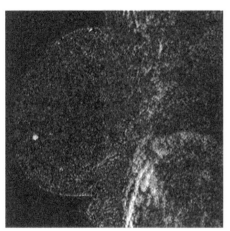
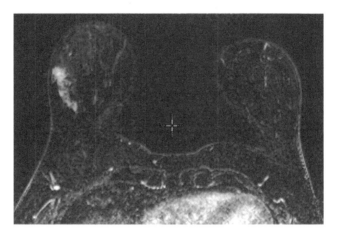

History: Four patients underwent MRI after receiving a diagnosis of invasive or intraductal malignancy on image-guided core biopsy.

1. What should be included in the differential diagnosis for the images shown? (Choose all that apply.)
   A. Atypical ductal hyperplasia
   B. Ductal carcinoma in situ (DCIS)
   C. Lobular carcinoma in situ
   D. Invasive ductal carcinoma

2. What is the best imaging tool for assessing extent of disease after DCIS is diagnosed on mammography?
   A. Mammography for additional sites of calcifications
   B. Ultrasound
   C. Positron emission mammography
   D. MRI

3. Which is more important in MRI assessment of DCIS—kinetics or morphology?
   A. Kinetics is more important because DCIS rarely forms a mass.
   B. Kinetics is more important because malignant disease relies on neovascularity, which results in brisk wash-in and wash-out on the time-intensity curve.

C. Morphology is more important because intraductal disease most commonly follows a duct and its branches.
D. Morphology is more important because DCIS may not enhance.

4. What is the most common presentation of DCIS on MRI?
   A. Small foci scattered throughout the breast
   B. Rim-enhancing masses in a ductal distribution
   C. Non-masslike enhancement in a segmental distribution
   D. Smooth linear enhancement

MRI of Ductal Carcinoma In Situ

1. A, B, and D
2. D
3. C
4. C

References

Liberman L, Morris EA, Lee MJ, et al: Breast lesions detected on MR imaging: features and positive predictive value. *AJR Am J Roentgenol* 2002;179(1):171-178.

Mossa-Basha M, Fundaro GM, Shah BA, et al: Ductal carcinoma in situ of the breast: MR imaging findings with histopathologic correlation. *Radiographics* 2010;30(6):1673-1687.

Orel SG, Mendonca MH, Reynolds C, et al: MR imaging of ductal carcinoma in situ. *Radiology* 1997;202(2):413-420.

Rosen EL, Smith-Foley SA, DeMartini WB, et al: BI-RADS MRI enhancement characteristics of ductal carcinoma in situ. *Breast J* 2007;13(6): 545-550.

Yamada T, Mori N, Watanabe M, et al: Radiologic-pathologic correlation of ductal carcinoma in situ. *Radiographics* 2010;30(5): 1183-1198.

Cross-Reference

Ikeda D: *Breast Imaging: THE REQUISITES*, 2nd ed, Philadelphia: Saunders, 2010, p 265.

Comment

The sensitivity of MRI in detecting DCIS has been reported to range from 40% to 100%. However, in more recent studies, the sensitivity was consistently approximately 90%. MRI is consistently better at detecting DCIS compared with the gold standard of mammography. The sensitivity of mammography for DCIS is approximately 27%. Mammography depends on microcalcifications to detect DCIS, and not all DCIS calcifies. Other presentations of DCIS include asymmetric density and focal mass. In a dense or heterogeneously dense breast, these manifestations are difficult to detect on mammography but are seen better on MRI, which is not affected by breast density.

The manifestations of DCIS on MRI are varied. Non-masslike enhancement is seen in 60% to 90% of cases and is more common than a mass (see the figures). Within this category, clumped enhancement in a linear or segmental distribution is most highly correlated with DCIS (see the figures). However, DCIS was seen as a mass in 30% of cases in one study (see the figures). MRI enhancement is related to neovascularity. In intraductal disease, the increased abnormal vascularity is present in the periductal region and in the stroma surrounding the abnormal ducts, not within the duct itself. It has been shown that high-grade DCIS, also known as DCIS with comedonecrosis, is more likely to enhance compared with low-grade or intermediate-grade DCIS. A study showed that not only the detection of DCIS but also the assessment of tumor size was affected by the DCIS grade. All of the patients illustrated here had grade II DCIS.

Morphology is more reliable than kinetics for detection in DCIS. Kinetics varies from brisk to slow initial uptake, with approximately 50% to 70% of cases having rapid initial uptake. Delayed kinetics can be wash-out, plateau, or persistent. In one study, the delayed kinetics was equally distributed among the three patterns; in another study, wash-out kinetics was seen in only 9% of DCIS. Using computer-assisted detection (CAD) systems, with color-coded information to draw the reader's attention to only lesions with wash-out, may cause DCIS, which is more likely to have persistent kinetics, to be missed.

It is important to assess extent of disease when DCIS is diagnosed. If DCIS is found on mammography as developing calcifications, MRI is better than mammography for assessing tumor size and multifocal and multicentric disease, which is important in surgical planning (see the figures).

Notes

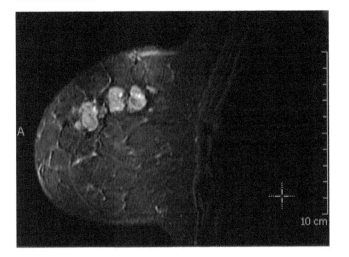

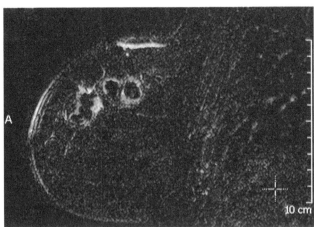

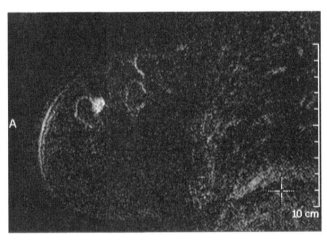

History: A 53-year-old woman found to have suspicious calcifications on screening mammogram underwent stereotactic biopsy of three sites in the right breast, with diagnosis of DCIS in all three sites. MRI is requested to evaluate for extent of disease.

1. What should be included in the differential diagnosis, based on MRI? (Choose all that apply.)
   A. Normal, expected enhancement at the seroma
   B. Residual ductal carcinoma in situ (DCIS) after biopsy
   C. Invasive malignancy adjacent to seroma
   D. Enhancing hematoma after biopsy

2. What is the reason for performing MRI after a malignant stereotactic biopsy?
   A. Not indicated because the area of cancer is documented, and the patient should have surgery first
   B. Not indicated because the patient may be unable to tolerate the examination, and it is expensive
   C. To document extent of disease and help guide surgical management
   D. Not indicated because mammogram performed after biopsy is a better tool for evaluating the presence of residual disease

3. How common is detection of additional ipsilateral disease after malignant image-guided biopsy?
   A. It is relatively uncommon, occurring in less than 10%.
   B. It is more common to find additional disease in the contralateral breast.
   C. It is very common, seen in more than 50% of patients.
   D. It is detected about 15% to 27% of the time.

4. Which pathology result on core biopsy is more likely to have additional disease detected on MRI (unsuspected on mammogram)?
   A. Mucinous carcinoma
   B. Tubular carcinoma
   C. Infiltrating lobular carcinoma
   D. Radial scar

CASE 139

MRI for Disease Extent after Biopsy

1. B and C
2. C
3. D
4. C

References

American College of Radiology: ACR practice guideline for the performance of contrast-enhanced magnetic resonance imaging (MRI) of the breast. Revised 2008.

Ciocchetti JM, Joy N, Staller S, et al: The effect of magnetic resonance imaging in the workup of breast cancer. *Am J Surg* 2009;198(6): 824-828.

Kuhl CK: Reviews and commentary—state of the art: current status of breast MR imaging. Part 2. Clinical applications. *Radiology* 2007;244(3):672-691.

Cross-Reference

Ikeda D: *Breast Imaging: THE REQUISITES*, 2nd ed, Philadelphia: Saunders, 2010, p 305.

Comment

Breast MRI is the most accurate tool for showing extent of disease in women who have undergone image-guided biopsy with a malignant result. The incidence of ipsilateral and contralateral cancer found on MRI that was unsuspected on conventional imaging ranges from 15% to 30% for the ipsilateral breast and 3% to 6% for the contralateral breast. This information is important to obtain before surgery so that all of the disease can be excised in a single operation. The finding of significant multicentric disease (cancer in multiple quadrants of the breast) may alter the surgical plan from breast conservation therapy to mastectomy. DCIS was upgraded to invasive carcinoma in 18% of patients in one series, as it was in the patient in the present case.

In this patient with dense breasts on mammography, there were suspicious calcifications in three sites in the right breast, and she underwent stereotactic biopsy of three sites, with histology on all core samples showing DCIS grade II. No masses were seen on mammography. MRI was performed (see the figures). The first figure shows the seromas from a recent biopsy on a T2-weighted image. The second and third figures show an enhancing mass adjacent to the seromas, suspicious for invasive carcinoma or additional DCIS on subtracted, T1-weighted, fat-suppressed images.

MRI has limited use in patients with calcifications. Biopsy should be performed of suspicious calcifications regardless of enhancement pattern (MRI is approximately 85% sensitive for detection of DCIS that is calcified on mammogram). However, MRI has a high negative predictive value for invasive cancer, according to the ACRIN trial 6667, so if MRI is negative in a breast with DCIS on stereotactic biopsy, it is highly likely that no invasive carcinoma would be found at excisional biopsy. However, if there is enhancement, as in this patient, invasion is more likely, and the surgeon can be directed to excise the area of enhancement. Excision appears to reduce the rate of local recurrence after breast conservation therapy.

Notes

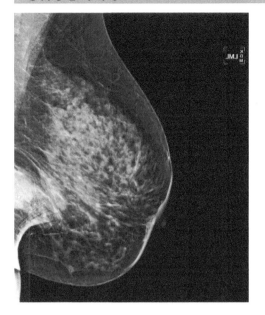
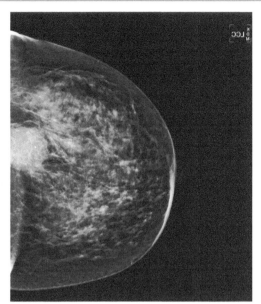
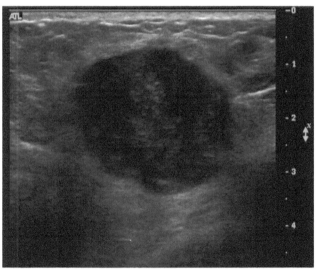
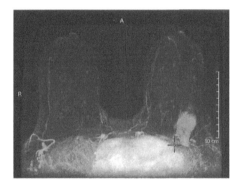

History: A 52-year-old woman presents for a baseline mammogram because of a palpable mass in the left breast.

1. What should be included in the differential diagnosis for the mammogram views shown? (Choose all that apply.)
   A. Ductal carcinoma in situ
   B. Invasive ductal carcinoma
   C. Desmoid tumor
   D. Invasive lobular carcinoma

2. What is the next step in evaluation?
   A. Ultrasound and ultrasound-guided biopsy
   B. Stereotactic biopsy
   C. MRI
   D. Surgical excision

3. What is a desmoid tumor?
   A. A malignant mass of the chest wall with malignant potential
   B. Related to diabetic mastopathy and likely related to inflammation
   C. Aggressive fibromatosis that may arise from the pectoralis fascia
   D. A mass related to fat necrosis

4. What is the management?
   A. Surgical excision with axillary node sampling should be performed.
   B. Close clinical follow-up is needed after diagnosis is made with core biopsy.
   C. Wide local excision should be performed.
   D. Surgery is unnecessary for this benign tumor, and the patient can return to screening mammogram annually.

C A S E   1 4 0

Desmoid Tumor

1. B, C, and D
2. A
3. C
4. C

References

Erguvan-Dogan B, Dempsey PJ, Ayyar G, et al: Primary desmoid tumor (extraabdominal fibromatosis) of the breast. *AJR Am J Roentgenol* 2005;185(2):488-489.

Glazebrook KN, Reynolds CA: Mammary fibromatosis. *AJR Am J Roentgenol* 2009;193(3):856-860.

Cross-Reference

Ikeda D: *Breast Imaging: THE REQUISITES*, 2nd ed, Philadelphia: Saunders, 2010, p 401.

Comment

Desmoid tumor is a rare, benign tumor of fibroblasts that can occur in the breast and in other organs. It is also termed *aggressive fibromatosis* or *extraabdominal desmoid*. Desmoid tumors account for less than 0.2% of all breast tumors. This tumor does not spread beyond the breast but is locally aggressive and can recur after local excision in 29% of cases. It has been reported to be associated with implants, perhaps arising in the fibrous capsule of the implant, or with prior surgery or trauma, although the etiology is uncertain. Desmoid tumor was initially reported in a patient with familial polyposis, or Gardner's syndrome, although few additional cases in that subset have been reported.

The presentation of desmoid tumor is similar to that of breast cancer, and because of its rarity, it should not be the first choice when a mass is seen in the breast. The tumor has irregular margins, is dense, and typically does not calcify. It is often posterior because it may arise from the pectoralis fascia (see the figures). On ultrasound, it is hypoechoic, with irregular margins, usually without posterior shadowing (see the figures). MRI is a valuable imaging tool after the diagnosis has been made by needle biopsy. Although signal characteristics may vary on T1-weighted and T2-weighted images, and variable enhancement characteristics have been reported, MRI remains the best way to evaluate the tumor relative to the chest wall and thus aid the surgeon in planning excision (see the figures).

In this patient, the mass was initially thought to represent a malignant mass until needle core histology revealed fibromatosis. The patient underwent wide excision, and the histology was concordant. No further treatment was needed, and the patient returned to routine mammography.

Notes

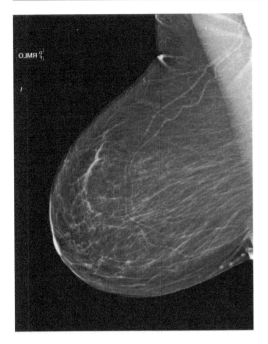

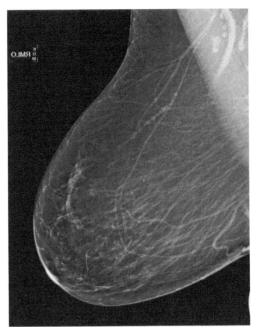

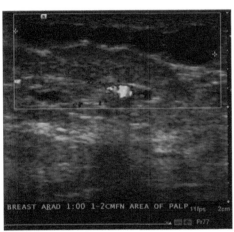

History: A 47-year-old woman presents with a palpable cordlike area in the axillary tail of the left breast. The first figure is the right mediolateral oblique (MLO) view from her mammogram 1 year earlier, when she was asymptomatic. The second figure is the right MLO view from the mammogram taken on the day she presented with her concern.

1. What is the differential diagnosis for the mammogram taken at presentation? (Choose all that apply.)
   A. Normal mammogram
   B. Ductal ectasia
   C. Varicose vein in the breast
   D. Superficial thrombophlebitis in the left breast

2. What is the next imaging exam to establish the diagnosis?
   A. Perform spot compression views.
   B. Perform ultrasound of the palpable concern.

   C. Perform MRI to evaluate for abnormal enhancement.
   D. Perform magnification views to check for microcalcifications.

3. What would an ultrasound exam show?
   A. A dilated, tubular, beaded vein with absence of blood flow
   B. No abnormality, only fat
   C. Abnormal lymph nodes
   D. Several cysts in a chain

4. What are the clinical signs of this disease?
   A. The skin typically is normal.
   B. There may be a palpable cord.
   C. The finding is usually in the lower outer quadrant of the breast.
   D. Both breasts are typically involved.

Mondor's Disease

1. C and D
2. B
3. A
4. B

Reference

Conant EF, Wilkes AN, Mendelson EB, Feig SA: Superficial thrombophlebitis of the breast (Mondor's disease): mammographic findings. *AJR Am J Roentgenol* 1993;160:1201-1203.

Cross-Reference

Ikeda D: *Breast Imaging: THE REQUISITES*, 2nd ed, Philadelphia: Saunders, 2010, p 399.

Comment

Mondor's disease is a focal, superficial thrombosis of a vein in the breast. It is typically in the upper outer quadrant or axillary tail of the breast, and it has a characteristic appearance, as is seen in the images presented in this patient (see the figures). When this typical beaded appearance is seen, the diagnosis is usually not in question. The patient can present with a tender, palpable cord in her upper outer quadrant. There can be skin dimpling along the cord, caused by retraction of the thrombosed vein. This condition can be associated with trauma, including surgery and needle biopsy, or with dehydration, but it can also be idiopathic. Because it is rarely associated with ipsilateral breast cancer, care should be taken to examine the mammogram, and the patient, for any sign of concomitant malignancy.

Ultrasound is useful in the diagnosis. When the ultrasound is targeted to the patient's palpable cord, the dilated vein, with a beaded contour, will be seen. Color flow Doppler will demonstrate the absence of flow in this thrombosed vein (see the figures). Low-level echoes of thrombus within the vein may be seen.

The condition is self-limited and resolves spontaneously or with the application of warm compresses. This is a benign condition and, in the absence of the rare associated malignancy, would be categorized as a Breast Imaging Reporting and Data System (BI-RADS) 2.

Notes

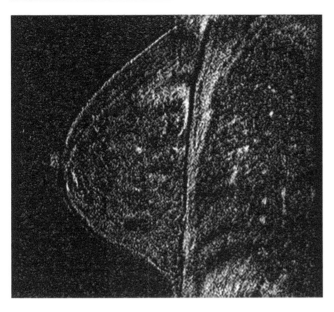

History: A 54-year-old woman with a personal history of Hodgkin's disease and mantle radiation 25 years ago.

1. What is the differential diagnosis of the imaging findings on the one sagittal subtraction image on her MRI? (Choose all that apply.)
   A. Newly developing invasive cancer
   B. Lymph node
   C. Benign mass
   D. Ductal carcinoma in situ (DCIS)
   E. Cyst

2. What is your recommendation?
   A. Continue routine annual screening with mammogram and MRI.
   B. Perform MR-guided biopsy.
   C. Refer her to a surgeon.
   D. Perform targeted ultrasound of the area of abnormality to see if this represents a cyst.

3. What constitutes a high-risk population?
   A. Women who have a personal history of breast cancer
   B. Women who have greater than 20% to 25% lifetime risk of breast cancer
   C. Women who are extremely anxious about breast cancer
   D. Women with a personal history of cervical cancer

4. What is pretest probability in interpreting breast cancer on imaging?
   A. The likelihood that a patient will survive her disease
   B. The likelihood that a woman will have a routine screening mammogram
   C. The likelihood that an imaging finding represents cancer in a certain population
   D. The likelihood that the patient will reject advice to have a biopsy

Screening High-Risk Women

1. A, B, C, and D
2. B
3. B
4. C

References

Berg WA: Tailored supplemental screening for breast cancer: what now and what next? *AJR Am J Roentgenol* 2009;192:390-399.

Saslow D, Boetes C, Burke W, et al; American Cancer Society Breast Cancer Advisory Group: American Cancer Society guidelines for breast screening with MRI as an adjunct to mammography. *CA Cancer J Clin* 2007;57:75-89.

Cross-Reference

Ikeda D: *Breast Imaging: THE REQUISITES*, 2nd ed, Philadelphia: Saunders, 2010, p 268.

Comment

In 2007, the American Cancer Society (ACS) published guidelines for screening high-risk women. The ACS advised adding MRI as an adjunct to mammography to increase the detection of early cancer in this population. They recommended MRI in addition to mammography in women who carried a lifetime risk of at least 20% to 25%. An individual woman's risk of breast cancer can be assessed with risk models such as the BRCAPRO, Tyrer-Cuzick, or BOADICEA models. Multiple trials of women at very high risk found that adding MRI to mammography significantly increased detection of cancer: mammography found only 36% of cancers present, whereas performing MRI in addition increased detection to nearly 93%.

Patients who are at very high risk include those who carry the *BRCA1* or *BRCA2* mutations; those with several first-degree relatives (mother, father, sister, brother, daughter, son) with breast cancer, particularly diagnosed at a young age; those who were treated with mantle radiation between the ages of 18 and 30 years, with the incidence of breast cancer beginning 8 years after treatment; and those who have Li-Fraumeni or Cowden's syndrome.

The presence of increased risk factors affects the pretest probability of the lesion, which is the probability that cancer is present in a certain population before the results of the biopsy are known. In this case, the lesion was tiny (see the figure), and morphology and enhancement characteristics were not particularly worrisome. However, the patient's high-risk status (prior mantle radiation) changes the likelihood that a new mass, however benign in appearance, is malignant. Thus, rather than 6-month follow-up, a biopsy was recommended. The MR-guided biopsy result was DCIS, nuclear grade III.

Notes

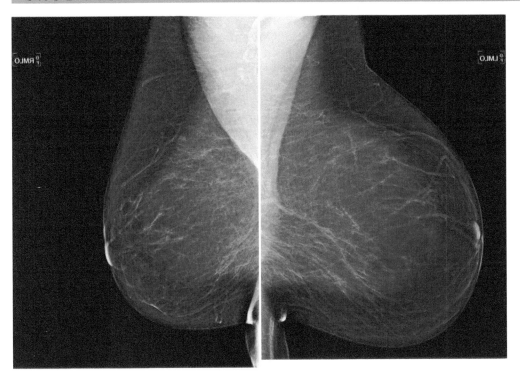

History: An asymptomatic 60-year-old woman presents for routine screening mammogram.

1. What is the differential diagnosis in this patient with asymmetric breast size? (Choose all that apply.)
   A. The breast bud was removed when the patient was a child.
   B. This is a normal variant, with one breast smaller than the other.
   C. Poor technique was applied, with one breast poorly positioned.
   D. Poland's syndrome should be considered.

2. What is the clinical significance of asymmetric breast size?
   A. It is never significant.
   B. It is not significant if it is long standing and the patient is asymptomatic.
   C. The larger breast is typically the normal breast.
   D. The smaller breast is typically the normal breast.

3. If this is a baseline mammogram, and you have no clinical history of palpable mass, what is the next best step?
   A. Obtain a history from the patient regarding her experience with breast size asymmetry.
   B. Recommend an MRI.
   C. Recommend short-interval follow-up.
   D. Recommend surgical consultation.

4. What is Poland's syndrome?
   A. It is breast hypoplasia in women from Poland.
   B. Only affecting women, it usually includes hypoplasia of pectoral muscle.
   C. It is a relatively common congenital defect of known origin.
   D. It is a rare congenital abnormality affecting the chest and arm on one side.

Asymmetric Size of Breasts

1. B, C, and D
2. B
3. A
4. D

References

Samuels TH: Poland's syndrome: a mammographic presentation. *AJR Am J Roentgenol* 1996;166:347-348.

Scutt D, Lancaster GA, Manning JT: Breast asymmetry and predisposition to breast cancer. *Breast Cancer Res* 2006;8(2):R14.

Cross-Reference

Ikeda D: *Breast Imaging: THE REQUISITES*, 2nd ed, Philadelphia: Saunders, 2010, p 408.

Comment

Breast asymmetry is usually considered a benign condition, although several features must be established to consider it benign. The condition should be of long standing. The patient herself is usually the best source for this information. The mammogram should be normal, with no evidence of developing mass or developing asymmetric tissue. If there are no prior mammograms for review, and one breast is denser or has skin thickening, further evaluation with ultrasound, physical exam, and perhaps MRI is indicated. The possibility of invasive lobular cancer, infection, or diffuse involvement of the breast with lymphoma must be considered.

History of prior breast cancer, with lumpectomy and radiation therapy, would cause a decrease in the size of the affected breast, so that history must be obtained. Benign surgery, particularly of a large volume of tissue, would cause breast asymmetry. The asymmetry can occur after pregnancy and breast-feeding, with one breast decreasing in size after pregnancy and lactation and the other breast failing to do so.

There are inherited conditions in which one breast may be smaller. One such condition is Poland's syndrome, which also may include unilateral absence of the pectoralis muscle. There may also be arm abnormalities on the ipsilateral side, as well as rib anomalies. There is also developmental hypomastia, which is not associated with other anomalies or syndromes.

This patient did not have any other anomalies, and the asymmetry was of long standing, possibly related to size change after lactation.

One author has published a series showing an increase in breast cancer in patients who have asymmetric breast size. However, in the absence of other mammographic findings, additional evaluation is not needed. Typically, if the asymmetry is stable and there is no mammographic abnormality (as in the figure), then this condition is given a Breast Imaging Reporting and Data System (BI-RADS) score of 1, and routine mammography is recommended.

Notes

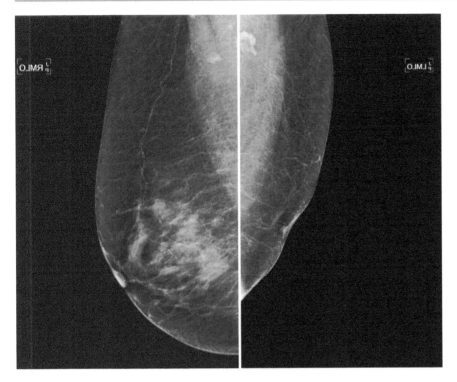

History: A 48-year-old asymptomatic woman presents for a routine mammogram.

1. What should be included in the differential diagnosis for this mammogram? (Choose all that apply.)
   A. Asymmetry of breast size
   B. Removal of left breast bud when the patient was a child
   C. Left breast that was badly burned in adulthood
   D. Poland's syndrome

2. What injury can cause this condition?
   A. Biopsy of the rudimentary nipple-areolar complex
   B. Radiation to the breast in adulthood
   C. Motor vehicle accident with seat belt trauma in a teen
   D. Reduction mammoplasty in a young adult

3. What is premature thelarche?
   A. Development of breast tissue before puberty
   B. Onset of menstruation earlier than age 8
   C. Presence of accessory nipples
   D. Precocious puberty

4. What BI-RADS (Breast Imaging Reporting and Data System) score would you give this case if you had no prior films for comparison?
   A. BI-RADS 0—need additional evaluation
   B. BI-RADS 4—suspicious, recommend biopsy
   C. BI-RADS 3—probably benign, recommend short-interval follow-up
   D. BI-RADS 2—benign

CASE 144

Breast Bud Removed

1. B and D
2. A
3. A
4. D

References

Bland KI: Copeland EM: *The Breast*, 2nd ed., Philadelphia: Saunders, 1998, p 214.

Chautard EA, Freire-Maia N: Poland's syndrome. *Br Med J* 1971;4(5790):812.

Pescovitz OH, Hench KD, Barnes KM, et al: Premature thelarche and central precocious puberty: the relationship between clinical presentation and the gonadotropin response to luteinizing hormone-releasing hormone. *J Clin Endocrinol Metab* 1988;67(3):474-479.

Cross-Reference

Ikeda D: *Breast Imaging: THE REQUISITES*, 2nd ed, Philadelphia: Saunders, 2010, p 150.

Comment

The patient in this case had surgery as a young child for a congenital heart abnormality. The incision was made at the fourth intercostal interspace and interrupted the anlage for the ipsilateral breast (the breast bud). This iatrogenic injury to the breast resulted in removal of the breast bud and in failure of development of the normal ducts and lobules of that breast. The contralateral breast developed normally (see the figure).

Premature thelarche is the enlargement of the breasts before sexual maturation and is usually seen at age 6 months to 2 years. The enlargement can be unilateral, and the prematurely enlarging breast can be removed because of suspicion for malignancy (although the actual chance of this is vanishingly small) or abscess. When the breast bud is removed, the breast fails to develop. Radiation to the chest may cause the same result.

If the pectoralis muscle is also missing or there are other anomalies of the chest or ipsilateral arm, a congenital syndrome may be present. Poland's syndrome is the most well-known congenital syndrome; patients present with variable features that are always unilateral and can include absence of the pectoralis muscles, absence of breasts, rib anomalies, and brachysyndactyly.

Notes

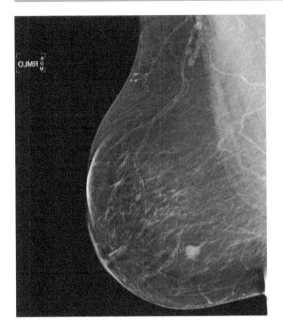

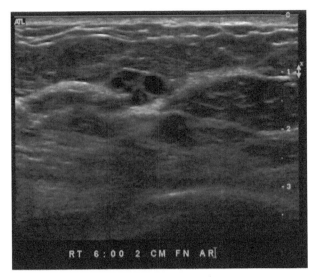

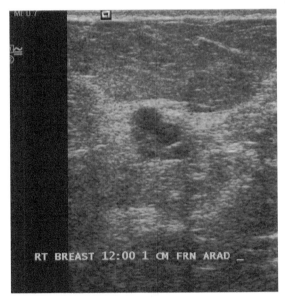

Ultrasound of a palpable mass in a different patient.

History: An 80-year-old patient has a new mass on mammogram.

1. What is the differential diagnosis for this mammogram? (Choose all that apply.)
   A. Complex cyst
   B. Solid benign mass
   C. Solid malignant mass
   D. Lymph node

2. What is the next stage of the work-up?
   A. Spot compression views and ultrasound
   B. No work-up needed for this benign-appearing mass
   C. MRI
   D. Galactography

3. What is a complicated cyst on ultrasound?
   A. A cyst that has been aspirated
   B. A cyst that contains debris but has a thin wall
   C. A suspicious cyst
   D. A cyst that recurs after aspiration

4. What is a complex cyst on ultrasound?
   A. A cyst that contains internal echoes, thick septations, or a mass
   B. A cyst that is painful
   C. A cyst that is palpable
   D. A cyst with low-level internal echoes

Complex Cyst

1. A, B, and C
2. A
3. B
4. A

References

Berg WA, Campassi CI, Ioffe OB: Cystic lesions of the breast: sonographic-pathologic correlation. *Radiology* 2003;227(1):183-191.

Doshi DJ, March DE, Crisi GM, Coughlin BF: Complex cystic breast masses: diagnostic approach and imaging-pathologic correlation. *Radiographics* 2007;27(Suppl 1):S53-S64.

Cross-Reference

Ikeda D: *Breast Imaging: THE REQUISITES*, 2nd ed, Philadelphia: Saunders, 2010, p 159.

Comment

A new mass is detected in the lower right breast in an 80-year-old, asymptomatic patient. On mammogram, the mass does not have completely smooth borders (see the figures). To further evaluate this new finding, the patient must be recalled for an additional view (spot compression) and ultrasound. Any new mammographic finding in the elderly must be viewed with suspicion because the malignancy rate is high, and typically the elderly breast is quiescent, not forming new benign masses or cysts, as is common in younger patients.

The ultrasound image is shown. Spot compression views in this patient are not shown, but the mass looked essentially unchanged from the standard images. The ultrasound exam demonstrates a mass that has anechoic areas, as well as thick septations. It is consistent with a complex cyst. Although most complex cysts are benign, there is a higher risk of malignancy in the complex cyst. Suspicious features must be sought, and the cyst must be judged by the most suspicious feature seen. Suspicious features include thick internal septations, mural nodules, fibrovascular stalk, and microlobulated margins. If any of these is seen, biopsy is indicated. Color flow Doppler is useful in determining the presence of blood flow within the cyst, either within the stalk, in the septations, or in the intracystic nodule. When blood flow is seen within the complex cyst, biopsy is indicated.

In two series, complex cysts with these features were malignant 23% to 31% of the time. In the majority of cases, these complex cysts are fibrocystic change, intraductal or intracystic papilloma, or atypical hyperplasia, either ductal or lobular. When malignant, the complex cyst can be ductal carcinoma in situ (DCIS) or infiltrating cancer, either ductal or lobular.

The last figure shows another complex cyst in a different patient, also malignant on needle biopsy.

Notes

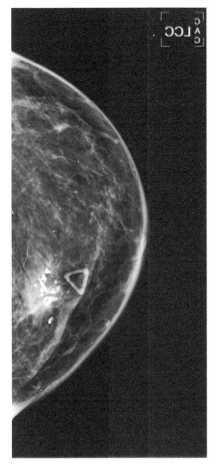 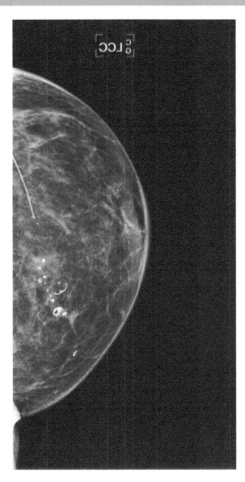 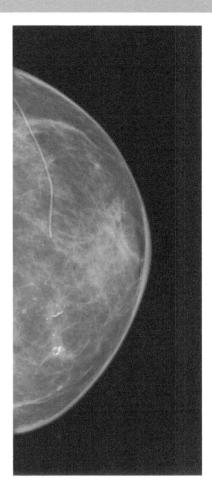

History: A 59-year-old woman presents with a palpable concern in her medial left breast. She had a benign excisional surgical biopsy 5 years ago. Left craniocaudal (CC) views from the current exam, as well as from 3 years ago and 2 years ago, are shown.

1. What is the differential diagnosis of the palpable finding on the current left CC view? (Choose all that apply.)
   A. Infiltrating carcinoma
   B. Fat necrosis
   C. Fibroadenoma
   D. Ductal carcinoma in situ (DCIS)

2. Is this mammographic appearance consistent with fat necrosis?
   A. No, fat necrosis does not appear as a spiculated mass.
   B. No, fat necrosis must have an oil cyst with rim calcifications.
   C. Yes, this is consistent with fibrosis increasing at an area of fat necrosis.
   D. No, fat necrosis effect decreases with time.

3. What is the next step in evaluation?
   A. A 6-month follow-up mammogram
   B. Image-guided needle core biopsy
   C. Routine annual mammography
   D. A return in 1 month to see if findings are related to trauma

4. If needle core biopsy is done, and histology is fat necrosis, what is the management?
   A. This appearance is nonconcordant with that histology, and surgery must be performed.
   B. This appearance is concordant with that histology, and the lesion can be followed.
   C. This is nonconcordant with fat necrosis appearance; recommend repeat image-guided biopsy.
   D. Histology is concordant, but the patient must have surgery to remove the lesion.

CASE 146

Fat Necrosis in an Unusual Presentation

1. A, B, and D
2. C
3. B
4. B

Reference

Taboada JL, Stephens TW, Krishnamurthy S, et al: The many faces of fat necrosis in the breast. *AJR Am J Roentgenol* 2009;192:815-825.

Cross-Reference

Ikeda D: *Breast Imaging: THE REQUISITES*, 2nd ed, Philadelphia: Saunders, 2010, p 109.

Comment

A 59-year-old woman presents with a palpable mass. She had a benign excisional biopsy of the breast 5 years ago. The work-up starts with a mammogram (the first figure shows a single view from this exam) demonstrating a spiculated mass in the medial right breast, corresponding to the palpable concern. When the mammogram is compared with the woman's previous mammograms, the spiculated mass has developed (see the figures). The work-up may then continue with an ultrasound exam to further evaluate the palpable and imaging abnormality (not shown). In this case, the mass was hypoechoic, with irregular margins and shadowing on ultrasound. The mammographic, ultrasound, and clinical findings are all consistent with malignancy. However, on review of the prior mammograms, elements of fat necrosis are seen, with fat lucency and rim calcifications, which coarsen in the interval between the two prior exams. The spiculated mass develops in the area of fat necrosis.

Fat necrosis has many appearances, depending on the histologic features of the injury. Fat cells (adipocytes) degenerate, forming a pocket of fat or oil (oil cyst). This is associated with hemorrhage, and degenerated red blood cells conglomerate in the area of necrotic adipocytes. Histiocytes and multinucleated giant cells infiltrate. Hemosiderin is deposited, and fibrosis develops. Varying degrees of these elements are seen in the individual area of fat necrosis. When an oil cyst is present on mammogram with rim-type calcifications, the appearance is pathognomonic for fat necrosis. However, when fibrosis develops or predominates, the spiculated appearance of fibrosis overlaps with the appearance of malignancy, and biopsy is needed.

Because needle core biopsy is a sampling procedure, sampling can be incomplete. If the diagnosis is a specific benign histology, such as fat necrosis in an area where fat necrosis was previously seen, as in this case, you may place the patient into a short-interval follow-up category, Breast Imaging Reporting and Data System (BI-RADS) 3. You may also seek a surgical opinion, although surgical excision is not mandatory. This patient consulted with her surgeon, who elected to follow. No excision was performed.

Notes

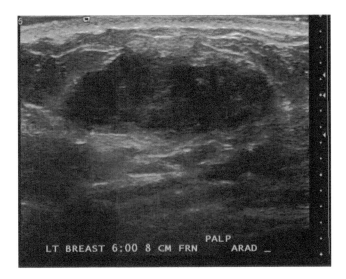

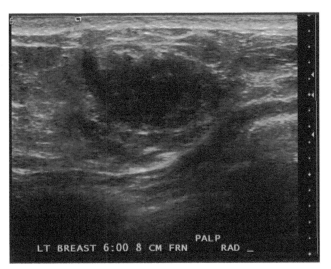

History: A 25-year-old woman has a palpable lump in the inferior left breast, which she reports has increased in size in the last 6 months.

1. What is the differential diagnosis, based on the ultrasound images presented? (Choose all that apply.)
   A. Normal glandular tissue
   B. Fibroadenoma
   C. Infiltrating ductal or lobular carcinoma
   D. Complicated cyst

2. What are the ultrasound features of this mass that suggest benign etiology?
   A. Angular margins, parallel alignment
   B. Hypoechoic, oval, smooth margins
   C. Angular margins, abrupt interface
   D. Parallel alignment, oval shape, abrupt interface with surrounding tissue

3. What are the ultrasound features of this mass that suggest malignancy?
   A. Angular margins, some posterior shadowing
   B. Vertical alignment, angular margins
   C. Angular margins, thick echogenic halo
   D. Oval shape, smooth margins, abrupt interface

4. Needle core biopsy yields histology of fibroadenoma. What is the next step?
   A. Result is concordant, follow in 1 year.
   B. Result is concordant, ask patient to monitor growth of mass and return if it increases in size.
   C. Result is concordant, recommend surgery because of young age.
   D. Result is noncorcordant, recommend surgical consultation.

Nonconcordant Biopsy

1. B and C
2. D
3. A
4. D

References

Mendelson EB, Baum JK, Berg WA, et al: BI-RADS: Ultrasound. In: D'Orsi CJ, Mendelson EB, Ikeda DM, et al: *Breast Imaging Reporting and Data System: ACR BI-RADS—Breast Imaging Atlas*, Reston, VA: American College of Radiology, 2003.

Raza S, Goldkamp AL, Chikarmane SA, Birdwell RL: US of breast masses categorized as BI-RADS 3, 4, and 5: pictorial review of factors influencing clinical management. *Radiographics* 2010;30:1199-1213.

Stavros T, Thickman D, Rapp CL, et al: Solid breast nodules: use of sonography to distinguish between benign and malignant lesions. *Radiology* 1995;196:123-134.

Cross-Reference

Ikeda D: *Breast Imaging: THE REQUISITES*, 2nd ed, Philadelphia: Saunders, 2010, pp 163, 229.

Comment

The ultrasound images of this young woman with a rapidly enlarging mass show a hypoechoic mass with irregular margins and an abrupt interface with the surrounding tissue. The mass is parallel to the skin surface (see the figures). The images shown are taken in radial and antiradial orientation, which is important in documenting the lesion.

There is an American College of Radiology (ACR) lexicon for the description of ultrasound findings, which includes descriptors for masses. It is helpful to use the language of the lexicon to aid communication to the referring physician and between imaging centers. Mass descriptors should include shape (oval, round, or irregular), mass orientation (parallel or vertical), mass margin (circumscribed or not circumscribed), lesion boundary (abrupt or echogenic halo), internal echogenicity, and posterior acoustic features (shadowing or enhancement).

This mass is oval and is parallel to the skin, with an abrupt interface. These features are consistent with benign mass. However, the margins are not circumscribed. When margins are not circumscribed, they can be defined as microlobulated, indistinct, angular, or spiculated (increasing level of suspicion). This mass has microlobulated and angular margins. The decision to biopsy and the Breast Imaging Reporting and Data System (BI-RADS) code given to the mass should be based on the most suspicious feature, so this should be assigned a BI-RADS 4. Core biopsy was performed with a 10-gauge, vacuum-assisted biopsy device, and histology was fibroadenoma.

The biopsy result is felt to be nonconcordant with the imaging findings. When this occurs, further action is needed. The patient should be referred to a surgeon for consideration of excising the mass. This mass was excised, and the histology on excisional biopsy was fibroadenoma.

Notes

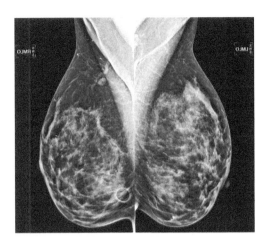

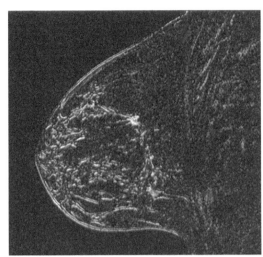

MRI of right breast.

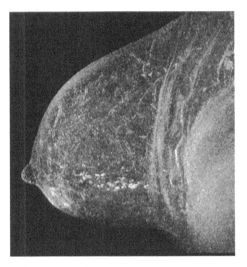

MRI of left breast.

History: A 51-year-old woman presents with a complaint of dimpling in her right upper outer breast. Mammogram, ultrasound, and ultrasound-guided needle core biopsy are performed.

1. What should be included in the differential diagnosis based on the mammogram? (Choose all that apply.)
   A. Architectural distortion from prior surgery in the right breast
   B. Architectural distortion caused by malignant mass in the right breast
   C. Radial scar in the right breast
   D. Suspicious microcalcifications in the right upper outer breast

2. The tissue diagnosis of the right upper outer breast mass is invasive lobular carcinoma (ILC). What is the next best imaging examination?
   A. Bilateral ultrasound
   B. Bilateral MRI
   C. MRI of the ipsilateral breast only
   D. MRI of the contralateral breast only

3. What is the one best diagnosis based on the MRI examination of the left breast?
   A. Ductal carcinoma in situ
   B. Pseudoangiomatous stromal hyperplasia (PASH)
   C. Mastitis
   D. Fibroadenomas

4. What is the next step in management of the left breast?
   A. The patient should be encouraged to undergo bilateral mastectomy.
   B. The surgeon should be instructed to excise a portion of the left breast in the area of enhancement.
   C. The patient should undergo definitive surgery of the right breast and 6-month follow-up of the left breast with MRI.
   D. The patient should undergo MRI-guided core biopsy of the left breast area of abnormal enhancement.

Contralateral Breast Screening with MRI

1. A, B, and C
2. B
3. A
4. D

References

Dedes KJ, Fink D: Clinical presentation and surgical management of invasive lobular carcinoma of the breast. *Breast Dis* 2009;30:31-37.

Hollingsworth AB, Stough RG, O'Dell CA, et al: Breast magnetic resonance imaging for preoperative locoregional staging. *Am J Surg* 2008;196(3):389-397.

Lehman CD, Gatsonis C, Kuhl CK, et al; ACRIN Trial 6667 Investigators Group: MRI evaluation of the contralateral breast in women with recently diagnosed breast cancer. *N Engl J Med* 2007;356 (13):1295-1303.

Teller P, Jefford VJ, Gabram SG, et al: The utility of breast MRI in the management of breast cancer. *Breast J* 2010;16(4):394-403.

Cross-Reference

Ikeda D: *Breast Imaging: THE REQUISITES*, 2nd ed, Philadelphia: Saunders, 2010, pp 104, 265.

Comment

This 51-year-old woman noted dimpling in her right breast and underwent mammography and ultrasound. Subsequent biopsy of the mass, seen best on ultrasound, showed ILC. MRI was recommended to establish the extent of disease in this woman with heterogeneously dense breast tissue.

ILC has a variable appearance on imaging, including mammography, ultrasound, and MRI. On mammography, ILC may appear as a noncalcified mass, with ill-defined or spiculated margins. Because its growth pattern is infiltrative, a focal mass may not be present at all. This carcinoma may cause only distortion, may be completely occult, or may be seen only on one view. ILC accounts for less than 10% of all breast cancers but is more commonly associated with bilateral disease and multicentric and multifocal disease (additional malignancy in the same breast) than is the more common invasive ductal carcinoma. In the ACRIN trial of MRI of the contralateral breast in women with breast cancer, occult contralateral cancer was identified in 6% of women with ILC versus 3% of women with invasive ductal carcinoma.

In this patient, MRI showed only one mass in the ipsilateral breast. In the contralateral breast, clumped enhancement was seen to extend posteriorly in a segmental distribution. No mammographic calcifications are present in this location. MRI-guided biopsy of two sites in the left breast yielded a diagnosis of ductal carcinoma in situ in both sites; this represents occult breast cancer in the contralateral breast, not suspected clinically or mammographically.

The mammographic sensitivity for detecting ILC is reported to be 34% to 81%, inversely related to breast density. MRI is reportedly 93% to 96% sensitive for the detection of ILC. Women with a diagnosis of ILC and dense breasts should consider undergoing bilateral breast MRI.

Notes

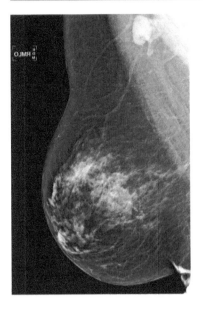
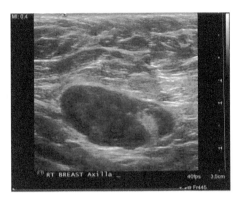
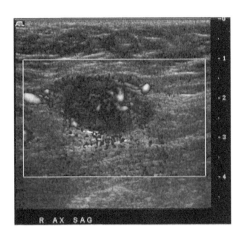

History: A 64-year-old woman whose left breast cancer was diagnosed in 2002 developed radiation-induced angiosarcoma of the left breast in 2009 and underwent left mastectomy. She now presents for routine annual evaluation of the remaining right breast.

1. What should be included in the differential diagnosis of the right mediolateral oblique view presented? (Choose all that apply.)
   A. Enlarged right axillary node, suspicious for metastatic breast cancer
   B. Enlarged right axillary node, possible metastatic angiosarcoma
   C. Sebaceous cyst in the right axilla
   D. Enlarged right axillary node, most likely lymphoma

2. What is RIS?
   A. Sarcoma that occurs immediately after the treatment of the breast with external beam radiation
   B. Sarcoma related to the type of breast cancer, more common in invasive lobular carcinoma
   C. Sarcoma that develops in the radiation field years after treatment
   D. An indolent process that is a complication of radiation therapy

3. What is the prognosis for RIS after treatment for breast cancer?
   A. The prognosis is good because RIS is not as aggressive as typical sarcoma.
   B. The prognosis is poor because it is usually detected late.
   C. The prognosis is dire, with nearly all patients dying of this complication within 1 year of diagnosis.
   D. The prognosis is very good because this is a routine complication of radiation therapy.

4. What imaging modality should be used to follow patients with breast cancer to detect RIS?
   A. All patients treated with radiation should have annual MRI.
   B. All patients treated with radiation should have annual mammograms, supplemented with ultrasound.
   C. All patients treated with mastectomy and radiation should have annual bilateral mammograms.
   D. All patients treated with breast conservation therapy should have annual bilateral mammograms.

CASE 149

Radiation-Induced Sarcoma

1. A and B
2. C
3. B
4. D

References

Blanchard DK, Reynolds C, Grant CS, et al: Radiation-induced breast sarcoma. *Am J Surg* 2002;184(4):356-358.

Kirova YM, Vilcoq JR, Asselain B, et al: Radiation-induced sarcomas after radiotherapy for breast carcinoma: a large-scale single-institution review. *Cancer* 2005;104(4):856-863.

Cross-Reference

Ikeda D: *Breast Imaging: THE REQUISITES*, 2nd ed, Philadelphia: Saunders, 2010, p 398.

Comment

Radiation-induced sarcoma (RIS) is a disease that develops in the radiated field 3 to 20 years after treatment. The incidence is related to the dose, with most reported cases occurring after a dose of 60 to 80 Gy. It is relatively rare, occurring in 0.07% of patients treated with radiation therapy for breast cancer 5 years after treatment in one large series. The incidence increases with time following therapy, with 0.048% risk after 15 years. RIS carries a poor prognosis, with 5-year survival rate of 36% in the aforementioned series.

Late detection is believed to be one reason for the poor prognosis. Although in one series most RIS developed in the breast, the lesions also were found in the chest wall, sternum, above the clavicle, in the scapula, and in the axilla, where they may go undetected.

The patient in the present case was diagnosed with RIS when she felt a lump in her treated breast 7 years after lumpectomy and radiation treatment for left breast cancer. The mass was surgically excised and revealed a high-grade angiosarcoma. She underwent mastectomy, and she presented 1 year later for routine evaluation of the contralateral breast. An enlarged node was seen in the right axilla (see the figures). Ultrasound was performed (see the figures) to guide biopsy. Increased blood flow within the node was noted on ultrasound (see the figures). Biopsy pathology was metastatic high-grade angiosarcoma.

Notes

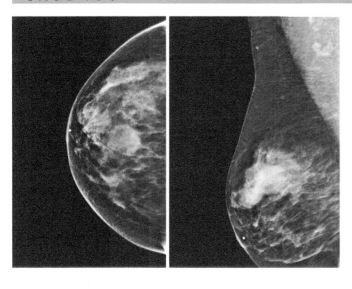

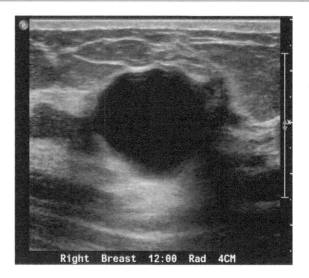

Right Breast 12:00 Rad 4CM

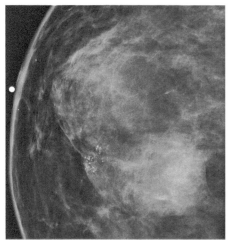

History: A 49-year-old woman who has a family history of breast cancer in her mother, diagnosed at age 52, presents with a palpable mass in the right upper breast.

1. What should be included in the differential diagnosis, based on the mammographic and ultrasound images shown? (Choose all that apply.)
   A. Simple cyst
   B. Ductal carcinoma in situ (DCIS) adjacent to a cyst
   C. Mucinous carcinoma, with adjacent DCIS
   D. Fibrocystic change, with benign calcifications and a cyst

2. After standard mammogram views and ultrasound, what additional imaging may help?
   A. Magnification views to evaluate the calcifications further
   B. Rolled craniocaudal views to evaluate the round mass better
   C. True lateral mediolateral view
   D. Spot compression view of the calcifications

3. Biopsy is indicated. How would you approach the biopsy?
   A. Stereotactic biopsy of the calcifications
   B. Ultrasound-guided core biopsy of the round mass
   C. MRI-guided biopsy of the mass
   D. Ultrasound-guided biopsy of the calcifications

4. What is the role of MRI in this patient?
   A. To evaluate the calcifications further before biopsy
   B. To evaluate for enhancement in the round mass
   C. To evaluate for extent of disease after malignant diagnosis is established by needle biopsy
   D. To evaluate only the right breast, for evidence of additional disease

CASE 150

Cancer Adjacent to Palpable Cyst

1. B and C
2. A
3. A
4. C

Reference

Venkatesan A, Chu P, Kerlikowske K, et al: Positive predictive value of specific mammographic findings according to reader and patient variables. *Radiology* 2009;250(3):648-657.

Cross-Reference

Ikeda D: *Breast Imaging: THE REQUISITES*, 2nd ed, Philadelphia: Saunders, 2010, pp 85, 95, 100, 271.

Comment

This case shows numerous important points in the diagnostic work-up of a palpable finding, as follows:

- A patient who has a family history, especially of a first-degree relative at a young age, must be evaluated very carefully.
- Mammogram should be performed because ultrasound alone may not show the full extent of the problem. In this case, the calcifications would have been missed.
- If a cyst is seen that corresponds with the palpable finding, other findings that are nonpalpable should not be ignored.
- If a suspected cyst on ultrasound does not have the characteristic features of a simple cyst, aspiration should be attempted.
- It is essential to establish concordance between the palpable finding and the imaging finding.
- Clinical breast examination is important, and palpable findings should not be ignored.

This 49-year-old woman has a family history of cancer in her mother at age 52. Clinical or mammographic findings should be viewed with suspicion because of this family history. Mammography (see the figures) shows a mass and adjacent clustered calcifications; this is suspicious for a round invasive malignancy with adjacent DCIS. Ultrasound and magnification views (see the figures) fail to clarify the mass as a simple cyst. The calcifications are pleomorphic and tightly clustered.

Biopsy was performed with stereotactic guidance and showed in situ and invasive ductal carcinoma, grade II.

Notes

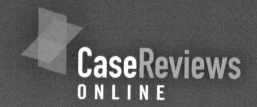

THE CASE REVIEWS YOU TRUST,
in a format you've been waiting for.

The most trusted radiology review book series is now online! With the new **Case Reviews Online**, you can review your way, with interactive features and customizable study tools that are accessible online, anytime.

Case Reviews Online allows you to:

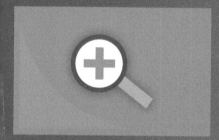

Accurately assess your board readiness with customizable tests that mimic the format of official exams.

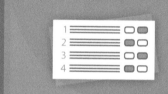

Test your understanding of each case with the four multiple-choice questions that accompany them.

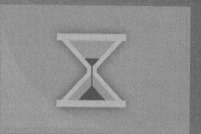

Spend more time reviewing and less time searching because cases are organized by radiologic subspecialty.

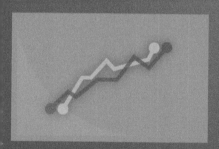

Confirm or challenge your diagnostic interpretations by selecting the label on/label off option.

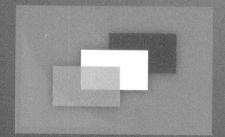

Track your progress by comparing your previous test results with your latest scores.

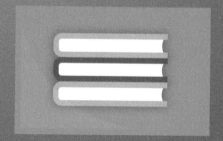

Review cases from a variety of subspecialties including Musculoskeletal, Thoracic, Interventional, Spine, Pediatrics, Brain, Head and Neck, and Emergency Medicine.

SEE WHAT **CASE REVIEWS ONLINE** CAN DO FOR YOU.

To learn more, visit **casereviewsonline.com**

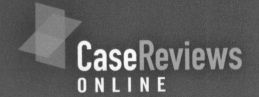

SEE WHAT **CASE REVIEWS ONLINE** CAN DO FOR YOU.

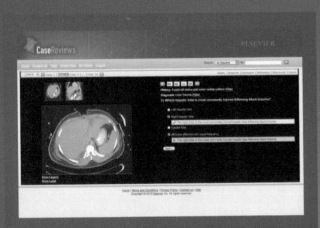

Practice Test questions on Case Reviews Online allow you to see rationale for both correct and incorrect questions as you take the test.

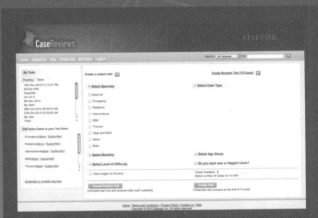

With Case Reviews Online, users can create a Practice Test with unlimited test time, or a "Real" Test that is timed and simulates the board-testing experience.

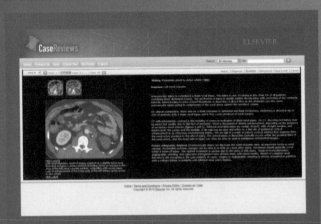

You can choose to take tests with or without help, with the ability to show or hide legends, labels, history, diagnosis, questions, discussion and review.

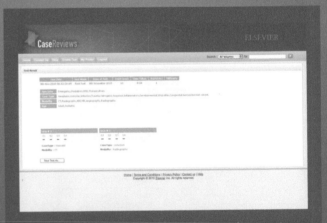

Results include full details on the test you took, along with test title, test mode, date and time, number of cases, score and difficulty.

To learn more, visit **casereviewsonline.com**

To inquire about Institutional Access contact
h.licensing@elsevier.com